THE SKIN TYPE SOLUTION

THE SKIN TYPE SOLUTION

*The Revolutionary Guide to Finding
and Caring for Your Skin Type*

DR LESLIE BAUMANN

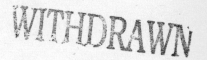

HODDER
MOBIUS

Copyright © 2005 by Dr Leslie Baumann

First published in Great Britain in 2006 by Hodder and Stoughton
A division of Hodder Headline

The right of Dr Leslie Baumann to be identified as the
Author of the Work has been asserted by her in accordance
with the Copyright, Designs and Patents Act 1988.

A Mobius Book

2

A CIP catalogue record for this title is available from the British Library

ISBN 9 780340 84116 7
ISBN 0 340 84116 8

Typeset in Adobe Garamond by Hewer Text UK Ltd, Edinburgh
Printed and bound by Mackays of Chatham Ltd, Chatham, Kent

Hodder Headline's policy is to use papers that are natural,
renewable and recyclable products and made from wood grown in
sustainable forests. The logging and manufacturing processes are expected
to conform to the environmental regulations of the country of origin.

Hodder and Stoughton Ltd
A division of Hodder Headline
338 Euston Road
London NW1 3BH

This book is dedicated to my wonderful family:
Roger, Robert, and Max Baumann

CONTENTS

ACKNOWLEDGMENTS

Many people contributed directly or indirectly to this book and I am extremely grateful for everyone's help. First, I want to thank my patients, friends, family, and colleagues who patiently answered questionnaire after questionnaire over the years until I got it right. The original version contained over two hundred questions, requiring quite a commitment on their part. I offer tremendous thanks to the questionnaire experts who gave me excellent advice about questionnaire development, including Dr David Lee in the Department of Epidemiology at the University of Miami and those at the Survey Research Office at the University of Illinois. Special thanks to Sharon Jacobs, MD, an expert on contact dermatitis at the University of Miami who helped me develop the questions covering skin allergies and sensitivity.

Thanks to all of the companies that sent skin care products to be studied and evaluated. I also thank my patients, family, and friends who used these skin care products and reported back to me about their experiences. Some of them suffered redness, acne, rashes, and itching in the name of Skin Type science. What troupers!

Thanks to Nikki at Brownes & Co. in Miami Beach for letting me spend hours looking at skin care products and for letting me use her beautiful store as a background in my picture in this book.

Thanks to my staff for putting up with me during the years leading up to the publication of this book. Thanks for being flexible, hardworking, and dependable. Susan Schaffer and Laura Black suffered the most and I can't thank them enough. Susan, you're a great friend and colleague. Tere Calcines was always there for me when I needed help. I'm also grateful to Denese, Marie, Franshely, Jussane, Jasmine, Vanessa, Conchita, Clara, Debra, Olga, and all the others who worked or volunteered in my office. My fellows – Esperanza Welsh, Lucy Martin, Monica Halem, Justin Vujevich, Anele Slezinger, and Melissa Lazarus – were terrific.

Special thanks to Joy Bryde, who organised my life and whose teachings helped shape the development of this book.

Many people mentored me in my career, but each of the following people selflessly taught me and guided me to this point: Ben Smith, MD; Francisco Kerdel, MD; William Eaglstein, MD; Larry Schachner, MD; Steve Mandy, MD; Jim Leyden, MD; Joseph Jorizzo, MD; and David Leffell, MD.

Thanks to Richard Pine and Catherine Drayton, my incredible agents at Inkwell Management, and Alison Rose Levy, a true pleasure to work with – you all are the best. I also want to thank Stephanie Golden for her help with the regimes. This book would not have happened without you. To my new friends at Hodder & Stoughton – I offer thanks for the opportunity and your enthusiasm. I hope that we have many more chances to work together.

And last, but certainly not least, I want to thank my loving family. My parents, Lynn and Jack McClendon, and in-laws, Josie and David Kenin, helped me on every level possible. My husband, Roger, who has been by my side for the last sixteen years, and my two sons, Robert and Max, who bring happiness, fun and tons of love to my life. I adore you all and wish you all a lifetime of great skin!

PART ONE

The Skin Type Revolution

CHAPTER ONE

Why Skin Typing?

INTRODUCTION

How many times have you gone to a cosmetic counter and spent £25 to £50 on products you never again use? Has a saleswoman or cosmetologist sold you a line that 'did wonders for me', but does nothing for you? Have you developed an allergy or irritation to a product without knowing the cause? Why does your best friend swear by a facial care product that makes your skin look and feel terrible? Should you or shouldn't you use soap? Why do you hate the feel of sunscreen, though you know you should use it? Is a chemical face peel right for you? Should you consider using Retin-A?

If you owned a Porsche, you wouldn't follow the maintenance procedures for a VW Golf. So if you happen to have dry, sensitive skin, why on earth would you use a moisturiser, cleanser and cosmetic procedure more suited to someone with oily, resistant skin?

The reason? You don't know what type of skin you have; therefore, you don't know how to care for your skin. Until the publication of *The Skin Type Solution*, the Baumann Skin Typing System was not widely known or available. While many people have a general understanding of their skin, most have relied on commonly known but imprecise, unscientific definitions that fall short of providing a true and complete picture.

My many years as a dermatologist, researcher, and associate professor of dermatology have convinced me that no one ever needs to have a 'bad skin day'. Knowing your Skin Type is the missing, essential step to finding your way to beneficial products and treatments – and beautiful skin. But if you're like the typical first-time patient at my bustling University of Miami clinic, I'll bet you:

- Don't know your Skin Type
- Don't know that it's essential to base skin care decisions on your Skin Type

- Use the wrong products for your Skin Type
- Spend much more than you should on those products
- Use the wrong procedures for your Skin Type
- Fail to take advantage of procedures that would benefit your Skin Type

When it comes to using skin care products and services, most people have been in the Dark Ages, wandering through a maze of product misinformation and overzealous marketing, lucky to stumble on anything that works.

Olivia's Story

Olivia, a forty-eight-year-old estate agent with dry, sensitive, wrinkle-prone skin, was embarrassed by facial redness and flaking around her nose and eyebrows. Before she came to see me, she had been using an over-the-counter hydrocortisone ointment to relieve this condition. But when we discovered through my diagnostic questionnaire that Olivia's skin was especially wrinkle prone, I warned her that long-term steroid use could worsen her Skin Type's natural tendency to thinness and wrinkles. Instead I switched her to the prescription product Elidel, which safely treated her redness and flaking without accelerating the skin thinning and wrinkling that bother people with Olivia's Skin Type.

Like Olivia, to properly care for your skin and prevent aging, you need a treatment model that describes and captures the very real and scientifically verifiable distinctions in skin physiology.

Skin Typing does just that.

Plus, you need a concrete programme specifically and individually tailored to the unique attributes of *your* Skin Type. *The Skin Type Solution* provides all of that vital information and guidance.

Once you've discovered your Skin Type (through answering a questionnaire in Chapter Three), you can go straight to the chapter on your Skin Type and find everything you need right there. There is a science to skin care, and once you know your Skin Type, it all gets a lot easier.

I've spent the last eight years defining and clinically testing my Skin Type solutions on thousands of patients at my University of Miami clinic to assure that my scientific criteria will work for everyone, of every skin colour, ethnicity, age and sex. And it does.

Perhaps you've already benefited from understanding your psychological type, your learning style, or your Ayurvedic type. If so, you'll appreciate how critical it is to get a handle on your Skin Type. This understanding lets you take control of your skin.

MY SPECIAL EXPERTISE

The guidance and gems I'll give you won't appear anywhere else. I launched, and currently direct, the University of Miami Cosmetic Center, the first university-run cosmetic research centre in the United States, where I treat thousands of patients every year. In addition to being an MD, I am an associate professor at the University of Miami and the chief of the Division of Cosmetic Dermatology, making me the first cosmetic dermatologist in the United States dedicated to the field of cosmetic dermatology who is also a full-time university faculty member, teaching and conducting research.

This unprecedented combination affords me a unique position. My academic responsibilities keep me right on the cutting edge of research, while my clinical work has been a proving ground for refining the recommendations that arise from my findings.

My clients – who range from gorgeous fashion models to topflight professionals, to fellow physicians, to all kinds of men and women concerned about aging – have reaped the benefits of my unique under-standing of the role of Skin Type in skin care.

As a scientist who is also a woman who loves to experiment with beauty and skin care products and routines, I'm tireless in seeking out and researching all beauty options because I use them myself. What's more, as a person who wants to look my best all my life, I can put myself in your shoes and figure out how to best serve your skin care needs.

DEFINING A NEW TYPOLOGY

Up until now, the field of dermatology lacked a rational model that people could learn to follow and apply for themselves. Prior to Skin Typing, the pre-existing mode of analysing skin differences dated back to the early 1900s, when cosmetic giant Helena Rubenstein first divided skin into four categories: normal, combination, dry and sensitive. While that was revolu-tionary for its time, today we can apply more accurate scientific criteria to the range of skin differences.

Before Skin Typing, even dermatologists felt frustrated, since we all want to understand skin better and offer our patients tailor-made solutions. But until now, the revolutionary classification of the sixteen Skin Types was not there to help.

Here's just one example of the kind of confusion that runs rampant, even among professionals. I recently was on the advisory board of a major company with two prominent dermatologists. One was an 'R' (someone with resistant, nonreactive skin) and the other one was an 'S' (someone with sensitive skin). Right there in front of the company president, the two had a huge argument, with the 'R' dermatologist claiming that there was no difference in skin care products and that it was all marketing hype. She could use anything on her facial skin, she told us, even soap, without a problem. The 'S' skin dermatologist was shocked. Almost everything made her skin turn red and sting, she retorted. These two skin professionals did not understand that their opposing points of view stemmed from their opposite Skin Types. I saw very clearly that something was missing and wanted to simplify skin care, once and for all.

As a clinician, I'd seen the damage caused by following an inappropriate skin care routine. As a caring doctor, I'd heard the frustration and confusion of people trying to make good skin care choices while barraged by a plethora of products and overwhelmed by conflicting and often misleading marketing claims. Because each person had particular skin care needs, I noticed that the same products did not work for everyone, so I tailored individualised skin care regimens for my clients. Over time a clear, consistent, and replicable typology emerged. The sixteen Skin Types are the keys to a complete diagnostic and treatment programme that covers every significant skin factor and that *really works*.

The Baumann Skin Typing System can help anyone determine their Skin Type and base their skin care decisions on what's best for their type. My system measures four factors in skin: oiliness vs. dryness, resistance vs. sensitivity, pigmentation vs. non-pigmentation, and tightness vs. wrinkling. Determining where you fall in each of the four categories serves as the foundation for typing your skin. Your Skin Type is more than the sum of the four different factors. Their interplay and expression is unique for each type. After seeing literally thousands of patients and refining the Baumann Skin Type Questionnaire over the last eight years, I can assure you that Skin Typing captures each Skin Type's unique qualities and shows you how to work with your type's strengths and weaknesses.

Once you understand your Skin Type, proper skin care isn't complicated or costly. You won't need to use a shelfful of products. Honing in on what your skin needs will actually simplify your beauty routine, making it easier to follow and more economical. Following the advice I'll extend in your Skin Type's chapter will end 'bad skin days' because it will end bad skin care decisions.

How to Use This Book

In reading the opening chapter of this book, you'll familiarise yourself with the underlying principles of Skin Typing. In Chapter Two, you'll learn my innovative vocabulary to help you understand the different factors that I take into account when determining your Skin Type. In Chapter Three, you'll take the Baumann Skin Type Questionnaire. Once you tabulate your results, you will know exactly which one of the sixteen types describes your skin. You can then turn directly to that chapter for a complete profile that will provide you with everything you need to take charge of your skin and give it the best possible care. Your chapter will overview your type's main characteristics as well as share stories of patients who've experienced and treated skin problems similar to the ones that may have troubled you. The bottom line is that by reading your chapter, you will get to know your skin. This will provide the foundation for following my subsequent advice.

Each chapter contains Daily Skin Care Regimens specifically designed to address your Skin Type's problem areas. To follow your type's regimen, you will need to use the kinds of products I recommend. I'll provide a list of suggestions for each type of product, as well as extra suggestions to use when you have specific skin problems. In most product categories, I also provide a selection called Baumann's Choice, a good option to simplify your purchasing decision.

If you currently use products that you find effective, you can also continue to use them, if you wish. However, if you decide to do that, I advise you to consult the lists of ingredients that define which ones are favourable or counterproductive for your Skin Type. Some ingredients may be helpful for one of your skin concerns, but exacerbate another skin problem. For example, genistein, a component found in soy, helps wrinkles, but also increases pigmentation. A Non-Pigmented, Wrinkled Skin Type could safely use it, but a Pigmented, Wrinkled Type should only use products that contain soy that has had the genistein removed. That's one reason why I advise that you double-check your current products to ensure that they do not contain any no-no's. If they do, I recommend that you change products, as you could be unwittingly causing a problem. And you may also find that some of your favourite products do indeed contain helpful ingredients for your type. Still, I can best guarantee results with the products I know and recommend.

This book should be your companion when you shop for skin care products. As you put my recommendations in place, monitor how well they are working for you to assess whether or not consulting a dermatologist would be of benefit. For some Skin Types, I provide one or more additional Stage Two Daily Skin Care Regimens, which address treating special skin problems via helpful prescription medications. Near the end of each chapter, I will point you towards your best options in cosmetic dermatology. A section of the book called 'Further Help' will follow each of the four main Skin Type groups to offer more specific advice on certain prescriptions and procedures. It will also contain lifestyle, nutritional, and supplemental suggestions for your special needs.

In the chapter on your Skin Type, you will find:

1. Understanding of:
   a. The basic qualities of your Skin Type
   b. Your Skin Type's issues and challenges
   c. Risk factors associated with your Skin Type
2. Guidelines for:
   a. Your Skin Type's Daily Skin Care Regimen
   b. Sun protection for your skin
   c. Makeup that will help improve your skin condition
   d. Types of prescription products helpful for your Skin Type
   e. Cosmetic procedures that can help your skin (where applicable)
   f. Cosmetic procedures that are not recommended for you (where applicable)
3. Specific Recommendations for:
   a. Skin care products for your daily skin care routine
   b. Skin care ingredients (to look for on product labels) that address your key skin issues
   c. Skin care ingredients (to look for on product labels) that you should avoid because they can worsen your skin

Instead of letting you waste valuable time and money tracking down and purchasing products that wind up in the bin, I will direct you to ones that will really help. My role in research and industry development gives me an unparalleled across-the-board knowledge of skin care ingredients.

I'll indicate the best way to cleanse your skin, reveal whether you need to use a toner or a moisturiser, diagnose whether exfoliation is advisable for you, and show you when you'd benefit from prescription skin medications. All of my product recommendations will include options at low, medium and high prices. As a result, whether you shop at Harrods, Space NK or Boots, whatever your budget, you can follow my recommendations to successful skin care. I have endeavoured to offer selections that are widely available in the UK, to make it easier for you to obtain them. However if you have difficulty locating any item, for your convenience, many of them can be found at www.Baumannstore.co.uk with a portion of the proceeds going to fund dermatological research.

Your Skin Type chapter will also help you to avoid products and procedures that – while recommended for other types – are either useless or potentially harmful for you. If you are curious about a cosmetic procedure, like Botox, your chapter will indicate whether, based on your Skin Type, it's something that you and your dermatologist should consider. That way you can make sure you choose the skin procedures most beneficial for your skin's particular needs.

WHEN TO CONSULT A DERMATOLOGIST

In addition to guiding you through the product maze, I will help you decide when to consult a dermatologist and reveal how to get the most out of your visit in a section of your Skin Type chapter called 'Consulting a Dermatologist'. Some types have very little need to see a doctor, while certain others really benefit from the prescription medications, light treatments, and other procedures doctors can provide. In fact, for certain Skin Types with increased skin issues, nonprescription products may not be sufficiently effective. People with highly resistant skin, for example, need higher-octane products, which only licensed physicians can prescribe.

Due to a shortage of qualified dermatologists, people can often wait for some time to get an appointment. As a result, most dermatologists cannot always spend the time necessary to address basic skin care needs. The resource section at the end of the book will help you find a qualified dermatologist in your area. By teaching you how to meet your basic skin care needs without a dermatologist and by helping you zero in on how he or she can best aid you, I'll ensure you make efficient use of your valuable appointment time.

Finally, I have launched a Web site, www.DrBaumann.co.uk, to track your responses to different products, so now you can join the patients who see me at my clinic in offering your feedback and experiences while following the Baumann Skin Type Solution. Once you've discovered your Skin Type and tried my recommendations, you may want to explore further and discover new products that contain ingredients recommended for your type. If so, I want to hear about your discoveries as well as how my favourites have worked for you. Log on to www.DrBaumann.co.uk and fill out the online questionnaire to share your skin care discoveries with me and other people who share your Skin Type. You can also visit www.skintypesolution.com for more information and upcoming events in your area.

WHAT YOU NEED TO KNOW
ABOUT SKIN CARE PRODUCTS

For you as a consumer in the booming international skin care industry, lack of information about products is costly, and you have to bridge the gap between what you *know* and *what you need to know*. Without accurate information, you are throwing your money away, because you are completely at the mercy of advertisers and marketing people. With the specific information about your skin's needs explained in this book, you can take control of your skin.

In 2001, the average American owned about five hundred dollars' worth of cosmetic products, and this amount has surely risen dramatically as more and more expensive product lines have been developed since that time. Do you really need to spend that much to get quality skin care? No. What truly matters is not your skin cream's price, but whether it's right for your Skin Type. No matter how glamorous its packaging or delicious its feel, that four-hundred-dollar cream is not right for everyone. (In fact, some types don't need to use any skin cream at all.)

This book will save you the expense, trouble, and waste of buying the wrong products – while directing you to the right ones. My recommendations are ingredient driven, and once you've learned my criteria, you too will be better able to read a cosmetic label and figure out if it's appropriate for you.

I have tried to incorporate into this book every kind of skin care product that I feel is useful, limiting the scope to facial care products. (The book would be three times this size if I included body care advice as well.) I have chosen the products recommended in this book based on their ingredients, manufacturing practices, and formulations.

I've reviewed the clinical trial data of the products, when available, to offer those proven effective. Finally, since my patients have used my recommendations, I've listened to their feedback and tracked their treatment results to guarantee the efficacy of the treatment approach and product selection for each Skin Type. All you have to do is take the test, determine your Skin Type, and choose from the products in your chapter. And at least when you splurge on products and procedures, you'll know you are getting your money's worth.

The recommendations are independent of any relationships that I have with the companies that manufacture them. Of course, when I work with a company, I know more about their products. However, I work with over thirty-seven companies and have approached many others for information while writing this book. In addition, when I find products with helpful ingredients from other sources, like stores or the Internet, I test them as well. After all, I test skin care products for a living – so why not?

All the products that I recommend:

1. Contain the right ingredients for your Skin Type
2. Contain sufficient amounts of active ingredients to be effective
3. Do not contain counterproductive ingredients
4. Are formulated effectively for your needs
5. Are packaged to maintain stability of the active ingredients
6. Are cosmetically elegant (smell good and feel good)
7. Got a thumbs-up from those who've used them
8. Are easily available for purchase

Finally, since all products meet all of the above criteria, I often pick the cheapest option (or a hands-down favourite) as a Baumann's Choice. This designates the best value to make your product selections easier.

Chloe's Story

Unaware that her freckles, dark spots, and dark under-eye circles indicated that she had pigmented skin (skin that freckles, or easily forms brown spots), Chloe had paid a steep price for a highly touted antiwrinkle cream that was dead wrong for her Skin Type because it contained soy (a common ingredient in skin care). Although soy can be great for dark spots, some forms of soy contain oestrogen-like substances. And with pigmented skin, it's vital to shun products that contain ingredients that act like oestrogen, which *increases* the formation of brown spots. While certain components of soy have this undesirable, oestrogenic effect, other components *prevent* brown spot formation, and therefore should be used by Chloe (or you, if you have pigmented skin).

Yet Chloe had no idea how to interpret the fine-print ingredients in her wrinkle cream. She was lured to purchase it by its pretty blue packaging and the rave reviews of it in *Vogue*. Even if she had read the ingredients, she would not have known what they meant or how that would affect her skin. She would never have guessed that this product was increasing her spots and skin discoloration.

What Chloe needed instead was a product in which the problematic oestrogen-like components had been removed, while the beneficial properties were retained, such as Aveeno Positively Radiant Daily Moisturizer, which contains soy without the oestrogenic components. This product is available for a modest price at Boots. Using a cream of true benefit to her Skin Type, Chloe could have saved herself a bundle.

Through the Baumann Skin Type Questionnaire, which you'll find in Chapter Three, you will learn whether and to what extent skin pigmentation is an issue for you. That information will be synthesised with other key skin characteristics to arrive at the final assessment, so that you know once and for all what Skin Type you have. Full guidelines and detailed product and procedure dos and don'ts will be spelled out in your chapter.

To give another example, let's say that (in contrast to Chloe) the test determines that you are *not* pigmented, and that your skin can also be classified as wrinkled. With that combination, it would be beneficial for you to use a soy-based product that includes the oestrogenic components. Two different Skin Types need two entirely different types of ingredients and, as a result, require highly individual product recommendations.

SKIN TYPING IS UNIVERSAL

One of the fascinating features of Skin Typing is that people of different ethnic or racial backgrounds can share a Skin Type. In most instances, all people with the same Skin Type will follow the exact same treatment plan, but sometimes skin colour can be a differentiating factor because of the way pigment (the factor in skin that produces colour) is produced in different racial and ethnic groups. For example, two best friends, Amelia, a medium-skin-toned brunette, and Grace, a dark-skinned woman, came in for back-to-back appointments. After they each took the questionnaire and tabulated their results, they were surprised to discover that they shared the same Skin Type. They were both 'P', Pigmented Skin Types, which gave both Amelia and Grace a tendency to develop pigmentation issues. And each of them *did* have a problem with pigmentation. That's why they came to my office.

Amelia had an area of dark skin discoloration (called melasma) on her cheek, and Grace had dark spots in areas where she had once had pimples. Although I recommended that they follow the exact same protocol and use the same kinds of products, there was one key difference. Amelia could benefit from an advanced cosmetic procedure that uses light instruments or lasers to treat pigment problems like hers, while Grace would benefit most from prescription products used daily and should not undergo laser treatment since this can cause discoloration in people with darker skin tones.

That's why, throughout the book whenever an adjustment based on skin colour is needed, I'll fine-tune recommendations so that you will know how to adapt them to your needs whether you have a light, medium or dark skin tone.

Mona's Story

M ona came to see me because of skin discoloration on her chin and cheeks. An Egyptian exchange student with oily skin, Mona never guessed that her skin scrub was causing this problem. Anyone with highly pigmented skin (like many dark-skinned people) must stay away from all ingredients and procedures that cause inflammation.

Yet, not knowing her Skin Type, Mona had no idea that her choice of skin product stimulated the inflammatory response, which in turn led to dark spots.

I taught Mona what to look for on product ingredient labels. Common ingredients, like vitamin C, AHA and alpha lipoic acid, can create inflammation, as do buff puffs and strong scrubs. She was surprised to learn that hair removal formulas, and hot wax products may also cause inflammation. In using wax or a chemical depilatory to remove facial hair, Mona wound up with unsightly dark patches that looked far worse than the hair she was trying to remove. Now she knew to avoid them. Once she became aware of the needs of her Skin Type, she was able to make changes that helped reduce the dark spots considerably. In addition, I recommended she use products containing oatmeal, feverfew, chamomile, or licorice extract, which are known to have anti-inflammatory properties.

SKIN CARE MYTHS

When people come into my office, I regularly have to deprogramme them of skin care *dis*-information. For example, do you buy into any of these common beauty myths?

Myth 1: *The way to find the right skin care product is by buying lots of different products until you find one that works for you (if you're lucky).*

Actually, this approach works well for the cosmetics industry, but it's not so good for you – unless you happen to have loads of money, tons of free time, and a desire to experiment on your skin. Yet, that's the way most people purchase skin care products and services. Without knowing your

Skin Type and being directed to the range of products that work well for it, you are at the mercy of marketing people and advertisers.

In this book, I will cut through the hype around skin products, and let you know what's worthwhile, or worthless, for your Skin Type's needs – and why. Because of the way that their products are regulated by governmental agencies, cosmetic companies cannot lay claim to any biological activity. If they did, their products would be regulated as drugs, with costly clinical trials needed to validate their claims. Instead they make vague marketing statements. No wonder people are confused. However, as a dermatologist, I can reveal the biological effects of different products to cut through the hype.

Myth 2: *The more expensive a product, the better it will work.*

What does the high price tag on that designer skin cream buy you? Not the ingredients in the bottle. Instead, most often you are footing the bill for the marketing and bottling of that product. In fact, if tomorrow someone invented the world's best skin cream, they could sell the rights to market it to different segments of the skin care marketplace, and very likely the only difference between the chemist's shop item, the department store brand-name version, and the special edition sold by dermatologists would be, you guessed it, the packaging and price. However, the creams contained therein could well be absolutely identical. Some day I'd love to see high-end lines that are really worth the extra expense because they are packed with ingredients that can deliver real results. In this book, you'll learn what products work well for your Skin Type's unique needs, without busting your budget.

Caitlin's Story

C aitlin was a thirty-seven-year-old interior designer with an impressive list of high-end clients. She preferred and could afford the very best. But paying top dollar hadn't helped her to find the right care for her dry, resistant, pigmented and wrinkle-prone skin.

'At one time or other, I've used every kind of cream and moisturiser, from the most expensive brands to stuff from the corner pharmacy,' she told me. But none of these products helped the crow's-feet that were forming around her eyes and on her forehead. Given her skin's resistance, Caitlin was fortunate that none of the products on her worldwide search for a moisturiser caused a reaction. But none of them were very effective either.

I recognised immediately that Caitlin was a candidate for Retin-A, which accelerates the skin's natural exfoliation process. This has a twofold effect. First, it increases collagen production, which slows the formation of wrinkles. Second, it also prevents the formation of brown spots since the cells that make colour cannot keep up with the accelerated cell turnover. As with most of my patients, I had Caitlin start slowly, at first using the product once every three nights to assure that she remained reaction-free. I advised her to mix it in with a little of her moisturiser, which is helpful in offsetting the dryness typical of her Skin Type.

'I love the way my skin looks with Retin-A,' Caitlin reported six months later. 'It's taken years off my face and prevented new wrinkles from forming.'

Another concern for someone with dry, wrinkle-prone skin, like Caitlin, was finding the right moisturiser. I advised her to look for moisturisers containing ingredients like glycerin, cholesterol, ceramides and fatty acids, as these restore hydration, always an issue for someone with her Skin Type. Some of my personal favourites are in the Dove Essential Nutrients line. Avoiding toners and gels that could dry her skin was another essential aspect of her skin care protocol, as was utilising hydrating creams rather than lotions.

Myth 3: *Fragrance-free products contain no perfume or fragrance.*

People with sensitive skin often buy products with this misleading labelling, hoping to avoid ingredients they react to. 'Fragrance-free' is no guarantee that the product does not contain perfumes or fragrances. It means that no fragrance is detectable by the average person's sense of smell.

In fact, fragrances are added to most face creams to neutralise their bad odour. Have you ever noticed that your old makeup foundation smells funny? That's because over time the fragrances evaporate, leaving the unpleasant smell unmasked. For most people, this doesn't matter so much, but if you have sensitive skin, you may need to find products completely free of these sensitising ingredients. My Skin Type guidelines and product recommendations will help you do that.

Myth 4: *Soap can be fine for sensitive skin.*

Any product that vigorously suds and foams contains detergent, a strict no-no for dry skin. One example is Pear's soap. Vigorously foaming soaps, like Pear's, are terrible for dry skin because they wash away the natural lipids that help your skin retain moisture. If you have dry skin, never use anything that makes a lot of bubbles, especially bubble bath. Thin foam and thin bubbles are all right. Never wash your face with shampoo no matter what your Skin Type. Instead use non-foaming cleansers or minimally foaming cleansers like Cetaphil, Dove, or certain Nivea products.

Georgina's Story

A fifty-four-year-old credit controller for a company, Georgina was also a mother and grandmother. 'Believe me, I've tried everything for my skin redness,' Georgina told me on her first visit to my office. Of English and Irish background, Georgina had creamy fair skin, but a red nose, red splotches and red marks on her neck.

'Once a friend recommended I use her favourite cleanser, which was Sisley Cleansing Milk. I got such a bad rash, the doctor thought I had a contagious disease,' Georgina reported. Even products labelled as mild or for sensitive skin caused her eyes to swell. Although many people love this product, with sensitive skin, there is always the risk of a reaction.

Georgina lived in a cold, dry climate. Because of her skin's tendency to wrinkle, moisturising and wrinkle prevention were key for her. Her skin thirsted for moisture, but reacted to nearly all moisturisers by burning, stinging, or turning red. Fortunately, I knew which products tended to be less irritating and had ingredients known to decrease facial flushing. I recommended Olay Total Effects with niacinamide, which has been shown to decrease facial flushing. Georgina was delighted that this inexpensive moisturiser worked for her. A procedure called Intense Pulsed Light, or IPL, was performed with a Lumenis light device to shrink her blood vessels, leading to decreased facial redness and flushing. In addition, I recommended that she add antioxidant vitamins and fish oils to her diet. Antioxidants help combat free radicals, which can lead to wrinkles. Fish oils do double duty: they add needed fatty acids to the diet and help build up the lipids in the skin, restoring the skin barrier and reducing skin sensitivity. Georgina says that she recently saw a picture of herself from a wedding and was thrilled that her face did not look red in the photo.

Myth 5: *The food I eat won't affect my skin.*
Your diet does impact your skin, and there's no doubt that going on a no- or low-fat diet can increase skin dryness. Studies have shown that patients on cholesterol-lowering drugs often suffer from dry skin. Cholesterol is actually an important part of the skin that helps it remain hydrated.

Samantha's Story

S amantha, a twenty-year-old model, consulted me because she was having trouble getting work due to excessive skin flakiness. When I questioned her, I learned that she had recently gone on a low-protein, no-fat diet, eating lots of vegetables and zero fats. Her dry skin suffered. Flaking and peeling, her skin looked dull and lifeless. Once I was able to persuade her to reintroduce healthy protein and fats into her diet, her skin softened as it regained its moisture and vibrancy. And Samantha experienced an energy boost as well. Her skin became so well hydrated that she was hired to model a new skin care line of products specially developed to treat dry skin.

Myth 6: *Paying attention to my skin is a waste of time.*

If you have one of the easier Skin Types, your recommended routine is not going to create unnecessary complexity. What's more, fine-tuning your skin care can only save you money and optimise your skin in the long run. On the other hand, if you have a challenging Skin Type, treating your skin right and preventing future problems is an absolute essential. Most skin problems are better addressed sooner rather than later. And whatever your age, skin condition or Skin Type, sooner is today.

READY, SET . . . SKIN TYPE!

I'm truly delighted to be able to share with you my discoveries and to help you manage your skin and treat it right. Try the regimens and products, and see how they work for you. Don't hesitate to see a dermatologist if you need to, as there are many advanced medications and procedures of real benefit. Finally, share Skin Typing with your friends, family and loved ones because there's a Skin Type Solution for everyone.

CHAPTER TWO

Understanding Skin Type Categories

In Chapter Three, you will take the Baumann Skin Type Questionnaire to identify the four dominant factors that determine your Skin Type. These factors are: oily vs. dry, sensitive vs. resistant, pigmented vs. non-pigmented, and wrinkled vs. tight. But first, in this chapter, I'll offer some basic wisdom about each of these factors, as well as provide the science behind them. The key factors interact to determine the skin's appearance, problems, needs and vulnerabilities, and therefore dictate the kinds of products, ingredients and treatments useful to address them. To get started, let me introduce you to some basics about the skin.

THE BIOLOGY OF THE SKIN

The top layer of the skin, called the epidermis, is made up of four distinct layers. When you look at someone's skin, you see the very top layer, made up of cells that reflect light. When that top layer is smooth, it reflects light evenly so that the skin looks more uniform and radiant than it does when the surface is rougher.

At the lowest portion of the epidermis are 'mother cells', called basal cells, which produce all the other skin cells. They divide into 'daughter cells', which rise up to the higher levels of the epidermis. As they travel, they age and eventually die, so that the top layer consists of dead cells which naturally exfoliate off in a process called the 'cell cycle', which can take anywhere from twenty-six to forty-two days. Between the third and eighth decades of life, the cell cycle slows from 30 to 50 percent of its pace in youth. That means that older skin renews itself much more slowly, forming a rough surface of cells, rather than a smooth surface.

The uppermost cells contain a natural moisturising factor (NMF), which holds moisture. The body responds to a dry environment by producing more NMF, but it takes several days for production to rev up, so your skin may become quite dehydrated before help comes. That's why it's important to moisturise your skin in any dry environment.

Substances released by the cells in the middle of the epidermis form a protective film made of lipids (fats) that surrounds skin cells and helps keep the skin hydrated. Your fingers and toes contain fewer lipids and are therefore not as 'watertight' as your legs, which is why your fingers and toes look shrivelled after immersion in water but your legs do not. Your skin cracks in cold weather because the chilled lipids become stiffer and less able to adjust to movement. The goal of the best moisturisers is to increase the amount of these important lipids, helping your skin to hold moisture.

FACTOR ONE: SKIN HYDRATION: OILY VS. DRY

With oily skin, your face may often look shiny, and you naturally avoid products that feel oily. You'll be more vulnerable to acne and breakouts than Dry Skin Types. People with dry skin will notice that their skin feels dry, and has a dull colour and/or rough texture.

Dryness and oiliness depend primarily on the condition of the skin barrier, the outer layer of skin, which helps the skin retain moisture, and the oil (sebum) production itself.

The barrier is like a brick wall, with each brick (or cell) held in place by mortar (fats called lipids). Harmful ingredients, cold, and dry weather can wear down these fats, eroding the mortar so that the 'bricks' are not secured in their proper place. A variety of outside agents, including detergents, acetone, chlorine and other chemicals, and even prolonged water immersion can harm the barrier, or the barrier may be deficient for genetic reasons.

The barrier's main components are ceramides, fatty acids and cholesterol, all different kinds of lipids. These must be present in the right proportion to keep the skin watertight. An impaired barrier will tend towards both dryness and sensitivity. Dryness results when skin moisture evaporates. Sensitivity results when a deficient barrier permits the entry of outside irritants.

Repairing the skin barrier with the right skin care products will help treat a variety of skin conditions. Incorporating key dietary nutrients, such as essential fatty acids and cholesterol, provides the necessary building blocks. Nutrient deficiencies can weaken your skin's ability to repair and rebuild, which is why people who take cholesterol-lowering drugs often have dry skin. In the 'Further Help' pages following each of the four sections of the book, I'll recommend supplements providing the necessary components of the skin barrier.

Oil Production

The skin has many oil (sebaceous) glands, which secrete oil that contains wax esters, triglycerides and squalene. These fats (or lipids) form a film that helps keep moisture in the skin. While increased sebum production results in oily skin, the opposite is not always the case, as dry skin can also arise from an impaired skin barrier. Oil production can be affected by diet, stress and hormones – as well as genetics. In a study of twenty pairs each of identical and nonidentical same-sex twins, identical twins had virtually identical amounts of oil production, while the nonidentical twins had significantly different amounts.

Your results on the O/D score portion of the questionnaire will reveal not only which factor is predominant but also, depending on your degree of oiliness and dryness, the skin issues you'll experience and the way you should address them.

FACTOR TWO: SKIN SENSITIVITY: SENSITIVE VS. RESISTANT

Resistant skin has a solid skin barrier that shields the skin cells, keeping allergens and irritating substances from the deeper skin layers. Unless sunburned, your skin rarely stings, reddens, or develops acne, allowing resistant types to use most products without reacting. However, the irony is that many products may not be potent enough to penetrate the 'thick' barrier and deliver results.

Sensitive skin, which is reported by over 40 percent of people, has a weaker barrier, making it vulnerable to many kinds of skin reactions. While many products target sensitive skin, there are four very different subtypes of sensitive skin, so your treatments and products must address your unique subtype:

Acne subtype: Develops acne, blackheads or whiteheads
Rosacea subtype: Develops recurring flushing, facial redness and hot sensation
Stinging subtype: Develops stinging or burning of skin
Allergic subtype: Develops redness, itching and flaking of skin.

All of these sensitive skin subtypes have one thing in common: inflammation. That's why all the treatments for S types are geared to reduce inflammation and remove its cause.

Lily's Story

A Hungarian chemist with blue eyes and pale blond hair, Lily always enjoyed easy, slightly dry skin, until one day, she noticed pimples dotting her jaw line. This prompted her to take a pregnancy test and the results were positive. As the acne worsened, Lily looked for acne products at the pharmacy but felt overwhelmed and decided to just hope the acne went away. By sixteen weeks into the pregnancy, her acne had worsened, and she also developed dark spots on her face for the first time in her life.

Lily came to see me in tears. I explained that hormonal changes had increased oil production, resulting in acne, while higher oestrogen levels activated her skin colour cells to make dark spots, an occurrence so common in pregnancy that it's called the 'mask of pregnancy'. Sun exposure exacerbated the problem. Whenever the skies looked overcast, Lily stopped using sunscreen because due to her skin's oiliness, sunscreen now made her skin feel too greasy. I gave her a gel sunscreen instead, and provided acne treatment safe for both Lily and the baby.

Lily came back when her baby boy was eight months old. By then, she'd reverted to her Dry Skin Type and needed new skin care recommendations.

Acne Subtype

Millions of people are troubled by acne, with eleven- to twenty-five-year-olds accounting for 70 to 80 percent of acne sufferers, while many adult women have acne resulting from hormonal imbalance. Adults are often more perturbed by acne than teens.

Three main factors contribute to acne: increased oil production, clogged pores, and a bacteria called P. acnes. Here's how they interact: oil causes the dead skin cells to stick together, leading to a clogged pore, which is called a blackhead or a whitehead. Bacteria then moves into the pore, producing inflammation, which manifests as redness and pus. Addressing acne requires medications that decrease oil secretion, unclog pores, and kill bacteria. I'll provide recommendations for specific treatments in the prescriptive sections of each type chapter.

Rosacea Subtype

Rosacea typically begins in adults over twenty-five years old. Its symptoms are facial redness, flushing, pimples and the formation of prominent blood vessels in the face. Prior to age twenty-five, people prone to rosacea may experience frequent blushing and facial redness with strong emotion. The same bacteria that causes ulcers (*H. pylori*) may contribute to rosacea, some studies show. Rosacea sufferers with inflammatory bumps and facial redness should be tested for *H. pylori*, which can be treated with oral antibiotics. If you suffer from rosacea, please see your dermatologist for the many effective prescriptive treatments.

Stinging Subtype

Stinging in response to products and ingredients is not due to allergies, but to more sensitive nerve endings. In dermatology, tests (like the lactic acid stinging test) can determine whether or not you're a 'stinger'. If you are, you may experience terrible stinging in response to benzoic acid, present in many products such as K-Y Jelly and vaginal yeast infection creams.

Skin stinging is not necessarily accompanied by redness or irritation, although it's more common in people who experience facial flushing as well. 'Stingers' should avoid products that contain the following ingredients:

Alpha hydroxy acids (glycolic acid)
Benzoic acid
Bronopol
Cinnamic acid compounds
Dowicil 200
Formaldehyde
Lactic acid
Propylene glycol
Quaternary ammonium compounds
Sodium lauryl sulfate
Sorbic acid
Urea
Vitamin C

Allergic Subtype

When the protective outermost layer of the skin breaks down or weakens, substances can seep around the skin cells and penetrate to deeper layers of the skin. Through these gaps, allergens, chemicals, and other irritants come in from the outside, invading inner levels of the skin tissue and bloodstream, and triggering an inflammatory response. While this is the mechanism for topical skin allergies, there can also be internal allergies to foods or other substances that trigger an inflammatory response expressed via the skin.

A recent epidemiological survey in Great Britain revealed that 23 percent of women and 13.8 percent of men experience an adverse reaction to a personal care product over the course of a year. While stinging is the most common reaction, allergies to cosmetic ingredients also occur. To identify cosmetic ingredient allergies, dermatologists perform patch tests, in which twenty to one hundred ingredients are taped to a person's back. Twenty-four to forty-eight hours later, when the tape is removed, reddened or swollen areas indicate allergies. Up to 10 percent of patients test allergic to at least one cosmetic-product ingredient, according to various studies. But many more may be allergic, as most people don't consult a physician; instead they simply discontinue using the products that bother them. However, whatever your type, due to the high rate of people who experience these allergies, there is no way to be absolutely certain that a given product is right for you, without patch testing. That's why I always recommend that people with sensitive skin try out a product sample, if possible, prior to purchase. If your skin reacts to many ingredients, you may need to consult a dermatologist to identify the specific ones that cause a problem, so you can avoid them.

The most common allergens are fragrances and preservatives. Recently the International Fragrance Association (IFRA) started an initiative to develop safe products that contain fragrances. Since the benefits of aromatherapy have been revealed in recent studies, it's important to find ways to harness the benefits of essential oils and fragrances without causing allergies. People who use a variety of skin care products are more likely to develop allergies because they have been exposed to more ingredients. People with dry skin (indicating an impaired skin barrier) will tend to have more topical or localised skin allergies. Allergies are most common in Dry, Sensitive Skin Types, which is why in Chapters Twelve to Fifteen, I'll show how to strengthen the skin barrier to alleviate this problem.

FACTOR THREE: SKIN PIGMENTATION: PIGMENTED VS. NON-PIGMENTED

The pigmented vs. non-pigmented scale in my questionnaire measures the likelihood of developing unwanted dark spots on the face or chest. Although the test will also take into account skin colour and ethnicity, that is not as important in my system as determining the tendency towards unwanted spots. That's why people of all ethnicities can score as any of the sixteen Skin Types. That being said, in some cases, the majority of those with a particular Skin Type may come from certain ethnic backgrounds, while people from a very different ethnicity might be in the minority for that particular type.

Why do I place such emphasis on unwanted dark spots? Twenty-one percent of visits to the dermatologist are for their treatment. Over eighty thousand people annually buy over-the-counter (nonprescription) skin care products to reduce their dark spots. Various kinds of dark spots cause cosmetic concern. In this book, I'll focus on those that are avoidable and removable without surgery. Birthmarks, moles, and scaling patches called seborrhoeic keratoses are outside of that scope. Instead I'll focus on melasma, sun spots (solar lentigos), and freckles, which can be prevented and treated with skin care products and procedures.

Dark Spots

Melasma, also known as the 'mask of pregnancy', consists of light or dark brown or grey patches ranging from the size of a 5p coin to large areas on the face or chest. Appearing in sun-exposed areas, it's more common in pregnant women or those on oestrogen therapy, whether birth control pills or hormone replacement. Melasma can be stressful and, in severe cases, even disfiguring. More commonly seen in darker-skinned people, such as those of Mediterranean, Asian, Latin-American, and African descent, melasma is difficult to cure but can be controlled with the right skin care products and procedures. Pigmented types with any combination of the other three factors can have melasma.

Solar lentigos are caused by sun exposure and sunburns. They're completely preventable with sun avoidance and sun protection. Popping up on people of all skin and hair colours, solar lentigos result from environmental factors, like excess sun, more than genes. I feel that they contribute to the appearance of aging as much or more than wrinkles, a view shared by Asians, who are often more concerned with dark spots than wrinkles.

My patients often tell me that they want 'skin like yours', referring to the fact that my complexion is free of spots and wrinkles, both of which contribute to an aged appearance. Yet many people focus more on wrinkles, not recognizing how spots detract from skin's youthfulness. On the first visit, I use a Wood's light (black light) or a UVB camera to reveal facial dark spots before they are visible in ordinary light. Most people are shocked by what they see in the mirror. Several patients dragged their teenage daughters in to look at their skin under the light in order to convince them to wear sunscreen. One broke down in tears when she realised how her skin would look in ten years.

People with many solar lentigos generally fall into the wrinkled category on the wrinkled-vs.-tight scale. If you do not come out with a wrinkled score on the questionnaire, consider yourself a borderline W and follow the recommendations in the corresponding pigmented and wrinkled chapter. For example, if you're an Oily, Resistant, Pigmented and Tight Skin Type (ORPT) with ample solar lentigos, follow the recommendations aimed at wrinkle prevention for Oily, Resistant, Pigmented and Wrinkled (ORPW) as a preventative. The good news is that my recommendations for products and procedures can make a dramatic difference in the way your skin looks.

Freckles, also called ephelides, are associated with red hair and fair skin, while solar lentigos are not, although their appearance is similar. The gene believed to be responsible for freckles is the MC1R gene, which is closely associated with fair skin and red hair. While you can't control your genes, you can control sun exposure. Freckles appear early in childhood, increase as a result of sunburn before the age of twenty, and partly disappear with age, while solar lentigos worsen with age. Because fair-skinned redheads, those most prone to freckles, frequently burn and cannot tan, they often end up avoiding the sun, resulting in less cumulative lifetime sun exposure than people with solar lentigos. However, these fair-skinned redheads are at a higher risk of melanoma, which increases with a history of frequent sunburns and sun exposure.

Unlike people with many solar lentigos, people with freckles can fall into the tight group if they've avoided sun exposure and followed good skin habits, such as eating an antioxidant-rich diet, not smoking, and using retinoids.

Ethnicity and Skin Tone

While people with a darker skin colour are more likely to fall into the pigmented category, not all dark-skinned people are pigmented types, with pigment problems. Those with even skin tones and no spots will be Non-Pigmented Skin Types, even though they have darker-toned skin. On the other hand, light-skinned people who freckle and get melasma or solar lentigos may fall into the P category. The P/N scale measures the tendency to develop unwanted dark spots, not ethnicity.

Skin pigment-producing cells (called melanocytes) produce skin pigment (melanin), which creates skin colour as well as all the forms of pigmentation I've mentioned. Skin pigment formation can be prevented by two main mechanisms. The first is to inhibit the enzyme tyrosinase, which prevents the formation of melanin. Many topical cosmetic ingredients such as, kojic acid, arbutin, and licorice extract are tyrosinase inhibitors. The second method of preventing the production of skin colour is to forestall the transfer of the colour into the skin cells. Studies show that niacinamide and soy prevent that transfer, which is why they are in skin lightening products.

Pigmentation and Skin Cancer Risk

Pigmentation contributes to your risks of getting the various types of skin cancer, which I'll detail in the specific Skin Types chapters. Melanoma skin cancers result when the pigment cells that produce colour become cancerous. Though curable if caught early, this form of cancer can metastasise very rapidly, making early detection essential. Non-melanoma skin cancers are cancers of the skin cells themselves. There are two varieties. Basal cell cancers occur at the basal skin level between the dermis and epidermis. These can be easily removed but may leave scars. Squamous cells grow on the top layer of skin, and although they can metastasise, they are less deadly than melanoma. All should be checked for regularly and treated promptly. Guidelines for detection can be found in 'Signs of Melanoma: The A, B, C and D' in Chapter Five, and 'How to Recognise a Non-Melanoma Skin Cancer' in Chapter Seven. When in doubt, consult a dermatologist.

Ultraviolet Light

When UV light hits the skin, it stimulates an increased production of skin pigment, which is what we call tanning. This is the skin's major defence against further UV damage. In addition to tanning skin, ultraviolet light worsens melasma and causes sun spots (solar lentigos). UVB rays cause an immediate sunburn; UVA rays cause long-term damage. Many sunscreens do not block both types of UV light. Even broad-spectrum sunscreens do not block 100 percent of the sun. Sun avoidance is the most important method of preventing skin pigmentation.

Light-skinned people with high P scores are likely to have freckles and may also be at a risk for melanoma. People of Middle-Eastern, Indian, Latin-American, Asian and Mediterranean ethnicity are often on the cusp of the P/N scale. In any event, if you have dark spots that bother you, call yourself a P. If not, call yourself an N. Though you are less likely to get skin cancer, with enough sun exposure you may get bothersome darks spots. Dark-skinned people with high P/N scores who are also a T are unlikely to develop skin cancer but often suffer from dark patches.

FACTOR FOUR: WRINKLED VS. TIGHT

The two main processes of skin aging are intrinsic and extrinsic. Intrinsic aging is your individual genetic programming, which unfolds over time. It's inevitable and beyond your control. Extrinsic aging results from external factors – such as smoking, pollution, poor nutrition and sun exposure – that can be changed.

Of these, the most universally experienced extrinsic factor is sun exposure, and that's why I place great emphasis on achieving adequate protection. Here I'll overview the basic principles of sun protection, while in the Skin Type chapters, I'll recommend the appropriate products to be employed.

Daily Sunscreen Use

Make it a habit to apply sunscreen every morning whether you plan to be indoors or out. UVA easily penetrates windows to send harmful sun rays into buildings, cars and aeroplanes. Keep your favourite sunblock in your car, desk and handbag in case you forget to apply it as part of your morning routine. Select a product with a minimum SPF of 15 for daily protection, when you will not be receiving prolonged sun exposure. You can also derive sun protection from a variety of skin care products, such as moisturisers, facial foundations and facial powders that contain SPF. Just make sure that you use a combination of products to assure a combined SPF of at least 15 when they are used together.

Sunscreen Application

To apply, squeeze a portion of the product the size of a 10p coin and apply it to your entire face, neck, hands and chest. Make sure to apply it to all exposed areas that give away your age. (I can almost always tell someone's age by looking at the hands, neck and chest.) Since there are no procedures that effectively turn back the clock for the neck, it's vital to protect these areas if you want to remain youthful looking.

If you plan to expose the rest of your body to the sun for more than fifteen minutes, apply sunscreen to your legs, shoulders, arms, back and feet too.

Increased Sun Exposure

If you swim, play sports, walk to work, drive in your car, or experience any other form of sun exposure, I recommend that you follow my precautions for avoiding the sun. Even on cloudy or overcast days, you can receive sun exposure, and should protect yourself. Don't think you can take the risk of getting a little sun when you go on vacation because you're indoors the rest of the time. That's when people are most likely to burn their skin, and even a single sunburn can create a lifetime of skin damage. Always do the following:

- Wear a broad-spectrum sunscreen of SPF 45–60 and reapply it every hour.
- Apply your sunscreen thirty minutes prior to sun exposure so it can adequately penetrate the skin.
- Confine your exposure to the times when the sun is less powerful, before ten AM, and after four PM.
- Stay under an umbrella when possible.
- Wear protective SPF clothing, available from www.sunprecautions.com and other suppliers.

In addition, apply sunscreen to your body, as clothes provide less protection than most people realise. A normal T-shirt only has an SPF of 5, while tighter weave fabrics offer more protection. You can apply sunscreen to the eye area unless you experience itching, burning or irritation. In very hot weather, or if you are involved in active sports, you may find that if you sweat, the sunscreen runs into your eyes, causing a burning sensation. If this occurs, bypass sunscreen on the eye area, and use a concealer or foundation with sun protective ingredients. Plus, don't forget to protect other family members, especially your children. I'm a Mum so I know how kids want to run out and play right away, but make sure they are well-coated with sunscreen, covered with protective clothing, and wearing a hat with a brim that shades their faces. They'll thank you when they are older!

Wrinkle Prevention

While sun protection is key to wrinkle prevention, there are some other factors. The epidermis, or top skin layer, makes the skin look radiant and smooth; wrinkles are caused by changes in the lower layer of the skin, the dermis. Unfortunately, many skin care ingredients cannot penetrate far enough into the dermis to affect wrinkles. But there are a few exceptions. Many studies have shown that retinoids can affect wrinkles and in fact Avage and Renova have received approval by the US government's Food and Drug Administration (FDA) for this purpose and are available with a prescription.

So, the best route is preventing the formation of wrinkles. Antioxidants, when used consistently on the skin, will likely prevent some of the extrinsic aging that occurs. The goal of 'wrinkle prevention' is to stop the loss of collagen, elastin and hyaluronic acid (HA), three important structural components that decrease with age and inflammation. Some antiaging products contain these ingredients and aim to put them 'back' into skin, but that is not possible because their molecules are simply too large to be absorbed topically. Although hyaluronic acid added in topical formulas may help hydrate the skin, it does not penetrate and replace lost naturally occurring HA. I wish I had a dollar for every collagen-containing skin cream claiming it would help replace skin collagen and every HA product that claimed it would increase skin HA levels. This is simply not possible!

Topical agents that stimulate the skin to make its own collagen, elastin and HA are more effective. Retinoids, vitamin C and copper peptide have been shown to increase collagen synthesis. A new cosmetic skin cream is being developed that stimulates your skin's elastin gene to make elastin tissue, increasing the skin's ability to bounce back. Retinoids have been shown to increase production of hyaluronic acid and elastin. Supplements that increase collagen, elastin and hyaluronic acid (such as oral vitamin C) may increase collagen synthesis. I do not know of any supplements that increase elastin synthesis. Glucosamine supplements increase levels of hyaluronic acid. Antioxidants may help prevent the breakdown of these three components by neutralising free radicals.

Injecting these components in a cosmetic dermatological procedure called dermal fillers or via a new superficial-level injection called meso-therapy is effective. I'll discuss these options in greater detail in the sections on 'Further Help'.

If you test out as a Wrinkled Skin Type, don't despair. This is the only Skin Type parameter that you can control. Wouldn't you rather know it now and take steps to prevent it? Of course, you cannot control the genetic, or intrinsic, component. However, the extrinsic component is completely under your control.

Sun exposure accelerates the aging process by causing:

- Breakdown of collagen, the supporting structure of the skin
- Breakdown of elastin, which gives skin its resilience and bounce
- Loss of hyaluronic acid, which holds water and gives skin its volume
- Damage to DNA, which can cause cells to go awry, leading to cancer
- Disintegration of enzymes necessary for production of important cell components

The sad fact is that once your skin structures have broken down, it's harder to put them back together again. That's why it's better to protect your skin now, rather than pay later. Avoiding sun exposure, using sunscreen, avoiding cigarette smoke and pollution, taking antioxidant supplements, and eating a diet high in fruits and vegetables can help reduce wrinkling.

In addition, regularly using prescription retinoids and skin care products with antioxidant activity can also help. Experience with patients has suggested to me that Botox and Reloxin injections can prevent wrinkles caused in areas of movement by decreasing movement in those areas. Changing your habits will change you from a W to a T. I am actually a W by nature and a T by choice. If you fall on the boundary between T and W, follow the recommendations for W to help you prevent wrinkles as much as possible. If you are a W and already have the wrinkles to show for it, remember, there are many solutions. Several types of dermal fillers currently available to fill in wrinkles can give you instant gratification. Many more are on the horizon. Light, laser, and radio frequency treatments are becoming more advanced and less invasive.

HOW THE FOUR FACTORS INTERACT

The way the four factors combine with each other produces certain commonly seen tendencies. For example, Pigmented, Wrinkled Skin Types often have a significant history of sun exposure manifested by wrinkles and solar lentigos. They would do well with retinoids and light treatments. Dry, Sensitive Skin Types have a higher tendency to develop eczema and should use barrier repair moisturisers.

Oily, sensitive types are more likely to develop acne. Lighter-skin OS types, especially those with wrinkles and a strong history of sun damage, have a higher tendency to develop wrinkles and rosacea. Non-Pigmented, Wrinkled Skin Types are more likely to have light skin that wrinkles. Pigmented, Tight types most commonly (but not always) have dark skin. Based on Skin Typing as well as these common patterns, my hope is that companies will one day quite soon develop products that focus on your specific needs.

Now it's time to discover your Skin Type by answering the questionnaire in the next chapter. Afterwards, you can refer back to this chapter to understand how the science of your predominant factors impacts your skin. Or you may prefer to go directly to your Skin Type chapter.

CHAPTER THREE

Discovering Your Skin Type

In this chapter, you will discover your Skin Type. To do this, you will be taking the Baumann Skin Type Questionnaire. Most people find it helpful to accurately understand the unique nature of their skin, and of course, this serves as the basis for all the recommendations in the book and for all your skin care decisions.

HOW I DEVELOPED SKIN TYPING AND THE QUESTIONNAIRE

Many people ask me if I can tell their Skin Type at a glance. Having looked at thousands of people's skin, often I can. However, I'm a scientist and I need to be certain. That's why, with my patients, I always double-check by having them answer the questionnaire. Also, in rare instances their answers will reveal something in their history that is not visible to me. This is more likely to occur with young people, whose faces do not yet reveal the results of their skin's genetics, care and sun exposure.

This questionnaire is truly comprehensive. Despite the short time needed to take it, it reveals more information than would be covered in a typical office visit. As a result, I can spend that valuable time getting to know my patients and their needs, and also providing dermal fillers and other cosmetic treatments. Since everyone's feelings about their face and looks are so personal I like to get to know my patients so that I can address both skin care and their worries, fears and frustration about their skin problems. Using this questionnaire gives me more time to do that and still get home to spend time with my two young sons and husband.

Since my patients know that I write a monthly column called 'Cosmeceutical Critique' on skin care ingredients in *Skin and Allergy News* (www.eskinandallergynews.com), every week a few dozen ask me to devise a specific skin care regimen right for them. And for many years, I did just that. That's how, over time, I saw a pattern emerge which evolved into my understanding that there are four factors in evaluating people's skin – and as a result, sixteen distinct Skin Types.

To identify my patients' Skin Types, I began asking the questions that evolved over time into the Baumann Skin Type Questionnaire. As my patients used my regimens and recommendations, and we saw their results, I was able to refine these further to assure that they were truly effective for the different Skin Types. In the process, I learned a great deal about which products and ingredients worked always, sometimes, or never, so that within each Skin Type, I could guide people to skin care that met the particular skin issues they experienced.

I further tested every single question with patients to assure that the questions would reveal the right results. In addition, numerous medical colleagues have offered their input as well. So in taking the questionnaire, you can be assured that it will accurately reveal your Skin Type.

OVERVIEW OF THE QUESTIONNAIRE

The questionnaire is in four parts, with each part offering key questions, which will cumulatively capture where your skin falls on the spectrum of the four factors, between oily and dry, sensitive and resistant, pigmented and non-pigmented, and wrinkled and tight. While some of the factors are familiar to you, some of them may not be. But that's fine. You don't need to understand them to respond. The questions themselves are simple and will prompt you.

In the previous chapter, I explained each of the four factors and the skin characteristics common to both ends of the spectrum within each of the factors. Further information about these factors and how they interact will be revealed in the chapters on the Skin Types.

In taking the test, all you have to do is answer as honestly as you can. Consider it a game. Where I ask you to go without moisturiser and check your skin, or wear foundation but not powder, do it (unless you're a guy)! Of course, you can always guess, but you'll get the most accurate results from following the directions as described. If you haven't really noticed the condition of your skin sufficiently to answer certain questions, take a day or so, and pay attention to how your skin appears, feels and reacts in the various common situations described, and then go back and retake the test.

Unless specifically focused on something in the past, all questions refer to how your skin is now, and should be answered accordingly. Do not leave any questions blank. If necessary, answer *e,* which will be scored as 2.5 points, making it a neutral answer that will not affect the outcome of your total score. You'll get the most accurate Skin Type results if you answer *a, b, c* or *d,* so don't pick *e* unless you really can't answer the question.

Baumann Skin Type Questionnaire

This section measures skin oil-production and hydration. Studies show that people's preconceptions about whether their skin is oily or dry are often inaccurate. Don't allow your preconceptions or what others think and say about your skin to bias your answers.

1. After washing your face, don't apply any moisturiser, sunscreen, toner, powder or other products. Two to three hours later, look in a mirror under bright lights. Your forehead and cheeks feel or appear:
   a. Very rough, flaky, or ashy
   b. Tight
   c. Well hydrated with no reflection of light
   d. Shiny with reflection of bright light

2. In photos, your face appears shiny:
   a. Never, or you've never noticed shine
   b. Sometimes
   c. Frequently
   d. Always

3. Two to three hours after applying makeup foundation (also known as base) but no powder, your makeup appears:
   a. Flaky or caked in wrinkles
   b. Smooth
   c. Shiny
   d. Streaked and shiny
   e. I do not wear facial foundation.

4. When in a low-humidity environment, if you don't use moisturisers or sunscreen, your facial skin:
   a. Feels very dry or cracks

b. Feels tight

c. Feels normal

d. Looks shiny, or I never feel that I need moisturiser

e. Don't know

5. Look in a magnifying mirror. How many large pores, the size of the end of a pin or greater, do you have?
   a. None
   b. A few in the T-zone (forehead and nose) only
   c. Many
   d. Tons!
   e. Don't know (Note: please look again and only answer *e* if you cannot determine this.)

6. You would characterise your facial skin as:
   a. Dry
   b. Normal
   c. Combination
   d. Oily

7. When you use soap that suds, bubbles, and foams vigorously, your facial skin:
   a. Feels dry or cracks
   b. Feels slightly dry but does not crack
   c. Feels normal
   d. Feels oily
   e. I do not use soap or other foaming cleansers. (If this is because they make your skin dry, pick *a*.)

8. If not moisturised, your facial skin feels tight:
   a. Always
   b. Sometimes
   c. Rarely
   d. Never

9. You have clogged pores (blackheads or whiteheads):
   a. Never
   b. Rarely
   c. Sometimes
   d. Always

10. Your face is oily in the T-zone (forehead and nose):
    a. Never
    b. Sometimes
    c. Frequently
    d. Always

11. Two to three hours after applying moisturiser your cheeks are:
    a. Very rough, flaky, or ashy
    b. Smooth
    c. Slightly shiny
    d. Shiny and slick, or I do not use moisturizer

Scoring of O vs. D:

Give yourself 1 point for every *a* answer, 2 points for every *b*, 3 points for every *c*, 4 points for every *d*, and 2.5 points for every *e* answer.

Enter your total O/D score here: _____

If your score is between 34–44, you have very oily skin.
If your score is between 27–33, you have slightly oily skin.
If your score is between 17–26, you have slightly dry skin.
If your score is between 11–16, you have dry skin.

If you scored between 27–44, you are an **O Skin Type.**
If you scored between 11–26, you are a **D Skin Type.**

PART TWO

SENSITIVE VS. RESISTANT

This section measures your skin's tendency to develop pimples, redness, flushing and itching, all signs of sensitive skin.

1. You get red bumps on your face:
    a. Never

    b. Rarely

    c. At least once a month

    d. At least once a week

2. Skin care products (including cleanser, moisturiser, toner, and make-up) cause your face to break out, get a rash, itch or sting:

    a. Never

    b. Rarely

    c. Often

    d. Always

    e. I don't wear products on my face.

3. Have you ever been diagnosed with acne or rosacea?

    a. No

    b. Friends and acquaintances tell me I have it.

    c. Yes

    d. Yes, a severe case

    e. Unsure

4. If you wear jewellery that is not 24-carat gold, how often do you get a rash?

    a. Never

    b. Rarely

    c. Often

    d. Always

    e. Unsure

5. Sunscreens make your skin itch, burn, break out or turn red:

    a. Never

    b. Rarely

    c. Often

    d. Always

    e. I never wear sunscreen.

6. Have you ever been diagnosed with atopic dermatitis, eczema or contact dermatitis (an allergic skin rash)?

    a. No

    b. Friends tell me I have it.

    c. Yes

    d. Yes, a severe case

    e. Unsure

7. How often do you get a rash underneath your rings?
   a. Never
   b. Rarely
   c. Often
   d. Always
   e. I do not wear rings.

8. Fragranced bubble bath, massage oil or body lotions make your skin break out, itch or feel dry:
   a. Never
   b. Rarely
   c. Often
   d. Always
   e. I never use these types of products. (Note: answer *d* if you don't use them because they cause the above-mentioned problems.)

9. Can you use the soap provided in hotels on your body or face without a problem?
   a. Yes
   b. Most of the time, I don't have a problem.
   c. No, my skin itches, turns red or breaks out
   d. I would not use it. I've had too many problems in the past!
   e. I carry my own, so I'm unsure.

10. Has someone in your family been diagnosed with atopic dermatitis, eczema, asthma and/or allergies?
    a. No
    b. One family member that I know of
    c. Several family members
    d. Many of my family members have dermatitis, eczema, asthma and/or allergies.
    e. Unsure

11. What occurs if you use scented laundry detergents or static-control sheets in the dryer?
    a. My skin is fine.
    b. My skin feels slightly dry.
    c. My skin itches.
    d. My skin itches and gets a rash.
    e. Unsure, or I've never used them.

12. How often do your face and/or neck get red after moderate exercise, and/or with stress or a strong emotion, such as anger?
    a. Never
    b. Sometimes
    c. Frequently
    d. Always

13. How often do you tend to get red and flushed after drinking alcohol?
    a. Never
    b. Sometimes
    c. Frequently
    d. Always, or I don't drink because of this problem
    e. I never drink alcohol.

14. How often do you get red and flushed after eating spicy or hot (temperature) foods or beverages?
    a. Never
    b. Sometimes
    c. Frequently
    d. Always
    e. I never eat spicy food. (Note: if you don't eat spicy or hot food because of facial flushing, pick *d*.)

15. How many visible red or blue broken blood vessels do you have (or did you have prior to treatment) on your face and nose?
    a. None
    b. Few (one to three on entire face, including nose)
    c. Some (four to six on entire face, including nose)
    d. Many (over seven on entire face, including nose)

16. Your face looks red in photographs:
    a. Never, or I never noticed it
    b. Sometimes
    c. Frequently
    d. Always

17. People ask you if you are sunburned, even when you are not:
    a. Never
    b. Sometimes
    c. Frequently
    d. Always
    e. I always *am* sunburned. (You bad thing!)

18. You get redness, itching or swelling from makeup, sunscreen or skin care products:
    a. Never
    b. Sometimes
    c. Frequently
    d. Always
    e. I do not use these products. (Note: answer *d* if you don't use them because of redness, itching or swelling.)

Scoring of S vs. R:

Give yourself 1 point for every *a* answer, 2 points for every *b*, 3 points for every *c*, 4 points for every *d*, and 2.5 for every *e* answer.

Enter your total S/R score here: _____

If you've ever received a diagnosis of acne, rosacea, contact dermatitis or eczema from a dermatologist, add 5 to your score. If another type of physician has diagnosed you with these conditions, add 2 to your score.

If your score is between 34–72, you have very sensitive skin. (Don't worry, I'll help!)
If your score is between 30–33, you have somewhat sensitive skin. Following my recommendations may move you into the R Skin Type.
If your score is between 25–29, you have somewhat resistant skin.
If your score is between 17–24, you have very resistant skin. (Lucky you!)

If you scored between 30–72, you are an **S Skin Type.**
If you scored between 17–29, you are an **R Skin Type.**

PART THREE

PIGMENTED VS. NON-PIGMENTED SKIN

This section measures your skin's tendency to form melanin, a skin pigment that produces darker skin tones as well as dark patches, freckles, and dark areas after trauma. Melanin also helps you tan rather than burn.

1. After you have a pimple or ingrown hair, it's followed by a dark brownish/black spot:
   - a. Never
   - b. Sometimes
   - c. Frequently
   - d. Always
   - e. I never get pimples or ingrown hairs.

2. After you cut yourself, how long does the brown (not pink) mark remain?
   - a. I don't get a brown mark.
   - b. A week
   - c. A few weeks
   - d. Months

3. How many dark spots did you develop on your face when you were pregnant, on birth control pills or taking hormone replacement therapy (HRT)?
   - a. None
   - b. One
   - c. A few
   - d. A lot
   - e. This question does not apply to me (because I am male, or because I have never been pregnant or taken birth control pills or HRT, or because I'm unsure whether I have dark spots).

4. Do you have any dark spots or patches on your upper lip or cheeks? Or have you had any in the past that you've had removed?
   - a. No

b. I'm not sure.

c. Yes, they are (or were) slightly noticeable.

d. Yes, they are (or were) very noticeable.

5. Do the dark spots on your face get worse when you go in the sun?
    a. I have no dark spots.
    b. Unsure
    c. Slightly worse
    d. A lot worse
    e. I wear sunscreen on my face every day and never get sun. (Note: if you use constant sun protection because you're afraid you might get dark patches or freckles, answer *d.*)

6. Have you been diagnosed with melasma, light or dark brown or grey patches, on your face?
    a. No
    b. Once, but it went away.
    c. Yes
    d. Yes, a severe case
    e. Unsure

7. Do you have, or have you ever had, small brown spots (freckles or sun spots) on your face, chest, back or arms?
    a. No
    b. Yes, a few (one to five)
    c. Yes, many (six to fifteen)
    d. Yes, tons (sixteen or more)

8. When exposed to sun for the first time in several months, your skin:
    a. Burns only
    b. Burns then gets darker
    c. Gets darker
    d. My skin is already dark, so it is hard to see if it gets darker. (You can't pick 'I never had sun exposure.' Think of childhood experiences!)

9. What happens after you have had many days of consecutive sun exposure:
    a. I sunburn and blister, but my skin does not change colour.
    b. My skin becomes slightly darker.

c. My skin becomes much darker.

d. My skin is already dark, so it is hard to see if it gets darker.

e. Unsure (Again, you can't pick 'I never had sun.' If you really have to pick *e*, first consider all childhood experiences.)

10. When you go in the sun, do you develop freckles (small 1–2 mm, pinpoint-sized flat spots)?

    a. No, I never develop them.

    b. I develop a few new small freckles each year.

    c. I develop new freckles often.

    d. My skin is already dark, so it is hard to see if I have freckles.

    e. I never go in the sun. (Good for you!)

11. Did either of your parents have freckles? If so, please indicate how many. If neither or one parent did, respond to the question. If both did, answer the question as it relates to the parent with the most freckles.

    a. No

    b. A few on the face

    c. Many on the face

    d. Many on face, chest, neck and shoulders

    e. Unsure

12. What is your natural hair colour? (If grey, state colour before greying.)

    a. Blond

    b. Brown

    c. Black

    d. Red

13. Do you have a history of melanoma yourself or in your immediate family?

    a. No

    b. One person in my family

    c. More than one person in my family

    d. I have a history of melanoma.

    e. Unsure

14. If you have dark spots on your skin in areas of sun exposure, add 5 points to your score.

Scoring of P vs. N:

Give yourself 1 point for every *a* answer, 2 points for every *b*, 3 points for every *c*, 4 points for every *d*, and 2.5 points for every *e* answer.

Enter your total P/N score here: _____

If you scored between 29–57, you are a **P Skin Type.**
If you scored between 13–28, you are an **N Skin Type.**

PART FOUR

WRINKLED VS. TIGHT

This section measures your tendency to wrinkle, as well as how wrinkled you are right now. Some of my patients confessed that they cheated on this section to come out as a T – *after* I caught them doing it. Don't do that! You're only cheating yourself out of using preventative therapies that could prevent wrinkles. Changing your habits now could change your score in the future from a W to a T. So be honest and get the right treatments if you need them.

1. Do you have facial wrinkles?
   a. No, not even with movement such as smiling, frowning or lifting my eyebrows
   b. Only when I move, such as smiling, frowning or lifting my eyebrows
   c. Yes, with movement and a few at rest without movement
   d. Wrinkles are present even if I'm not smiling, frowning or lifting my brows.

In answering questions 2–7, please respond according to how you would compare yourself and other family members to *all* other ethnic groups, not just your own. For family members who you may not have known, please ask other family members or refer to photographs, where possible.

2. How old does/did your mother's facial skin look?
   a. Five to ten years younger than her age

b. Her age

c. Five years older than her age

d. More than five years older than her age

e. Not applicable; I was adopted or I cannot remember.

3. How old does/did your father's facial skin look?
     a. Five to ten years younger than his age
     b. His age
     c. Five years older than his age
     d. More than five years older than his age
     e. Not applicable; I was adopted or I cannot remember.

4. How old does/did your maternal grandmother's facial skin look?
     a. Five to ten years younger than her age
     b. Her age
     c. Five years older than her age
     d. More than five years older than her age
     e. Not applicable; I was adopted, never knew her, or cannot remember.

5. How old does/did your maternal grandfather's facial skin look?
     a. Five to ten years younger than his age
     b. His age
     c. Five years older than his age
     d. More than five years older than his age
     e. Not applicable; I was adopted, never knew him, or cannot remember.

6. How old does/did your paternal grandmother's facial skin look?
     a. Five to ten years younger than her age
     b. Her age
     c. Five years older than her age
     d. More than five years older than her age
     e. Not applicable; I was adopted, never knew her, or cannot remember.

7. How old does/did your paternal grandfather's facial skin look?
     a. Five to ten years younger than his age
     b. His age
     c. Five years older than his age
     d. More than five years older than his age
     e. Not applicable; I was adopted, never knew him, or cannot remember.

8. At any time in your life, have you ever tanned your skin on an ongoing basis for more than two weeks per year? If so, for how many total years did you do this? Please count tanning from playing tennis, fishing, playing golf, skiing or other outdoor activities. The beach is not the only place you can get a tan.
   a. Never
   b. One to five years
   c. Five to ten years
   d. More than ten years

9. At any time in your life, have you ever engaged in seasonal tanning of two weeks per year or less? (Yes, summer vacation counts!) If so, how often?
   a. Never
   b. One to five years
   c. Five to ten years
   d. More than ten years

10. Based on the places you've lived, how much daily sun exposure have you received in your life?
   a. Little; I've mostly lived in places that are grey and overcast.
   b. Some; I've lived in less sunny climes at times, but also in places with more regular sun.
   c. Moderate; I've lived in places with a fair amount of sun exposure.
   d. A lot; I've lived in tropical, Southern, or very sunny locales.

11. How old do you think you look?
   a. One to five years younger than your age
   b. Your age
   c. Five years older than your age
   d. More than five years older than your age

12. During the last five years, how often have you allowed your skin to tan either intentionally or unintentionally through outdoor sports or other activities?
   a. Never
   b. Once a month
   c. Once a week
   d. Daily

13. How often, if ever, have you been to a tanning bed?
    a. Never
    b. One to five times
    c. Five to ten times
    d. Many times

14. Over your entire life, how many cigarettes have you smoked (or been exposed to)?
    a. None
    b. A few packs
    c. Several to many packs
    d. I smoke every day.
    e. I've never smoked but I've lived with, been raised by, or worked with people who regularly smoked in my presence.

15. Please describe the air pollution where you reside:
    a. The air is fresh and clean.
    b. For part of the year, but not all of the year, I reside in a place with clean air.
    c. The air is slightly polluted.
    d. The air is very polluted.

16. Please describe the length of time that you have used retinoid facial creams such as retinol, Renova, Retin-A, Tazorac, Differin or Avage:
    a. Many years
    b. Occasionally
    c. Once for acne when I was younger
    d. Never

17. How often do you currently eat fruits and vegetables?
    a. At every meal
    b. Once a day
    c. Occasionally
    d. Never

18. Over your lifetime, what percentage of your daily diet has consisted of fruits and vegetables? (Note: don't count juices unless they are freshly squeezed.)
    a. 75–100 percent
    b. 25–75 percent

c. 10–25 percent
d. 0–10 percent

19. What is your natural skin colour (without tanning or self-tanners)?
    a. Dark
    b. Medium
    c. Light
    d. Very light

20. What is your ethnicity? (Please choose best answer.)
    a. African/African-American/Aboriginal/Maori/Caribbean/Black
    b. Asian/Indian/Mediterranean/Other
    c. Latin-American/Hispanic/Middle-Eastern
    d. Caucasian

21. If you are sixty-five years or older, add 5 points to your score.

Scoring of W vs. T:

Give yourself 1 point for every *a* answer, 2 points for every *b*, 3 points for every *c*, 4 points for every *d*, and 2.5 points for every *e* answer.

Enter your total W/T score here: _____

If you scored between 20 and 40, you are a **T Skin Type.**
If you scored between 41 and 85, you are a **W Skin Type.**

To define your final Skin Type results, please take all the factor indications that you have scored (in the order of your test responses) and write them in here:

My O/D score is _____, which equals _____.

My S/R score is _____, which equals _____.

My P/N score is _____, which equals _____.

My W/T score is _____, which equals _____.

Put them together and now you know your Skin Type!

WHAT YOUR TEST REVEALS

Now that you know your Skin Type, you may want to go back and reread the previous chapter, so that you understand where your skin's characteristics place you in each of the four factors. Next, you can turn to your Skin Type chapter and learn all that you need to know about caring for your skin. Here I'll go a little further into your results to explain more about your skin.

YOUR OILY VS. DRY SCORE

If your O score is 11–16, you have very dry skin.

With very dry skin, you may be deficient in natural moisturising factor (NMF), which is decreased by exposure to UVA light; avoiding sun exposure may help. If your skin is both dry *and* resistant, you may lack NMF, which cannot be replaced.

Hyaluronic acid (HA), which holds skin moisture, decreases with age. People who are dry *and* wrinkled may have less HA.

If you have dry skin, small pores and minimal acne, you may have decreased oil secretion. Oil production decreases with age (and menopause) and is most common with the Dry, Resistant (DR) Skin Type.

With dry skin, if you suffer from frequent redness and itching, you may have a damaged skin barrier. In this category, you've a higher risk for rashes and eczema, which may run in your family.

With a score of 17–26, you have slightly dry skin.

Your Oily/Dry score and your Sensitive/Resistant score can interact. If you score 30 or greater on the S/R scale, you may suffer from *occasional* skin itching, flaking and redness, indicating a less than perfect skin barrier. The recommendations I'll offer in the chapters for dry, resistant skin will help tackle this range of issues.

If you score less than 25 on the S/R questionnaire, then you probably have an intact skin barrier. Your skin dryness is more likely due to lower levels of natural moisturising factor (NMF) and/or sebum.

With a score of 27–33, you have slightly oily skin.

If your S/R score is 30 or below, you have the ideal degree of skin hydration. You likely have an intact skin barrier, good NMF levels, and enough sebum secretion without having too much to cause such problems as acne. However, if you score 34 or above on the S/R scale, you probably suffer from acne or rosacea.

With an O/D score over 34, you have very oily skin.

If you score 30 or below on the S/R scale, you suffer from skin oiliness but only rarely acne, and usually during times of stress or hormonal fluctuations. If so, figuring out what triggers the acne will help you address it.

However, if you score 34 or above on the S/R scale, you probably suffer from acne or rosacea. Your skin's oiliness will help you tolerate products that the drier S types cannot use. The OS chapters will offer recommendations.

YOUR SENSITIVE VS. RESISTANT SCORE

With an S/R score over 34, you are very likely to experience the more severe problems of one or more of the sensitivity subtypes described in Chapter Two.

With a score between 25–33, you are likely to experience some problems typical of several of the sensitivity subtypes, or have significant problems within one subtype.

With a score of 24 or less, you rarely suffer from the skin sensitivities detailed in Chapter Two. Even if you have a low S/R score, and are a Resistant Skin Type, you still may have occasional acne breakouts or redness; however, they're not the norm. If that occurs, temporarily follow the recommendations for your corresponding Sensitive Skin Type. For example, if you're usually a DRNW but as a result of recent stress, you develop acne, follow the recommendations in the DSNW chapter until your skin returns to its usual state.

I'll not go further into your scoring in the categories of pigmented vs. non-pigmented and wrinkled vs. tight, because your treatment needs and options for skin problems arising from these factors will depend on the issues you actually experience.

THE SKIN TYPE CHAPTERS

I could probably have written an entire book about each Skin Type, so I have tried to pack as much information as possible about skin, skin care and various treatments into each chapter. While your chapter will contain all the essential information you'll need, you may also find related information in the chapters of Skin Types that are similar, though slightly different, from yours. So if you'd like to know a little more, you can read these related chapters as well. Still you may find additional stories or scientific information that also applies to your Skin Type elsewhere in the book.

Which types are closest to yours? For starters, if you're an OSPT, then an OSPW would be pretty close to you – except that you would not be concerned with wrinkling. People with oily, sensitive skin share common problems, as do people with dry, resistant skin, so if you have the time and interest, you could read those related Skin Type chapters.

If you scored very near the changeover number between the two sides of the spectrum in any of the categories, you might choose to read both types. For example, people who score between 26 and 28 on the Oily/Dry questions have combination skin. While I provide additional options for combination skin in both the Oily and Dry Skin Type chapters, if you scored a 27 and were an ORPT, you might want to read DRPT as well, since you're pretty close. What's more, when you are borderline between factors, other influences can impact you, resulting in a temporary or permanent change in type.

For example, let's say that you have scored as an OSNW type, but are borderline dry. You have no problem with skin dryness – until the winter. At that time, you could follow the recommendations for Dry Skin Type, DSNW, switching back to your original type's regimen and products when warm weather returns. On the other hand, suppose you moved to a very dry climate. In that case, ongoing drying conditions could result in your turning permanently into a Dry Skin Type. To prevent that, read the related dry type chapter and take the precautions recommended to preserve your skin's moisture.

Here's another example: you may be an R type who has never experienced acne or skin rashes – until a stressful situation occurs. That stressful situation can make your skin *behave* like an S type. If that happens, follow the recommendations for your related Sensitive Skin Type, to calm your sensitivity and reduce your stress.

The category of pigmentation is primarily genetic. But if you were borderline between N and P, with a score between 25 and 30, and you are concerned about dark spots, you can follow the P recommendations for preventing and treating them.

Finally, many environmental influences impact people's T/W scores. If you're a tight type, such as a DRPT, but are close to the borderline for wrinkled, you could follow the recommendations for your corresponding wrinkled type, DRPW. That way, you can do everything right to help your skin preserve its tightness.

Now that you know your Skin Type, you can go directly to your Skin Type chapter. There you'll find everything you need to care for your skin with the certainty that when it comes to product choices and treatments, you've finally got it right.

Many people mail me their photos, asking if I can identify their Skin Type and prescribe a regimen for them. If only it were that easy! The sole way to guarantee an absolutely authentic Skin Type designation is by taking the questionnaire you've just completed. That being said, using a combination of photos, information reported on the media or the Internet, and guesswork, I can often come pretty close to divining a celebrity's Skin Type. However, unless I consult with that person, or they fill out the questionnaire, there is always the possibility that I may be mistaken. With that in mind, I hope that in reading your own and others' Skin Type chapters, you enjoy my 'guesses' about celebrities and their Skin Types.

PART TWO

Skin Care for Oily, Sensitive Skin

CHAPTER FOUR

Oily, Sensitive, Pigmented and Wrinkled: OSPW

THE SUN WORSHIPPER SKIN TYPE

'I love the sun, and the sun loves me. I always feel better with a tan. I think it helps my acne. I just don't see why there's such a fuss about avoiding the sun. Are we all supposed to walk around like pale ghosts?'

ABOUT YOUR SKIN

Many people with an Oily, Sensitive, Pigmented and Wrinkled Skin Type are the first ones on the beach in the morning and the last ones off it at sundown. The envy of all the other types, OSPWs tan to a perfect bronze. You are the surfer guys, the beach bunnies, the jet-setting socialites with the permanent tan, and the ever-bronzed CEOs. And let's not forget the bikini (or mono-kini) clad Frenchwomen that bake on the beach at Cannes, St Tropez, and St Bart's. You are all OSPWs and I see a lot of you in my Miami office when you fly in before (or after) your sun-filled Caribbean vacation.

Unlike non-pigmented folks, who don't tan very well, your pigmented skin turns to gold. And unlike many resistant types who prize their flawless complexions and flee the sun, you believe that there's nothing like an overall tan to diminish the appearance of the many tiny imperfections, including pimples, acne scars, brown spots, freckles, and other minor blemishes to which your type is prone. A tan shifts attention from blemished face to shapely legs. But it's a myth that the sun helps control acne. In fact, studies show that sun exposure increases breakouts by intensifying oil production.

If the questionnaire revealed you as an OSPW, but you are *not* a sun worshipper, you may be a common OSPW subtype with fair hair, fair skin, and freckles.

OSPW CELEBRITY

Suave, debonair, and eternally tanned, Hollywood icon Cary Grant married five times but had a lifelong love affair with the sun. Grant was the epitome of the OSPW. His slick hair and bronzed face revealed him as an oily type. His naturally dark skin indicated a high melanin content, while the tender heart hidden behind the trace of irony shading his performances showed him to be a sensitive man and, most likely, a sensitive type – although he may have had a low S/R score, because he rarely showed the acne and acne scars common to this type.

'Everyone wishes they were Cary Grant, even *I* wish I was Cary Grant,' he wittily commented. Like many OSPWs, Grant felt better eternally bronzed, and it suited his active, athletic lifestyle. As a hobby, Grant liked to play golf, and he also flew planes. But the cockpit and the golf course are prime spots for excess sun exposure.

Like many OSPWs I see in my practice, Cary Grant was a smoker (which contributes to skin aging), although he was able to quit in his middle years by undergoing hypnosis. Pictures of him in his later years (he lived to the age of eighty-two) show the toll that he paid for his decades of sunbathing, with wrinkles radiating from his eyes and mouth, lines creasing his forehead, and wrinkled jowls sagging from his manly jawline. Luckily for him, he *was* Cary Grant – and none of his fans seemed to mind the extra wrinkles.

But we mere mortals mustn't expect the same breaks. Instead it pays to safeguard skin against the natural aging process by avoiding the factors that accelerate it; and among them, sun exposure is number one. Harvey Keitel, Ray Liotta, Tommy Lee Jones, Mel Gibson, Roger Moore, Dennis Farina, Laurence Fishburne, and Harry Connick Jr are likely OSPWs as well.

SUN EXPOSURE: THE BAD NEWS

The fact is, with a tan these actors, like many OSPWs, just look *marvellous*. But I'm sorry to be the one to break the bad news that if you follow their lead you are ruining your skin.

I see OSPWs at every stage of the lifespan, and I can testify that the very same golden tan that makes you look great in youth is going to turn you into a dried-up prune as you age. Every day, younger OSPWs parade through my office, convinced that the sun is good for them, and I always wish I could let them eavesdrop on my visits with older OSPWs as they despair over wrinkles, sags, and other signs of aging, frequently forking over a small fortune to make things look right. It's much better to minimise, or at least moderate, your sun exposure now, to avoid paying such a steep price later. What's more, you run the risk of paying an even steeper price than premature aging.

Jake's Story

Carefree, action-oriented, fun-seeking Jake had been the golden god of the beach in his native habitat, Australia's Airlie Beach. As a teenager, he grew up diving by day and enjoying the adulation of his many female admirers by night. His blond hair was bleached white by the sun, while his skin was baked with a deep, permanent tan. That much sun exposure for a blond, freckled type is both aging and a potential health danger, but Jake never found that out because he was the last person on earth to consult a dermatologist. Girly stuff. Not for him.

In his late twenties, Jake launched a successful sailing business that kept him out on deck for long hours every day. He'd had more sunburns than he could count on his weathered fingers and toes. His tanned torso and sea-blue eyes melted the hearts of many. But by his forties, after three divorces, Jake decided to hide his freckled body under a baggy sweatshirt and the baby blues under an ever-present pair of sunglasses. Safer that way. Unfortunately, he didn't employ the same protection for the skin on his face, neck and hands.

By the latter part of his fifth decade, Jake's skin had turned to leather, with deeply etched lines and angry reddish freckles. His heart was equally hidebound. After too many women he'd had too easily, both cynicism and aging had caught up with him, and Jake lived alone. He took refuge in a few too many cigarettes and a few too many beers. In the end, the woman who noticed the ugly, asymmetrical mole on his back was not a paramour but Emma, his daughter with Wife Number Two. Jake had come to visit Emma and her new husband in Miami.

Emma, a resident in dermatology, immediately recognised the signs of a melanoma skin cancer. She reached for her cell phone and called me. I ran to my treatment room in time to meet them a half hour later. On a Saturday afternoon, I excised Jake's mole. A biopsy showed that it was a Clark's level I melanoma. When caught at that stage, the chances of the cancer spreading are minimal, but if left unattended, it could prove fatal. The old charmer was lucky. His daughter's discerning eye and swift action saved his life.

Melanoma is very definitely a risk factor for your Skin Type. Dermatologists take all melanomas extremely seriously, and we're trained to recognize them. On a number of occasions, I have spotted them on the arms of people in the supermarket queue and told them to see a dermatologist at once. Please turn to 'Signs of Melanoma: The A, B, C and D' in Chapter Five, and 'How to Recognise a Non-Melanoma Skin Cancer' in Chapter Seven for an explanation of how to spot the different kinds of skin cancer. When in doubt, consult a dermatologist.

AGING AND YOUR SKIN: GETTING REAL

Part of my job is persuading people like Jake that excess sun exposure is harmful. When words alone don't suffice, I tell the tale with pictures. In my clinic, as in many dermatologists' offices, we have a Wood's light, which is a black light that reveals the photoaging caused by sun-activated pigment, thus showing how your skin will appear in about ten years. Even though the light does not reveal future wrinkles, most people don't like what they see. Often a little trip to the black light room is a better motivator than I am.

Although genes govern a lot about your Skin Type, when it comes to wrinkling, genetic tendencies interact with lifestyle choices to determine whether your skin is wrinkled or tight. For example, a patient of mine named Janet has dark-toned, oily, resistant, thick skin that is much less prone to wrinkle than that of my former nurse Lisa, who has light, tissue-fine, dry and sensitive skin. Beyond genetic givens like their physical differences, people can increase or decrease their skin's native tendency through behaviour and lifestyle.

Protect your skin and consume antioxidants, and you'll get the best from your skin. Do the opposite, and you'll wind up in my office. When Janet baked in the sun year after year, she lowered the impact of her 'good' genes, even though they had kept both her mother and grandmother wrinkle-free into their eighties. On the other hand, Lisa, who regularly wore sunscreen and cared properly for her skin, aged much better than her chain-smoking mother.

That's why, if you fall into this category, it's very likely that your behaviour is the prime cause of your skin's wrinkling. However, a small percentage will fall into this category due to genetics. In either case, follow my recommendations to care for and protect your skin.

Genevieve's Story

A successful interior designer with an international following, Genevieve came into my office for a consultation about some antiaging options, while her handsome young man friend remained in the waiting room, flirting with some of the medical students in my clinic.

Tanned and rail slim, with long dark hair, Genevieve was about fifteen years older than I. She was elegantly attired in a back-baring silver wrap dress that I'd seen in Vogue. Confident, sensuous, a woman of a 'certain age', Genevieve had everything she'd ever dreamed of, except for one little problem: the wrinkles on her face. 'First, it was the lines between the eyebrow,' Genevieve pouted in her French-accented English. 'Now, it comes these and these.' A well-manicured nail pointed to 'puppet lines' around her mouth and crow's-feet creeping out of the corners of her eyes. 'And the ones I really, really cannot stand, are these,' she intoned emphatically, pointing to narrow lines crisscrossing her lips.

'Do you smoke?' I asked, though I knew the answer. Dermatologists call those lines on the upper lip 'smoker's lines'. Genevieve shrugged and raised her eyebrows. 'Mais oui, I smoke,' she admitted. How many times before had I seen women of a certain age (to be precise, it's usually their early to mid-forties) reaching their moment of truth? Fortunately, she'd come to the right place.

Many French, Italians, and other Europeans of Mediterranean background are OSPWs with dark hair, dark eyes and pigmented skin. Their culture and lifestyle are geared towards an appreciation of life, with a two-hour lunch break and August vacations on the beach, sunbathing in bikinis, mono-kinis or less. Perhaps it was a Frenchwoman who famously said, 'After the age of forty, a woman must choose between her figure and her skin.' With their svelte figures, it's pretty clear what most have chosen. But of course, Genevieve wanted to have it both ways.

The decades of tanning and smoking were totally disastrous for Genevieve's sensitive, pigmented skin, which not only had lines but also spots of brown and white pigment, especially on her arms, hands and chest. Antioxidants in the coffee and wine, which the French regularly consume, may have helped; however, consuming antioxidants was not enough. Time to trade her halter-top for a turtleneck.

How to tell a Frenchwoman to give up smoking and the beach, all in one day? The only way was with an estimate for cosmetic services to undo the damage, using every trick in my arsenal to help Genevieve hit the nightspots with her man friend without looking like his grandmère.

Genevieve tallied up the treatments and their costs: Intense Pulsed Light treatments, for existing brown spots and broken blood vessels on the face; Botox and dermal fillers, for her many wrinkles; and an ongoing protocol with daily retinoid use. Then she shrugged and commented, 'Cheaper and quicker than plastic surgery.' She gave me a smile.

After we scheduled her first treatments, I warned Genevieve that all my hard work (and her treatment expenses) would do no good unless she changed her habits. I gave her a clear list of dos and don'ts. Genevieve's dos: always use sunscreen and follow the daily skin care routine, loaded with antioxidant ingredients and retinoids to heal the sun damage, dark spots and wrinkles. Next, bypass cigarettes and increase antioxidants via healthy fruits and vegetables and supplements. And no more sunbathing!

'A little sunset beach walk, if I wear sunscreen?' she asked timidly. I agreed.

Five years later, I ran into her at an art gallery in Paris, still with her man friend and still looking fabulous, literally years younger. 'You changed my life,' she told me, flashing that dazzling smile.

A CLOSE-UP LOOK AT YOUR SKIN

If your questionnaire results reveal you to be an OSPW, like Genevieve, you may experience any of the following:

- Signs of sun damage
- Red or brown patches
- Areas with dappled brown and white pigment
- Skin spottiness on chest and face
- 'Fisherman's face' with broken facial capillaries
- Frequent acne breakouts
- Redness, stinging and burning in response to many skin care products
- Sunscreens feel oily and make your face appear shiny.
- Regular makeup wears off too easily but ColorStay and other long-lasting makeup brands cause skin redness and itching.
- Wrinkles begin in the late twenties or early thirties.
- Dark spots in areas of trauma such as cuts, burns, bruises, scrapes and breakouts
- Dark patches on cheeks
- Lipstick bleeds through edges of lips.
- Dark circles under the eyes

Your skin's oiliness can lead to acne, with breakouts triggering pigmentation. Acne scars can often result. For most OSPWs, higher levels of pigment increase the risk of developing unsightly dark spots, which spring up suddenly and take a while (if ever) to improve. Beyond pimples, many other minor skin irritants can stimulate the production of brown spots, including inflammation, wounds, nicks and cuts. Hormonal shifts arising from oral contraceptive use and pregnancy can raise oestrogen levels, also contributing to brown spots. In addition, sun exposure accelerates your skin's natural tendency to produce the pigment that creates dark spots, sun spots and freckles.

In fact, nearly all of the symptoms OSPWs typically experience are worsened by sun exposure. Yet due to your skin's sensitivity, it can be hard to find a sunscreen that does not cause burning or redness.

Claudia, a bank branch manager with medium-toned skin, was a native Floridian. But our sunny climate was hard on her pigmented, wrinkle-prone skin. Like many OSPWs, Claudia needed to be vigilant in using sunscreens, but her skin was reactive to a wide range of ingredients. If the product contained benzophenone, she'd flare up with redness, especially around the eyes and between her eyebrows. What's more, like many OSPWs, Anita hated oily sunscreens because they increased breakouts. 'My skin is oily enough already,' she complained.

I recommended that Claudia try a barrier sunscreen product containing micronised zinc oxide, which won't irritate most OSPWs. It's also perfect for people with oily skin. 'At last, I can wear sunscreen!' Claudia enthused after trying it.

Although I advise against sunbathing, moderate- to darker-skinned OSPWs usually tan well, with minimal sunburn. Frequent sun exposure can cause a natural buildup of melanin, the pigmenting factor in the skin. Although this contributes to aging and the formation of brown spots, and is therefore not advisable, there is one benefit. Pigmented cells surround the cellular DNA, protecting it from degrading into cancerous cells. Because of the dark-skinned OSPWs' ability to form pigment, this type may be less likely to develop non-melanoma skin cancers. However, those of you who are fair-skinned redheads are at an *increased* risk of both non-melanoma and melanoma skin cancers. Sunburns should be avoided at all costs. To learn how to identify a non-melanoma skin cancer, please consult 'How to Recognise a Non-Melanoma Skin Cancer' in Chapter Seven.

Are any levels of sun exposure safe? Even if you wear a broad-spectrum sunscreen of SPF 15 or more as I recommend, some minimal sun exposure will occur. That's why to assure you are protected, please follow my advice for sun protection in 'Daily Sunscreen Use' in Chapter Two.

ANTIAGING MYTHS

Because of skin wrinkles, often OSPWs want to use antiaging creams, but many contain ingredients too intense for your sensitive skin. Others are simply not that effective. One bestselling cream contains hyaluronic acid (HA), a sugar found in the skin that decreases with aging and sun exposure, causing skin to lose its volume. In fact, a highly popular cosmetic dermatological treatment (that I perform on a near daily basis) involves injecting hyaluronic acid to plump up facial wrinkles and sags.

That's why people assume that a cream with HA would deliver the same benefits. But it doesn't, since hyaluronic acid cannot be absorbed into the skin from a cream; it must be injected. Since hyaluronic acid helps hydrate the skin by holding water, applying it via a cream on the outer layer of the skin may actually be counterproductive because in a low-humidity environment it draws water from the skin and dries the skin out. Even people with oily skin, like OSPWs, won't benefit from dehydrating their skin. Reducing oil that causes acne and reducing water that gives the skin its volume are two different things.

You may also be tempted by popular antiaging creams or other skin care products that contain alpha lipoic acid and DMAE (dimethylaminoethanol). While these ingredients can be effective in treating wrinkles for resistant types, sensitive types often don't tolerate them well.

As a Christmas gift from her mother-in-law, Mia, a patient of mine with sensitive skin, received an expensive jar of 'soothing' facial cream. Unfortunately, from the moment she applied it, it was anything but. Red blotches appeared around the area of contact, followed seconds later by an intense burning sensation. She immediately washed the cream from her face and hands, saving herself from what could have turned into an ugly red rash that persisted for days.

A high price and pretty packaging don't guarantee a quality product. Next time you receive a skin care gift, carefully read the ingredient list. If you find it contains a no-no, don't open the jar. Instead, consider it a gift certificate and take it back to the store where it was purchased for a refund or exchange it for a product that suits your Skin Type.

Since antiwrinkle creams can cost hundreds of pounds for a tiny jar, I can't stress enough how important it is to be aware of exactly what you're allowing to contact your sensitive skin. Fortunately, certain antiaging ingredients really work for you, such as salicylic acid (SA), which decreases skin sensitivity, oiliness, and wrinkles. In addition, products containing nonprescription retinol or prescription retinoid are great for both minimising and preventing wrinkles. My recommended products contain these ingredients and will deliver them in your daily regimen.

THE SENSITIVE SKIN DILEMMA

Extreme skin problems, like wrinkling and dark spots, seem to call for powerful measures, so many OSPWs purchase and try products with strong ingredients, only to find their sensitive skin will not tolerate them. Like Anita, many OSPWs have trouble finding a sunscreen that they can use without redness or irritation. Skin lighteners that contain bleaching ingredients commonly cause reactions as well.

In the next section of this chapter, I'll teach you how to work with your skin's sensitivity. I'll offer a skin care routine that protects your skin from sun exposure while treating brown spots and wrinkling with products you can safely use. You need ingredients that calm rather than inflame your skin. Learn to recognise and avoid ingredients too irritating for you.

Decrease the reactive combination of oiliness, sensitivity and pigmentation (preventing breakouts and brown spots) by first avoiding sun exposure and, second, following the protocols I'll offer in the next section of this chapter.

In midlife, after menopause, both oil production and hormonal levels naturally decrease. This change provides relief for many of the skin problems you suffer in youth. However, since your skin tends to wrinkle, the aging process is not that kind to you. That's why I will offer wrinkle prevention strategies you can use when wrinkles start to appear in your twenties and thirties. In addition, you're a good candidate for the advanced skin prescription medications and procedures used to minimise the visible signs of aging. Currently, there are quite a few excellent options, with new innovations to be expected in the next few years.

Dr Baumann's Bottom Line: Your gorgeous tan is actually a sign of sun damage. Protect your skin and treat wrinkles and dark spots as early as possible.

EVERYDAY CARE FOR YOUR SKIN

The goal of your skin care routine is to address oiliness, brown spots and wrinkles with products that deliver antioxidant and anti-inflammatory ingredients. All the products I'll recommend do one or both of the following:

• Prevent and treat wrinkles
• Prevent and treat dark spots

In addition, your daily regimen will also help to address your other skin concerns by:

• Preventing and treating pimples
• Preventing and treating inflammation

Anything strong enough to help your wrinkles and dark spots may irritate your skin. I'll recommend products that are strong enough to have an effect while containing antioxidant ingredients (like green tea) and anti-inflammatory ingredients (like licorice extract) that both protect your skin and calm its sensitivity. Although wrinkles are your number-one skin problem, dark spots come in a close second. For that reason, I'll provide a two-stage protocol. In the first stage, outlined here, you'll undertake a foundation regimen that will show immediate results in lessening brown spots. Please look over your nonprescription regimen and then you can select the products you'll need from those I recommend in each category later in this chapter.

After two weeks to two months on this regimen, I recommend that you 'graduate' to my prescription protocol, detailed in 'Consulting a Dermatologist' later in this chapter, for a more advanced treatment plan to prevent wrinkles. There you will find more advanced prescription procedures for antiaging and other skin concerns. You can proceed to Stage Two right away, if you would like to, or you can use this less potent nonprescription regimen, if you choose. Remember, since you may need to wait for an appointment, always call a dermatologist at least two months in advance.

DAILY SKIN CARE

STAGE ONE: NONPRESCRIPTION REGIMEN

For dark spots

AM	PM
Step 1: Wash with a cleanser	Step 1: Wash with same cleanser used in AM
Step 2: Apply a skin lightener	
Step 3: Apply eye cream (optional)	Step 2: Apply a skin lightener
Step 4: Apply SPF facial lotion	Step 3: Apply a retinol-containing product or sunscreen regimen
Step 5: Apply foundation	Step 4: Apply eye cream (optional) with SPF
Step 6: Apply oil-absorbing (optional) powder	Step 5: Apply moisturiser

In the morning, clean your face with a cleanser containing salicylic acid to decrease acne and clean pores while easing pigmentation problems without irritating your sensitive skin. Next, apply a skin lightener to your entire face to help reduce brown spots. If you suffer predominantly from acne rather than skin redness and irritation, or if you have a lower S/R score (25–30), you can mix your skin lightener with a vitamin C powder, such as Philosophy Hope and a Prayer vitamin C powder. For application instructions, see box below.

After applying the lightener, you can use an eye cream, if you'd like to. Next, apply sunscreen and follow with makeup foundation and facial powder, if desired.

In the evening, cleanse and remove all makeup with a recommended cleanser. Next, in your hand mix a pea-size portion of the same skin lightener used in the morning with the retinol product (Steps 2 and 3) and apply them together. The retinol product should be applied only in the evening, and will help control acne and dark spots while preventing wrinkles. If you wish, you can apply an eye cream to the eye area and a light moisturiser to dry skin areas.

STAGE ONE: NONPRESCRIPTION REGIMEN

For red, inflamed skin with dark spots

AM	PM
Step 1: Wash with a nonfoaming gentle cleanser	Step 1: Wash with same cleanser used in AM
Step 2: Apply a skin lightener to spots	Step 2: Apply a skin lightener to spots
Step 3: Apply eye cream (optional)	Step 3: Apply a serum
Step 4: Apply a facial lotion (optional)	Step 4: Apply a retinol-containing product
Step 5: Apply a facial foundation or powder with SPF	

In the morning, wash with a nonfoaming gentle cleanser such as Cetaphil. Use a soft wash cloth and avoid vigorous rubbing. Do not use a toner. Your skin may not tolerate the skin lighteners that contain Vitamin C, so choose one with kojic acid and arbutin instead such as SkinCeuticals Phyto+. Apply an eye cream (optional).

If you have a lower O/D score, apply a facial lotion. Although an SPF containing lotion is best for sun protection, sometimes people with very sensitive skin can be allergic to certain sunscreen ingredients. If you experience sensitivity to sunscreens, look for products that contain z-cote such as Quintessence Sunshade SPF 30 or those by Skinceuticals. Apply a facial foundation or powder with SPF if you choose not to use a facial lotion.

All of the foundations and powders on the list of recommendations are right for you.

In the evening, wash with the cleanser and apply the skin lightener to dark spots. Cover the entire face and neck with a serum such as Olay Regenerist Daily Regenerating Serum (Fragrance Free) and follow with a retinol-containing product.

Using Vitamin C Powder

Vitamin C can help to prevent both pigmentation and wrinkles. Philosophy Hope and a Prayer vitamin C powder contains a scoop you can use to pour powder into the palm of your hand along with a 5p-size portion of skin lightener. Mix and apply. If you suffer from redness and facial flushing or have a high S/R score (34 or greater), eliminate this product and follow the rest of the morning regimen. Serums such as Laura Mercier Multi Vitamin Serum are also a good source of vitamin C.

Choosing and Using Cleansers

When removing makeup, use a nonirritating cleanser containing ingredients such as salicylic acid, aloe vera, cucumber, feverfew, chamomile or niacinamide, which will reduce redness, inflammation and acne and help to unclog pores. The products I recommend will help your skin retain its natural lipids, a key to controlling skin sensitivity. If a cleanser, soap, shampoo or bath product produces intense suds and bubbles, it contains detergent. Stay away from it. Read ingredient lists to assure you avoid irritants such as sodium lauryl sulfate, a detergent commonly used in shampoos, conditioners and other skin care products.

RECOMMENDED CLEANSING PRODUCTS

£ Cetaphil Daily Facial Cleanser for Normal to Oily Skin
£ Clean & Clear Blackhead Clearing Cleanser
£ Clean & Clear Continuous Control Acne Wash
£ Clearasil Face Wash
£ Dermalogica Anti-Bac Skin Wash
£ Eucerin Gentle Hydrating Cleanser
£ Jason D-Clog Naturally Balancing Cleanser
£ Neutrogena Visibly Clear Wipes
£ Olay Daily Facials Lathering Cloths for Combination/Oily SkinTotal Effects Cleanser
£ Paula's Choice One Step Face Cleanser
£ Stiefel Acne-Aid Cleansing Bar
££ Aesop Amazing Face Cleanser
££ B. Kamins Hydrating Acne Wash
££ Jan Marini Bioglycolic Oily Skin Cleansing Gel
££ Korres Hamamelis Cleansing Tonic Lotion
££ La Roche-Posay Effaclar Purifying Foaming Gel
££ Laura Mercier Oil Free Gel Cleanser
££ MD Formulations Facial Cleanser Oily and Problem Skin
££ Ren Balancing Facial Wash-Combination
£££ Dr Brandt Pore Effect
£££ Jurlique Cleansing Lotion
£££ Rodan & Fields Unblemish Wash Facial Cleanser

Baumann's Choice: Ren Balancing Facial Wash-Combination (which contains cucumber extract) for red inflamed skin or B. Kamins Hydrating Acne Wash for acne.

Toner Use

Although toners are unnecessary for you, some oily types enjoy their refreshing feeling. You can use a toner after cleansing. If you wish to add this extra step, the anti-inflammatory and pigment- and oil-control ingredients in the recommended toners remain on your skin longer, delivering ingredients better than cleansers that are rinsed off. However, if you have either a high S/R score (34 or greater) or dry or combination skin (an O/D score of 27 to 35), don't use toners. Also, if any skin products cause redness or stinging, avoid them.

RECOMMENDED TONERS

£ Dove Essential Nutrients Toner
£ Neutrogena Visibly Refined Facial Toner
£ Pond's Clear Solutions Pore Clarifying Astringent, Oil-Free
££ Citrix Antioxidant Toner by Topix
££ D.R. Harris Mild Skin Tonic
££ Joey New York Pure Pores 1-Step Toner and Moisturizer
££ Peter Thomas Roth Glycolic Acid 10% Clarifying Tonic
£££ N.V. Perricone M.D. Firming Facial Toner
£££ Rodan and Fields Unblemish Medicated Toner

Baumann's Choice: Dove Essential Nutrients Toner

Pimples

Above all, don't steam your face, apply a hot washcloth, or place an ice cube on a pimple. All of these actions cause rapid changes in temperature, which is strictly a no-no for types prone to inflammation – and that means you. While I don't recommend squeezing pimples, if you can't restrain yourself, please follow the guidelines in 'The Proper Way to Pop' in Chapter Five. As previously discussed, some people believe that sun exposure will help clear up acne, but since acne typically worsens in summer, I don't believe that it's helpful. The products in your daily regimen should help prevent pimples and acne and, in addition, you can treat breakouts with some of the blemish medications listed below.

If you like, these products can be added to concealer to both treat and cover blemishes. Directly after cleansing or toner application, mix the concealer (in an amount equivalent to one third the size of a pea) with medication and apply to the pimple. Other treatment products or moisturisers should only be applied afterwards.

RECOMMENDED SPOT TREATMENTS
FOR PIMPLES

£ Benzac AC Gel

£ Clean and Clear Extra Strength Invisible Blemish Treatment Gel

£ PanOxyl Acne Gel by Stiefel

££ B. Kamins Medicated Acne Gel 5% benzoyl peroxide

£££ Clinique Acne Solutions Spot Healing Gel

£££ Philosophy Hope in a Bottle or On a Clear Day H_2O_2

£££ Jurlique Blemish Cream

Baumann's Choice: PanOxyl Acne Gel or B. Kamins Medicated Acne gel because they contain benzoyl peroxide. (They are only sold at pharmacies.)

Treating Dark Spots

Apply skin-lightening products to your dark spots only after cleansing and toning but before applying other recommended products. The products listed below should be used as soon as the dark spot appears, and until the spot has completely disappeared. Hydroquinone-containing products are very common in the USA. However, they are not available in many European countries. If you find that over-the-counter remedies don't work, ask your dermatologist about prescription lighteners.

RECOMMENDED NONPRESCRIPTION
SKIN LIGHTENERS

££ B. Kamins Skin Lightening Treatment

££ L'Occitane Immortelle Brightening Serum

££ Laura Mercier Multi Vitamin Serum

££ Philosophy A Pigment of Your Imagination (Philosophy Hope and a Prayer mixed with vitamin C powder)

£££ DDF Intensive Holistic Corrector Swabs

£££ Dr Brandt Lightening Gel

£££ Dr Michelle Copeland Skin Care Pigment Blocker 5

£££ Pevonia Lightening Gel

£££ Rodan and Fields Reverse Prepare Skin Lightening Toner

£££ Thalgo Unizones

Baumann's Choice: I prefer hydroquinone-containing products which are not available in the UK. Visit www.DrBaumann.co.uk to learn where to find the products on this list.

Moisturisers

Moisturisers are unnecessary for most oily types; however, if you have a lower O/D score (27–32), feel free to use my recommended moisturisers on dry facial areas. Serums often contain healing ingredients in even higher concentrations, which results in better skin penetration. Contained in a dropper-style bottle, serums are thicker in texture than other products, so a little goes a long way. Use only a few drops and spread over your face as indicated in the regimen. You can apply a moisturiser over the serum if you wish. When you get to Stage Two and incorporate prescription antiaging products, you will use the serum as a delivery system. This is a highly effective combination for wrinkled skin, much more so than many pricey antiwrinkle creams, which are often too oily – and ineffective.

When using a retinol or retinoid product, light moisturising can help offset the flaking that may accompany its use and is helpful if you tested slightly lower on oiliness, from 24 to 30 on the O/D Score.

RECOMMENDED MOISTURISERS

£ Eucerin Q 10 Active Antiwrinkle Fluid SPF 15
£ Dove Essential Nutrients Protective Moisturising Lotion SPF 15
£ Dove Fresh Radiance Brightening Moisturiser
£ Olay Total Effects 7x Visible Anti-Aging Vitamin Complex
££ Aesop Mandarin Facial Hydrating Cream
££ Elizabeth Arden Ceramide Time Complex Moisture Cream SPF 15
££ Jan Marini Recover-E
££ Ultraceuticals Ultra C Sheer Facial Cream – 20%
£££ Jurlique Day Care Face Lotion
£££ Ole Henriksen Vitamin Plus Balancing Crème
£££ Peter Thomas Roth Power Rescue Facial Firming Lift
£££ Thalgo Ultra-Matte Moisturising Fluid

Baumann's Choice: Eucerin Q 10 Active Antiwrinkle Fluid SPF 15 because Co Q10 is a strong antioxidant to prevent wrinkles.

RECOMMENDED SERUMS

£ Roc Retin Ox anti-wrinkle serum- soft
££ Alchimie Forever Diode 1 and Diode 2 serums
££ Aveda Balancing Infusion for Oily Skin/Acne
££ Dr Andrew Weil for Origins Plantidote Mega-Mushroom Face
Serum
££ Elizabeth Arden Bye Lines Anti-Wrinkle Serum
££ L'Occitane Immortelle Elixir For The Face
££ La Roche-Posay Toleriane Facial Fluid
£££ Jurlique Herbal Recovery Gel
£££ SkinCeuticals Serum 15

Baumann's Choice: Dr Andrew Weil for Origins Plantidote Mega-Mushroom Face Serum because it helps relieve redness, and prevents dark spots and wrinkles.

RECOMMENDED RETINOL - CONTAINING PRODUCTS

£ Roc Retin Ox anti-wrinkle serum- soft
££ Philosophy Help Me
££ Sothy's Retinol 15
££ Skinceuticals Retinol 0.5
££ Topix Replenix Retinol Smoothing Serum 3x
£££ Clarins Renew Plus Night Lotion
£££ Estée Lauder Diminish Anti-Wrinkle Retinal Treatment
£££ Jan Marini Factor A Plus Lotion
£££ Lancôme Resurface
£££ Prescriptives Skin Renewal Cream

Baumann's Choice: Philosophy Help Me and the Roc product because they are properly packaged and readily available.

Eye Creams

For dark circles under eyes, use eye creams (like Roc Retin Ox Correxion Intensive Eye Care or Clarins Extra-Firming Eye Contour Serum), which contain retinol and/or vitamin K to address the blood congestion that causes them. Do not apply a full-strength prescription retinoid to the eye area, as it will convey too strong a dose to the delicate skin there. If you choose to use a prescription retinoid around the eye area, dilute it by mixing it with an equal amount of moisturiser.

RECOMMENDED EYE CREAMS

- £ Nivea Anti-wrinkle Q 10 Eye Cream
- £ Olay Total Effects Eye Transforming Cream
- £ Revlon Eye Contour Cream
- £ Roc Retin Ox Correxion Intensive Eye Care
- ££ Aesop Parsley Seed Anti-Oxidant Eye Serum
- ££ Aveda Brightening Moisture Treatment
- ££ D.R. Harris Crystal Eye Gel
- ££ Elizabeth Arden Good Morning Eye Treatment
- ££ Fresh Soy Eye Cream
- ££ Laura Mercier Eyedration
- ££ Philosophy Eye Believe
- £££ Clarins Extra-Firming Eye Contour Serum
- £££ Dr Brandt Lineless Eye Cream
- £££ Skyn Iceland Icelandic Relief Eye Cream with Biospheric Complex

Baumann's Choice: Laura Mercier Eyedration because it contains mulberry root and licorice extract with Vitamin C to brighten the under-eye area.

Masks

Because they deliver concentrated ingredients to your skin for an extended time period, masks can be beneficial. Once or twice a week apply a mask with exfoliating and depigmenting properties, such as MD Formulations Vit-A-Plus Illuminating Masque. You can use it in the evening, immediately after cleansing. Follow the instructions on the package, and once you have rinsed it off, you can proceed to Step 2 (applying skin lightener). Or go to a spa or salon for a mask treatment by a spa therapist, making sure to ask for masks for sensitive skin with the depigmenting and anti-inflammatory ingredients I recommend.

Exfoliation

OSPW skin benefits from retinoid use. And though retinoids can cause flaking, they don't cause dryness. Instead, the flakes signify beneficial skin exfoliation, a process that helps your skin slough off dead cells.

The product Buf-Puf is a small deep-cleaning and exfoliating facial sponge, which I sometimes recommend to OSPWs. When I met a friend of the inventor at a medical convention, I told him to compliment the inventor and let him know that they were an excellent idea and quite useful. When he told me how the product came into being, I was even more impressed.

While the inventor was absentmindedly watching two janitors buffing a hospital floor – large round pads rotating to bring it to a shine – inspiration struck. He noticed that a large metal hose connected the round, buffing surface to the main body of the machine. A small cutout in the buffers accommodated this attachment. What about those middle pieces? Where were they? And wouldn't they be the perfect size for . . . He soon made contact with the manufacturer of the pads and arranged to purchase all of the leftover circular cutouts. The rest, as they say, is history.

SHOPPING FOR PRODUCTS

By reading labels, you can also widen your choice of products, selecting those that contain beneficial ingredients for your type while avoiding ones that increase allergic reactions, stinging, burning, redness, acne, inflammation or oiliness. Take the list below with you when you go shopping so that you can read labels, identify the common culprits, and avoid products containing them. If you find additional products beyond the ones I recommend, please tell us at www.DrBaumann.co.uk so that you can share your find with others of your Skin Type.

SKIN CARE INGREDIENTS TO USE

To lessen acne:

- Benzoyl peroxide
- Retinol
- Salicylic acid (beta hydroxy acid or BHA)
- Tea tree oil
- Zinc

To reduce inflammation:

- Aloe vera
- Arnica
- Calendula
- Chamomile
- Colloidal oatmeal
- Cucumber
- Dexpanthenol (provitamin B$_5$)
- Evening primrose oil
- Feverfew
- Green tea
- Licochalone
- Perilla leaf extract
- Pycnogenol (a pine bark extract)
- Red algae
- Trifolium pretense (red clover)
- Thyme
- Epilobium angustifolium (willow herb)
- Zinc

To prevent or lighten dark spots:

- Arbutin
- Bearberry extract
- Cucumber
- Glycyrrhiza glabra (licorice extract)
- Mulberry extract
- Niacinamide

To prevent wrinkles:

- Alpha lipoic acid
- Basil
- Caffeine
- Carrot extract
- Copper peptide
- Coenzyme Q$_{10}$
- Cucumber
- Curcumin (tetrahydracurcumin or turmeric)
- Ferulic acid
- Feverfew
- Ginger
- Ginseng
- Grape seed extract
- Green tea, white tea
- Idebenone
- Lutein
- Lycopene
- Pomegranate
- Pycnogenol (a pine bark extract)
- Rosemary
- Silymarin
- Trifolium pretense, fabaceae (red clover)
- Yucca

SKIN CARE INGREDIENTS TO AVOID

If you are acne prone:

- Cinnamon oil
- Cocoa butter
- Cocos nucifera (coconut oil)
- Isopropyl isostearate
- Isopropyl myristate
- Peppermint oil
- Sodium laurel sulfate

Each person with sensitive skin reacts to different ingredients, so selectively test products with suspicious ingredients, and notice how your skin responds. If possible, try products at a beauty counter or obtain samples before you purchase them to make sure that they work for you. As not every reaction is instantaneous, allow twenty-four hours to pass before making your decision. Making that extra effort will save you money and help you treat your skin right.

Sun Protection for Your Skin

OSPWs are vulnerable to sun damage, making daily sunscreen use an absolute necessity. However, since nearly all sunscreens contain oil, they can make your skin look shiny and cause your foundation and other makeup to streak. In addition, certain sunscreen ingredients can irritate your skin, leading to acne flare-ups.

I recommend using physical blocking sunscreens that contain micronised zinc oxide and titanium dioxide. If you have darker skin, look for tinted products so you do not get the violet hue associated with the white cream products. And rather than creams, look for gel or foam sunscreens or powders containing SPF.

While I don't recommend tanning, much less burning, I know many of you are sun worshippers, and if you do wind up with a sunburn, take an Advil (ibuprofen) or aspirin every four hours to decrease inflammation and prevent redness. Using an over-the-counter 1 percent hydrocortisone cream may help heal sunburn as well.

RECOMMENDED SUN PROTECTION PRODUCTS

£ Eucerin Q 10 Active Anti-wrinkle fluid SPF 15
£ Neutrogena Visibly Refined Moisturiser SPF 15
££ Dr Michelle Copeland SPF-40 Lotion Mist Sun Block
££ Elizabeth Arden First Defense Anti-Oxidant Lotion SPF 15
££ La Roche-Posay Anthelios Fluid Extreme

££ Origins Sunshine State SPF 20 Sunscreen
£££ DDF Daily Protective Moisturiser SPF 15
£££ Dr Brandt SPF 15 Chemfree
£££ SkinCeuticals Physical UV Defense SPF 30

Baumann's Choice: Origins Sunshine State SPF 20 Sunscreen

SUNSCREEN INGREDIENTS TO AVOID

If you have sunscreen sensitivity:

- Avobenzone
- Benzophenones (such as oxybenzone)
- Methoxycinnamate (often found in waterproof sunscreens, can cause a reaction)
- Para-aminobenzoic acid (PABA)

If your skin is very oily, you can protect it while decreasing shine by mixing an equal portion of an oil control product in with your sunscreen and applying them together. OC Eight lotion decreases shininess and prevents your make up foundation from streaking.

Your Makeup

Powders containing sunscreen are made for OSPWs since they cover dark spots, control shine and protect skin from the sun. If you use foundation to cover dark spots, look for an oil-free product with some of the anti-inflammatory ingredients I recommend.

RECOMMENDED POWDER/ FOUNDATIONS AND FOUNDATIONS

£ Boots Brand No 7 Uplifting Foundation SPF 15
£ L'Oréal Air Wear Powder Foundation SPF 17
£ Maybelline Pure Stay Powder & Foundation SPF 15
£ Maybelline Wonder Finish Foundation SPF 15
£ Revlon Skin Perfecting Makeup for Oily Blemish Prone Skin
££ Bare Escentuals Minerals SPF 15 Foundation
££ Bloom Compact Foundation with SPF 12
££ Bloom Pressed Powder

££ Dermablend Acne Results Treatment Foundation
££ Elizabeth Arden Flawless Finish Skin Balancing Makeup
££ Mirenesse Emulsion Pact with SPF 25

Baumann's Choice: Revlon Skin Perfecting Makeup for Oily Blemish Prone Skin because it contains aloe and chamomile.

CONSULTING A DERMATOLOGIST

PRESCRIPTION SKIN CARE STRATEGIES

Along with the cleansers, gels and other products you use in your non-prescription regimen, my Stage Two Regimens add retinoids to more intensively treat both dark spots and wrinkles, which are often your biggest concern. I provide two options for prescription regimens. The first both treats and prevents dark spots and wrinkles, while the second will prevent them. If you are experiencing pigmentation issues, begin with the first, and use the second as a maintenance programme once the issues have cleared. If dark spots or pigmentation are not problems for you, go straight to the second regimen. Don't hesitate to ask your dermatologist for a prescription for the products that are right for you. He or she will be delighted that you're well-informed and using your appointment time productively.

DAILY SKIN CARE

STAGE TWO: PRESCRIPTION REGIMEN

To treat and prevent acne, dark spots and wrinkles:

AM	PM
Step 1: Wash with cleanser	Step 1: Wash with same cleanser as in the morning
Step 2: Apply antioxidant serum	Step 2: Apply eye cream serum (optional)
Step 3: Apply a skin lightener	Step 3: Apply prescription retinoid to entire face
Step 4: Apply an acne medication to entire face (optional)	Step 4: Apply moisturiser (optional)
Step 5: Cover with sunscreen and/or an SPF-containing powder	

In the morning, after your cleanser, use an antioxidant serum to increase the antiwrinkling action of this regimen. Apply a prescription lightener to dark spots, if present. If you have acne, apply a prescription acne medication, such as Duac, to your entire face. Apply a sunscreen. A makeup powder can provide additional sun protection.

In the evening, follow the same regimen, omitting sunscreen, but adding eye cream, if desired, and including the prescription retinoid product for brown spots and wrinkles, and, if needed, a moisturiser. For those of you that suffer from acne, ask your dermatologist for Isotrexin which contains an antibiotic and a retinoid and can be used as Step 3 in the evening.

STAGE TWO: MAINTENANCE

To prevent acne and dark spots and to prevent and treat wrinkles:

AM	PM
Step 1: Wash with cleanser	Step 1: Wash with salicylic acid-containing cleanser
Step 2: Apply antioxidant serum	
	Step 2: Apply eye cream (optional)
Step 3: Apply a gel sunscreen or an oil-free foundation with sunscreen	Step 3: Apply a retinoid to entire face
Step 4: Cover with oil-control powder	Step 4: Apply a moisturiser (optional)

Use the recommended cleanser to wash your face in the morning. Next, apply the antioxidant serum. Then, apply sunscreen and oil-free foundation, topping it off with the oil-control powder.

In the evening, follow the same regimen, omitting sunscreen and including the retinoid for reducing oil and pigmentation problems. If you suffer from acne, I suggest using Isotrexin because it contains an antibiotic and a retinoid.

Treating Wrinkles and Dark Spots

When it comes to prescription products, gel retinoids containing adapalene, tretinoin or isotretinoin are ideal for OSPWs. Derived from vitamin A, but with a different chemical structure, retinoids may limit oil production, reduce skin oiliness, and prevent acne and the pigmentation that results in dark spots. Some common retinoid products include Retin-A, Differin Isotrex, and Isotrexin, all of which require a prescription. Though retinoids can be expensive, they are far more reliable than antiaging creams you might find over the counter. For instructions on their use, please go to 'Further Help for Oily, Sensitive Skin Types'.

RECOMMENDED PRESCRIPTION PRODUCTS

Retinoids to combat wrinkles and dark spots:

- Aknemycin Plus (contains an antibiotic as well)
- Differin gel or cream
- Isotrex
- Isotrexin (contains an antibiotic as well)
- Retin-A gel, lotion, or cream
- Retinova

Antibiotics to combat acne:

- Aknemycin Plus (tretinoin and erythromycin)
- Benzamycin (benzoul peroxide and clindamycin)
- Dalacin T (clindamycin)
- Duac (Benzoyl peroxide and Clindamycin)
- Isotrexin (Isotretinoin and erythromycin)
- Stiemycin (erythromycin)
- Topicycline (tetracycline hydrochloride and 4-epitetracycline hydrochloride)
- Zindaclin (erythromycin and zinc)
- Zineryt (erythromycin and zinc)

Baumann's choice: Ask your dermatologist to recommend the product right for your needs.

Is it safe to continue using retinoids when they cause redness and flaking? The redness comes about because of increased blood flow to the skin. And, though it might be disconcerting, the flaking isn't harmful either. It's actually a sign of cell regeneration, which is needed for you to see results. Retinoids actually thicken your skin, even though they may appear to be doing just the opposite. A moisturiser with antioxidants may help prevent some of the redness and flaking. If dark spots are a big problem, ask your dermatologist about prescription skin lighteners.

Other Options

While following the Stage Two Daily Skin Care Regimen will prevent and address all your major problems, I will also include some options for treating each specific problem if you prefer to do that. Nonprescription products are not quite as strong as prescription ones, but they can be effective in lightening dark spots and often contain additional ingredients that help improve acne or reduce skin inflammation. If they don't work, however, graduate to prescription products.

PROCEDURES FOR YOUR SKIN TYPE

Fortunately, the right prescription products can address *all* of your skin care needs. And, if desired, you can also augment their efficacy with some simple cosmetic procedures. Due to the wrinkling to which this type is prone, OSPWs may wish to consider going for botulinum toxins and dermal fillers. For a complete description of these procedures and what to expect if you opt for them, please consult 'Further Help for Oily, Sensitive Skin Types'.

Light Treatments

Intense Pulsed Light (IPL) can be used by your dermatologist to erase blood vessels and brown spots on the skin with minimal downtime. Although several of the companies that make these devices claim they are effective on wrinkles, this has not been proven. I happen to use the IPL by Lumenis in my practice, but there are other types available. In addition, there are other devices utilizing blue light or red light, which can be used alone or with a photosensitising agent called Metvix to treat acne and brown spots, and to shrink the size of the oil glands. More information on light treatments can be found in 'Further Help for Oily, Sensitive Skin Types'.

Chemical Peels

In addition to the over-the-counter cleansers containing salicylic acid that I've recommended, OSPWs can also benefit from chemical peels performed in the dermatologist's office. These peels contain higher concentrations of salicylic acid (approximately 20–30 percent) than those found in consumer products (typically 0.5–2 percent). Peels are helpful for unclogging pores, clearing acne, and improving brown spots.

Light-skinned OSPWs will also benefit from deeper peels, such as the TCA or Obagi Blue Peel, which act on both dark spots and wrinkles. Costing between £150 and £300 per peel, they can be done every six months, and depending on the severity of the spots and wrinkles, you may need anywhere from two to four treatments.

Another option is facial masks performed at a salon or spa. Choose masks that are antioxidant, depigmenting, skin lightening, anti-inflammatory, or oil-decreasing.

Dark-skinned OSPWs can also benefit from *superficial* skin peels, such as those performed at salons or spas, while some of the deeper chemical peels are not right for dark-toned skin.

Microdermabrasion

Instead of deep peels and light treatments, OSPWs with darker skin can use microdermabrasion, a process that blows aluminum, clay, or other types of particles against the skin to 'sandblast' it. By taking off your skin's dead surface, microdermabrasion speeds up natural exfoliation, allowing the dead pigment-containing skin cells to flake off, so that brown spots disappear. Used in conjunction with retinoids, microdermabrasion may help the retinoid penetrate further, increasing its effectiveness in removing brown spots. You will benefit from microdermabrasion or light chemical peels with salicylic acid when you are following either the prescription regimen or the nonprescription regimen for combating dark spots. These treatments are not needed once you have moved forward to the Stage Two Maintenance prescription regimen.

Many salons and spas offer a series of ten weekly treatments at a cost of about £60 per session. Microdermabrasion was one of the top five non-surgical procedures performed in 2003. Currently, at-home microdermabrasion kits have become available. These permit you to receive a similar benefit at a much lower cost.

ONGOING CARE FOR YOUR SKIN

Changing your habits can do a lot to slow down the slippery slope that leads to premature aging. First, come in from the sun. Next, use the Daily Skin Care Regimen I've designed for you. Because of your skin's tendency to wrinkle, I highly recommend that you move up to the prescription products sooner rather than later, as they will make a big difference. If you follow my lifestyle suggestions – increasing antioxidants while quitting smoking – you'll also help yourself a lot. And finally, OSPWs can really benefit from the best that cosmetic dermatology has to offer. If you can afford it, consider what advanced procedures like Botox and wrinkle fillers can offer.

CHAPTER FIVE

Oily, Sensitive, Pigmented and Tight: OSPT

THE FRUSTRATED SKIN TYPE

'I never get a break! Between breakouts and brown spots, there's always something ugly on my face. How I envy people who have clear skin!'

ABOUT YOUR SKIN

If you have an OSPT Skin Type, your skin's unique characteristics combine to create a vicious cycle of blemishes, followed by brown spots, followed by blemishes. Some people get acne and others get dark spots. OSPTs get both. You may feel overwhelmed because you are always battling one kind of outbreak or another. Nor will simple solutions aimed at one of your skin's problems resolve the situation. You need to understand and address all of them.

Pigmentation, sensitivity and oil production are your skin's three dominant features. In this chapter, I'll first reveal how each factor affects your skin, and then I'll show you how they interact. Yours is a complex type in which your skin cycles through one form of skin reaction after another. But don't worry, you can intervene and take charge of your skin.

OSPT CELEBRITY

Multitalented Vanessa Williams is a successful singer, actress, and first black Miss America. She is also, most likely, an OSPT. In spite of having a difficult Skin Type, her beautiful, medium-toned skin looks utterly fabulous, one of the benefits of well cared for skin. She has stated that her skin is oily and sensitive, leading to lifelong acne, a signature of this type. On her pigmented skin, acne could lead to dark spots that take anywhere from weeks to months to resolve.

Although her skin is gorgeous now, Vanessa has had her share of skin problems, with acne persisting even into her thirties. 'Acne is a drag. You're self-conscious; it's embarrassing. You just want to be normal,' Vanessa Williams has revealed. I'm not telling confidential secrets because Vanessa herself has publicly admitted that troubling acne, redness and bumps were resolved by using skin care products that contain many of the same kinds of ingredients I'll recommend later in this chapter.

While the acne–inflammation–dark spot cycle troubles all OSPTs, it's more disturbing when you're in the public eye. Along with her outstanding talents as a singer, performer and actress, Vanessa's beautiful classically featured face was her ticket to starring roles in movies like *Soul Food* and *Shaft*, as well as her Tony Award-nominated performance on Broadway starring in the Stephen Sondheim hit *Into the Woods*. When acne strikes or redness crops up on a day when a Grammy-nominated singer, like Williams, is slated to pose for an album cover, there's nowhere to hide. Fortunately, there *is* a solution even for the challenging, frustrating OSPT Skin Type – as lovely Vanessa Williams has obviously discovered.

ONE PROBLEM AT A TIME

Let's begin with oil, your biggest concern. Your skin's oiliness can lead to acne, especially during your adolescence and early twenties, with breakouts continuing well into your thirties, and sometimes beyond. Although many people expect acne to end with youth, for OSPTs, it doesn't!

You may also find that your skin's pigmentation produces dark spots and melasma, dark patches on the skin. They too are worse in your twenties and thirties. Why? Because at that age, more women become pregnant or take birth control pills, or do both in turn, leading to hormone fluctuations, which stimulate oil production and pigmentation. Certain birth control pills will help acne by decreasing oil secretion, but can make more colour and worsen melasma, due to their hormonal effects. Light-skin-toned OSPTs can often tolerate them, but those with darker skin tones may get undesirable pigmentation. In any event, the increased symptoms caused by hormonal levels will pass with time.

Address your challenges, or they can worsen. If you have acne, rosacea, or skin allergies, treatment is a necessity. You can decrease the reactive combination of oiliness, sensitivity, and pigmentation by following the protocols I'll offer later in this chapter. If you act to prevent breakouts and brown spots, you'll find that you can successfully manage your skin. Fortunately, many female OSPTs find that their skin improves after menopause, when oil production and hormones naturally level off.

By the time you get to your fifties and sixties, if you have protected your skin, your skin's good qualities will come to the fore. The oil production that has been your bane in youth becomes a balm as you age, preserving your skin's hydration. From midlife on, with minimal wrinkles, decreased oiliness, and reduced tendency to form dark spots, you enjoy skin that resists aging better than many other types. As others reach for the wrinkle creams (or other more advanced antiaging procedures), you will mature into the benefits that oily, tight skin confers over time.

PIGMENT AWAY

Your second major challenge is pigmentation. Higher pigment levels can lead to unsightly dark spots that spring up suddenly and don't fade for weeks or even months. Pigment-producing cells in the skin can produce several different kinds of dark spots, which I detailed more fully in the section on pigmentation in Chapter Two.

Depending on your skin colour and ethnic origin, you will get certain forms of pigmentation, but not others. Therefore, throughout this chapter, I'll discuss the best treatment options for the different types of pigmentation.

Dark spots of all types can develop from a wide range of factors, including inflammation, wounds, nicks and cuts, as well as increased oestrogen levels. In addition, sun exposure accelerates your skin's tendency to produce the pigment that creates dark spots, melasma, sun spots and freckles.

SPECIAL CHALLENGES OF YOUR SKIN TYPE

First, your skin's innate oiliness leads to a pimple, which is one form of inflammation. Next, the inflammation increases pigmentation at the site of the breakout, producing an unsightly dark spot in the exact location of the breakout.

This pattern of successive skin problems is frustrating. Whether your problem is acne, cuts, rashes or allergic reactions, you breathe a sigh of relief that you've finally cleared it up, only to notice that you now must contend with dark spots. You may notice that these spots look worse and last longer than the original problem! Dermatologists call this condition post-inflammatory pigmentation alteration (PIPA). Fearing these spots will become permanent, people often refer to them as 'scars.' But your dark spots are not permanent, nor are they scars. By preventing inflammation, you can intervene in the vicious cycle, once and for all.

This sequence of skin problems can also appear anywhere on the body. People come to my office complaining they feel too embarrassed to wear skirts because a cut on their leg has turned into an unsightly dark area. This is a common experience for many OSPTs.

OSPTS AND INFLAMMATION

Added to the above factors, the third element in your skin care challenge is your skin's sensitivity, which makes you more susceptible to inflammatory reactions that lead to dark spots. That's why it's essential to identify and avoid inflammatory triggers, so I'll identify a range of them for you here.

Inflammation is caused by the increased presence of red or white blood cells that rush to the site of an injury to aid in recovery. Pimples, burns, insect bites, bruises, rashes and allergic reactions are common ones, but any type of inflammation, even blood cells concentrated at the site of a cut, can trigger the formation of brown spots. Any heat source outside the body can also increase inflammation *inside* the body.

Lee, an Asian man, who was a chef in an upscale nouvelle French-Asian restaurant, consulted me about a large area of melasma covering his cheeks and forehead. We tried several topical treatments, but none of them worked. Even though he was stressed and embarrassed by these patches, he refused to wear makeup to cover them, curtly informing me that doing so 'would be even more humiliating'. Finally, I told him that the only cure was to get out of the kitchen. That's what you have to do if you can't stand the heat! And there was no doubt that his ongoing exposure to heat and steam was a major contributing factor. Lee followed my advice, and his melasma resolved. Sadly, South Beach lost a very fine chef, and I certainly miss his lemongrass chicken.

External heat contributes to inflammation, which is why burns, hot wax applications, sunburns or irritating skin care ingredients that cause redness can all lead to the OSPT vicious cycle. Sunning and burning on a hot day can also result in inflammation. Although skin pigmentation will prevent sunburns in dark-skinned OSPTs, the *heat* from sun can still be a problem.

Avoid sun exposure, hot weather, burns and excess heat from all sources. Elective services, including waxing, saunas, steam rooms, peels or other treatments that heat or irritate the skin can all provoke the inflammation cycle. So can these common cosmetic treatments:

- Plucking facial hair with tweezers can traumatise skin.
- Chemical depilatories that remove hair, like Nair, often contain strong chemicals that can irritate your skin.
- Hot waxes can create inflammation.
- Strong chemical peels are too harsh.
- Razors that promise a close shave increase the risk of developing ingrown hairs, which lead to inflammation.
- Hot, spicy food, drinks, and climate can cause inflammation.
- Saunas, body wraps, and hair treatments involving heat or harsh chemicals such as colouring, perming or straightening can cause a problem.

Make sure that you avoid these procedures. A prescription product called Vaniqa can slow the growth of hair so that you need hair removal less often. Bypass anything that causes skin trauma.

SKIN SENSITIVITY AND OSPTS

As a sensitive type, you're also more likely to develop redness, burning, stinging, rashes, or allergies in response to some skin care ingredients.

Maria, a twenty-nine-year-old estate agent, came from a large Italian family with the dark hair, olive skin, flashing black eyes, and lively personality to prove it. She also had the oily, pigmented skin common in people from Mediterranean backgrounds. Because she was always in contact with the public, she wanted her skin to look great; so she followed the advice of a cosmetologist and used a chemical peel, which turned her skin bright red and led to brown patches. 'The cosmetologist told me that this would *clear* my skin,' she told me. 'But look what happened! This is a disaster.'

Most people, including many skin service professionals, don't have a clue about which ingredients cause allergies or inflammations, so it's up to you to protect your skin from products and procedures that do more harm than good. Even products labelled hypoallergenic may contain fragrances or preservatives to which sensitive types react. Read the fine print and steer away from ingredients that might provoke a reaction. Later in this chapter, I will alert you to sensitising ingredients and steer you towards skin care products and ingredients that will help calm, rather than provoke, inflammation.

In addition to the risk of product reactions, you may suffer from enhanced sensitivity to reactive agents from other sources. Although the topic is outside the scope of this book, it's not uncommon for allergic individuals to react to certain foods, fabrics, or chemicals present in clothing, furnishings, or buildings. For example, Maria, an attractive woman with freckles and green eyes inherited from her German grandmother, had also inherited Granny's allergy to strawberries. When Maria ate them, she developed a small rash that disappeared within a few hours. Another type might have tolerated this passing reaction in order to enjoy a favourite fruit, but as an OSPT, Maria didn't have that luxury because the allergic reaction triggered an inflammatory–brown spot cycle. Some allergies are not as obvious as Maria's immediate reaction to strawberries, but can trigger a response hours or days later. If allergic reactions persist in expressing via your skin, consider working with a specialist in allergies to identify your triggers and avoid them.

Mukta's Story

A beautiful forty-two-year-old Indian woman, Mukta was an on-air personality on a local news show who felt exasperated by recurrent bouts of acne followed by dark spots that would last for three months or more. 'In my line of work, it's embarrassing to always have blemishes and discoloration dotting my face!' she complained.

She'd found that the professional on-camera makeup covered both the acne and the dark spots. But Mukta felt self-conscious wearing this heavy stage makeup off the set, and normal consumer foundation couldn't mask her skin problem. Concerned that her stage makeup was instigating breakouts, she wished to find a better alternative.

The pressure to look as beautiful in her everyday life as she did on camera made Mukta anxious. When she met people in person, she worried that they would talk behind her back about how much makeup she wore. In desperation, Mukta had purchased and tried at least ten different expensive 'lightening creams', spending over two hundred dollars on these products.

While they were somewhat helpful in slowly lightening her spots, inevitably the acne would return, followed by more spots. 'I just want to hide,' Mukta confessed.

Fortunately, I had a different strategy. Instead of trying to get rid of the spots, our main focus would be to prevent them. To do that, I recommended a three-pronged approach: First, use a retinoid to prevent acne and to increase her exfoliation rate so the dark spots would slough faster. Second, use a sunscreen to prevent activation of the cells that make colour and thus dark spots. Third, use a special topical product that prevents PIPA.

This approach would place Mukta ahead of the game instead of always playing catch-up by dealing with spots once they had appeared. Since acne occurs in an eight-week cycle, it would take longer than that to see results; so I suggested covering her pimples and dark spots with a foundation and facial powder that contained an acne-clearing ingredient like salicylic acid.

When Mukta returned for a follow-up visit, she looked radiant. Wearing no foundation, she had no acne and no dark spots! She'd started working out at a popular yoga studio, feeling relaxed and confident about being seen in public without makeup. I reminded her to remain vigilant by continuing her regimen, since this was an ongoing prevention strategy, not a permanent cure.

A CLOSE-UP LOOK AT YOUR SKIN

The OSPT Skin Type is quite common among people with medium and darker skin colour, like Mediterraneans, Middle-Easterners, Indians, and Caribbean, Latin-American, and Asian people. Lighter-skinned people from other ethnic backgrounds, like the English, Irish, Scottish, Welsh, or Germans, as well as people of those ethnic backgrounds residing in Australia and New Zealand, can all be OSPTs too. And so can a redhead with freckles, which are a form of pigmentation. If the questionnaire revealed that you're an OSPT, but you don't experience all the symptoms I'll cover, your test result isn't wrong. OSPTs share many common problems, but there are some differences, so throughout this chapter, I'll discuss the various symptoms, tendencies and treatment options typical for dark, medium, and light-toned OSPTs.

All OSPTs are likely to experience:

- Acne, rashes, skin allergies
- Dark spots or patches in areas of sun exposure
- Shininess from sunscreen use
- Stinging or irritation from many skin care products

With dark-toned OSPT skin, you may also experience:

- Dark spots in areas of previous acne, irritation or trauma (such as cuts, nicks, scrapes and burns)
- Sunscreen appears white or purple when applied to skin
- Difficulty finding a facial foundation in the right shade in a product that your sensitive skin can tolerate
- Makeup used to cover dark spots causes oiliness, shine or acne
- Ingrown hairs with resulting dark spots
- Dark circles under the eyes

Medium-toned OSPTs of Italian, French, Spanish, Indian, Middle-Eastern, Latin-American, Asian or other ethnicity may also experience:

- Oiliness, shine, or acne caused by makeup used to cover dark spots
- Dark circles under the eyes

Light-skinned OSPTs may also experience:

- Facial freckles
- Sun spots on hands, arms and legs
- Increased risk for melanoma skin cancer, especially if you have red hair or freckles

Finding the right treatments is easier for light-skin-toned OSPTs whose freckles and sunspots are easily improved by sun avoidance and sunscreen use in combination with skin care treatments that I'll discuss in this chapter. Skin-bleaching agents are helpful for all OSPTs, but those with light skin tones can also use stronger treatments, such as lasers and light treatments. However, I never recommend those treatments for darker skin tones as they can lead back to that same vicious cycle of inflammation. If you are Asian, beware. Although your skin colour may appear light, your skin may react to inflammation just like people with a darker skin tone. Follow the treatment recommendations for the dark- or medium-skin-toned OSPT groups.

Light-skinned OSPTs are at increased risk for melanoma skin cancers, especially if you have freckles and a history of sunburns. And if you have sunburned in the past, take steps to avoid sun exposure now so that you do not further harm your skin. It's important to check moles yourself and also to have regular checkups by a dermatologist.

SIGNS OF MELANOMA: THE A, B, C AND D

- Asymmetry: One side of the mole is not a mirror image of the other side.
- Borders: The borders are not distinct. It is hard to tell where the mole starts and stops.
- Colour: The presence of more than one colour or black, white, red and yellow hues
- Diameter: Larger than a quarter-inch

There is no way to prevent melanoma, although you can reduce your risk by avoiding sun exposure. Your best chance is to catch it early while it's curable. It you notice a suspicious mole, immediately see a dermatologist. It may save your life. Waiting even one day can make a difference.

RECOMMENDATIONS FOR OSPT SKIN

You can prevent acne, redness and rashes by using my recommended products, which walk the tightrope between avoiding potentially reactive ingredients and providing helpful oil-reducing and anti-inflammatory benefits. Second, sun exposure increases pigmentation, making regular sunscreen use essential. Third, manage stress and avoid all activities and skin care interventions that provoke inflammation. Taking the steps discussed below can make all the difference. Luckily for you, most of your type's key issues *are* preventable.

Dr Baumann's Bottom Line: Prevention is key! Lessen skin irritation and the pigmentation that follows it by using a consistent anti-inflammatory prevention strategy.

EVERYDAY CARE FOR YOUR SKIN TYPE

Depending on where you are in the inflammation–breakout–dark spot cycle, choose the appropriate treatment application.

The products I'll recommend act to do one or more of the following:

- Prevent and treat pimples
- Prevent and treat dark spots

In addition, some of the products will help in:

• Managing redness

Skin lightening and oil treatment products can help manage a wide range of typical OSPT symptoms, most of which are caused by pigmentation and overactive oil production. Please look over the various regimens and determine which one is right for your needs. Depending on whether your skin is more oily or combination, you can use or omit optional products like toners and moisturisers.

If after using this regimen for six weeks to two months, you find you need further help, go to 'Consulting a Dermatologist', where you'll find prescription medications for your problems. If your symptoms are acute, schedule an appointment at once, as there's often a waiting list.

I've provided different Daily Skin Care Regimens to address the different kinds of problems OSPTs experience. Select the right one, and then refer to the specific product recommendations that can be used with it.

Consider all the nonprescription regimens as the Stage One in a two-stage protocol. In the first stage, outlined here, you'll undertake a foundation regimen. After six weeks to two months, if you find that your skin problems have not resolved, I recommend that you 'graduate' to my prescription protocol for a more advanced treatment plan, detailed in 'Consulting a Dermatologist.'

Make it your daily habit to use the products that prevent your key problems. To this basic program, you can add supplementary treatment options when you have the specific problem they address.

DAILY SKIN CARE

STAGE ONE: NONPRESCRIPTION REGIMEN

For acne and dark spots:

AM	PM
Step 1: Wash with cleanser	Step 1: Wash with cleanser
Step 2: Apply a toner (optional)	Step 2: Apply a toner (optional)
	Step 3: Apply pimple medication

Step 3: Apply a skin lightener when you have dark spots (optional)

Step 4: Apply a benzoyl peroxide product to acne-prone areas

Step 5: Apply an eye cream (optional)

Step 6: Apply sunscreen (non-optional!)

Step 7: Apply SPF-containing makeup

when you have pimples (optional)

Step 4: If needed, apply a skin lightener to dark spots (optional)

Step 5: Apply an eye cream (optional)

Step 6: Apply a moisturiser to dry areas if you have combination skin (optional)

In the morning, clean your face with a cleanser containing either salicylic acid (if redness is a concern) or benzoyl peroxide (if acne but not redness is a concern). Complete facial cleansing with a toning product if your skin feels oily. (If your skin is less oily, you can omit this step). If dark spots are present, apply a skin-lightening gel to them. If you are prone to acne or when you have active breakouts, apply a benzoyl peroxide-containing gel directly to the pimples. You can also use an on-the-spot pimple treatment product, which can be applied periodically during the day. Use an eye cream if you'd like to.

Next, apply your obligatory sunscreen, and makeup, if desired.

In the evening, follow the same regimen, omitting the benzoyl peroxide gel and sunscreen and adding an eye cream and moisturiser if needed. To determine if moisturisers are right for you, please read the advice and product recommendations in the product sections following these regimens.

STAGE ONE: NONPRESCRIPTION REGIMEN

For skin redness and dark spots without acne:

AM	PM
Step 1: Wash with cleanser	Step 1: Wash with cleanser
Step 2: Apply a toner (optional)	Step 2: Apply a toner (optional)

Step 3: Apply a skin lightener when you have dark spots (optional)

Step 3: If needed, apply a skin lightener to dark spots (optional)

Step 4: Apply an eye cream (optional)

Step 4: Apply an eye cream (optional)

Step 5: Apply sunscreen (non-optional!)

Step 5: Apply a moisturiser to dry areas if you have combination skin (optional)

Step 6: Apply SPF-containing makeup

In the morning, cleanse your face with a cleanser that contains ingredients right for your condition. For facial redness, use an anti-inflammatory cleanser. If your skin has a high O/D score (34 or greater), follow with a toner. If dark spots are present, apply a skin-lightening gel to them. Apply eye cream, if you wish to.

Next, apply sunscreen. If your O/D score is less than 34, use a moisturiser or makeup foundation with sunscreen. If your O/D score is greater than 34, skip the moisturiser and use a sunscreen alone or makeup powder that contains sunscreen.

In the evening, follow the same regimen, omitting sunscreen and makeup, again including an eye cream and moisturiser if needed.

STAGE ONE: NONPRESCRIPTION REGIMEN

For skin redness and dark spots with acne:

AM

PM

Step 1: Wash with cleanser

Step 1: Wash with cleanser

Step 2: Apply a skin lightener when you have dark spots (optional)

Step 2: If needed, apply pimple medication to pimples (optional)

Step 3: Apply a pimple spot treatment to pimples (optional)

Step 3: If needed, apply skin lightener to dark spots (optional)

Step 4: Apply sunscreen (non-optional!)

Step 5: Apply SPF-containing makeup

Step 4: Apply a moisturiser to dry areas if you have combination skin (optional)

In the morning, use a salicylic acid cleanser to clean your face. If dark spots are present, apply a skin-lightening gel to them. If you are having acne or active breakouts, apply a pimple-control product to pimples, and take it with you to use if needed during the day. Next, apply sunscreen and makeup if desired.

In the evening, follow the same regimen, omitting the sunscreen, and including a moisturiser if needed.

Cleansers

Choose a nonirritating cleanser to remove makeup without stripping your skin's natural oils. This helps decrease or control skin sensitivity. If your cleanser is drying your skin, use it every other day, alternating with a cleanser designed for sensitive skin, like Aveda's All Sensitive Cleanser. Avoid cold creams and cream cleansers, which are too heavy for your oily skin.

Here I provide several different categories of cleansers: choose a cleanser from the category that matches your chosen Daily Skin Care Regimen.

RECOMMENDED ACNE CONTROL CLEANSERS

- £ Bioré Blemish Fighting Ice Cleanser
- £ Clearasil Face Wash
- £ Stiefel Panoxyl Wash 10%
- £ Clean & Clear Blackhead Clearing Cleanser
- £ Neutrogena Clear Pore Wash
- £ Stiefel Acne-Aid Cleansing Bar
- ££ Dermalogica Anti-Bac Skin Wash
- ££ Donell Super-Skin Beta Hydroxy Acne Cleanser
- ££ La Roche-Posay Effaclar Purifying Foaming Gel
- £££ Rodan & Fields Unblemish Wash Facial Cleanser (acne)

Baumann's Choice: Stiefel Panoxyl Wash 10% for acne. (Only available in pharmacies.)

RECOMMENDED GENTLE CLEANSERS
FOR OILY SKIN

£ Eucerin Gentle Cleansing Milk
££ Aesop Amazing Face Cleanser
££ Aveda's All Sensitive Cleanser
££ Dermalogica Ultra-Calming Cleanser
££ Elizabeth Arden Sensitive Skin Calming Foamy Cleanser
££ Jan Marini Bioglycolic Oily Skin Cleansing Gel
££ Korres White Tea Fluid Gel Cleanser
££ La Roche-Posay Toleriane Foaming Cleanser
££ Laura Mercier Oil Free Gel Cleanser
££ MD Formulations Facial Cleanser Oily and Problem Skin
£££ B. Kamins Booster Blue Rosacea Cleanser
£££ Dr Brandt Pore Effect
£££ Jurlique Cleansing Lotion

Baumann's Choice: La Roche-Posay Toleriane Foaming Cleanser for redness or stinging.

Toner Use

Oily types typically enjoy the clean and refreshing feeling that toners can provide. Also, anti-inflammatory, pigment- and oil-control substances in toners remain on the skin to deliver ingredients. However, if you have combination skin, avoid using toner on dry areas. If you experience redness or stinging when using skin care products such as moisturisers or sunscreens, omit toners and use a facial gel with anti-inflammatory ingredients. If your daily regimen gets too complicated, omit toner use.

RECOMMENDED TONERS

£ Bioré Triple Action Toner
£ Natural Collection Tea Tree Facial Cleanser & Toner
££ Exuviance Soothing Toning Lotion
££ Skin Medica Acne Toner with Tea Tree Oil and Salicylic Acid
£££ Dr Brandt Lineless Tone
£££ Erno Laszlo Conditioning Preparation Toner for Oily to Extremely Oily Skin
£££ Rodan and Fields UnBlemish Medicated Facial Toner

Baumann's Choice: Erno Laszlo Conditioning Preparation Toner. I usually don't pick the expensive ones but the resorcinol in this product makes it exceptional for OSPTs. If you suffer from redness and stinging, it may be too strong, but it's great for acne and dark spots.

Handling Breakouts

Oily, sensitive types are vulnerable to breakouts, which may leave scars, especially if you pick at them or squeeze them incorrectly. The products in your daily regimen should help prevent them, and you can treat breakouts with some of the products listed below, and then allow your body's natural healing process to resolve them.

Above all, don't steam your face, apply a hot washcloth or place an ice cube on a pimple. All of these actions cause rapid changes in temperature, which is strictly a no-no for types prone to inflammation. Some believe that sun exposure will help clear up acne, but since acne typically worsens in summer, I don't believe that it's helpful.

The best thing to do is to leave a pimple alone and apply a pimple medication that contains salicylic acid or benzoyl peroxide. Products with benzoyl peroxide can be found in pharmacies.

RECOMMENDED ACNE PRODUCTS

£ Clearasil Active Treatment Cream Cover Up
£ Clean and Clear Quick Clear Treatment Gel
££ Aesop Chamomile Concentrate Anti-Blemish Masque
££ Botani Rescue Acne Cream
££ D'Arcy Anti-Acne Serum
££ Dermalogica Medicated Clearing Gel
££ Eve Lom Dynaspot
££ Jo Malone Blemish Control Solution
££ MD Formulations Adult Anti-Blemish Kit
££ Ultraceuticals UltraClear Oily/Acne-Prone Gel
£££ Rodan & Fields Unblemish Regimen

Baumann's Choice: Eve Lom Dynaspot because it has chamomile and tea tree oil.

RECOMMENDED ACNE CONTROL PRODUCTS
WITH BENZOYL PEROXIDE

£ Brevoxyl Cream
£ Oxy 5 Acne Vanishing Cream
£ Oxy 10 Acne Vanishing Cream
£ Panoxyl Wash 10%
£ PanOxyl AquaGel 2.5%, 5% or 10%
£ Thursday Plantation Tea Tree Medicated Gel
££ Jan Marini Benzoyl Peroxide 5%
££ MD Formulations Benzoyl Peroxide 10%
££ Proactiv Repairing Lotion
£££ Ole Henriksen Roll-On Blemish Attack
£££ Zirh Fix Blemish Control Lotion

Baumann's Choice: Panoxyl AquaGel. Start with 2.5%. If you do not experience redness and continue to have acne, progress to 5%, and then to 10%, if needed.

The Proper Way to Pop

Though I prefer that you leave your pimples alone, I know that some of you will not rest until you've popped the pimple. That's why I offer instructions on the *correct* way to do it. Use this technique when the pimple is ready, as I'll describe here.

What You'll Need:

Soap and water
Alcohol
Cotton wool
Matches and needle
Sterilised glass medicine dropper (cooled)
or
cotton-wool ball

Knowing When It's Ready:

Your body responds to inflammation by walling off all the dead cells, pus and bacteria, and making them into a discrete little pustule ready to be popped. If the pimple has a little white head, showing that all the pus has gathered into a little pocket and can be released, you may proceed. Otherwise, stop, the pimple is not ready and messing with it will only make matters worse. You could wind up enlarging it or turning it into a cyst.

What to Do:

First, wash the area and your hands with soap until clean. Pass the needle through the flame of a match to sterilise it. Then use a cotton-wool ball soaked in alcohol to wipe the needle clean and remove all traces of black.

Use a second alcohol-moistened cotton-wool ball to wipe over and sterilise the pimple and surrounding area. Now, take the needle and very gently press it over the area of pimple where the white pus ball is visible, making one tiny prick to open it up. One little prick and that's it. If nothing happens and the pimple does not open up, then please leave it alone, and wait six hours. Believe me, if it's ready to pop, it will do so easily. If not, let it go.

If ready, you can next use a cotton-wool ball to put gentle, even pressure all around the outside of the pimple.

Alternatively, you can use a medicine dropper. Position it so that the centre of the pimple is at the hole in the dropper and the glass supplies pressure on all sides. Press gently until the pus is released.

Post Popping Treatment:

Wipe the area clean with the cotton-wool ball and apply an antiseptic drying lotion or stick made with alcohol, witch hazel, benzoyl peroxide or salicylic acid. Clinique makes acne sticks useful for drying out pimples.

Leave it to dry without bandaging or covering. You can cover the blemish with a stick or concealer made with anti-inflammatory and drying ingredients, like benzoyl peroxide, tea tree oil or salicylic acid, such as my recommendation, Eve Lom Dynaspot. Or you can opt for a prescription concealer made with sulphur.

If your pimple is not coming to a head, cover it with an acne-control product containing witch hazel, benzoyl peroxide or salicylic acid. Or if it persists, you can go to a dermatologist for a steroid injection that will remove the pimple but can temporarily leave a dent that looks like a scar.

RECOMMENDED SPOT TREATMENTS
FOR PIMPLES

- £ Boots Tea Tree & Witch Hazel Spot Wand
- £ Clean and Clear Extra Strength Invisible Blemish Treatment Gel
- £ PanOxyl Acne Gel by Stiefel 5% or 10%
- £ Pond's Overnight Blemish Reducers
- ££ Biotherm Acnopur Emergency Anti-Marks Concealer for Blemish Prone Skin
- ££ Clinique Acne Solutions Concealing Stick
- ££ Eve Lom Dynaspot
- ££ Jo Malone Blemish Control Solution
- ££ Jurlique Blemish Cream
- ££ Paula's Choice Blemish Fighting Solution
- £££ Clinique Acne Solutions Spot Healing Gel or Concealing Stick
- £££ Gatineau SOS Stick
- £££ Guerlain Issima Crème Camphréa

Baumann's Choice: Clinique Acne Solutions Concealing Stick helps hide the pimple as well as heal it.

Treating Dark Spots

For dark spots, apply skin-lightening products, making sure to use them after cleansing and toning but before other recommended products. Begin to use these products at the very first sign of darkening, and continue use until the spot has completely disappeared. You can also use them on dark spots you've had for some time. If you find that these nonprescription skin lighteners are not sufficiently effective, go to 'Consulting a Dermatologist' for prescription lighteners.

RECOMMENDED SKIN-LIGHTENING GELS

- ££ Peter Thomas Roth Potent Skin Lightening Gel Complex
- ££ Skin Doctors Fade Away Pigmentation Lotion
- ££ SkinCeuticals Phyto Corrective Gel
- £££ DDF Fade Gel 4
- £££ DDF Intensive Holistic Corrector Swabs
- £££ DDF Intensive Holistic Lightener

£££ Dr Brandt Lightening Gel
£££ Dr Michelle Copeland Skin Care Pigment Blocker 5
£££ Philosophy A Pigment of Your Imagination Gel
£££ Philosophy When Lightening Strikes

Baumann's Choice: I could not find any £ choices, but I love Philosophy A Pigment of Your Imagination Gel.

Moisturisers

Unnecessary or disadvantageous for most OSPTs, moisturisers can clog your pores and increase oiliness. In most cases, your own naturally occurring oil is all you need. However, if you have some dry areas, around the eyes, cheeks or jaw (or an O/D score between 27 and 35), apply a light moisturising product with ingredients that work against inflammation, acne, and dark spots to the dry areas only or, if needed, to the entire face. Antiaging preparations such as stronger night creams with fruit acids, alpha lipoic acid and DMAE can irritate and are unnecessary.

RECOMMENDED MOISTURISERS

£   Boots brand No 7 Uplifting Day Cream
£   Eucerin Q 10 Active Antiwrinkle Fluid SPF 15
£   Neutrogena Moisture Facial Day Cream SPF 15
£   Olay Total Effects 7x Visible Anti-Aging Vitamin Complex
    (Fragrance-Free)
££ Anthony Logistics Oil Free Facial Lotion
££ Jo Malone Protective Lotion Daily SPF 15
££ MD Formulations Glycare Lotion
£££ Caudalie Vinopure Matte Moisturizing Fluid

Baumann's Choice: Neutrogena Moisture Facial Day Cream SPF 15 because it contains active soy which improved dark spots.

Eye Creams

For dark circles under your eyes, use eye creams containing vitamin K, which may address the blood congestion that is thought to cause them.

RECOMMENDED EYE CREAMS

£ Eucerin Q 10 Active Antiwrinkle Eye Cream

£ Olay Regenerist Eye Lifting Serum

£ Roc Retin Ox Correxion Intensive Eye Care with retinol

££ Aveda Tourmaline Charged Eye Cream

££ Clarins Extra-Firming Eye Contour Serum

££ Elizabeth Arden Ceramide Eyewish SPF 10

££ Laura Mercier Eyedration

££ Origins A Perfect World For Eyes

££ Relastin Eye Cream

Baumann's Choice: Roc Retin Ox Correxion Intensive Eye Care because it has retinol, which has been shown to decrease under-eye circles. It may be too strong for those with very sensitive skin.

Exfoliation

Using a facial scrub helps certain types, but it's not beneficial for OSPTs because vigorous exfoliation can lead to inflammation and dark spots. If you use retinoids, you'll find that they naturally exfoliate the skin.

SHOPPING FOR PRODUCTS

Widen your choice of products by reading labels to determine product ingredients, so that you can select those that contain beneficial ingredients while avoiding ones that increase inflammation or oiliness. If you find products that you like that are not listed here, please visit www.DrBaumann.co.uk and tell me your favourites so I can pass them along to others of your Skin Type. Check the ingredients in your shampoos, conditioners, bubble baths and shaving products as well, as these contact your skin and can cause irritation.

SKIN CARE INGREDIENTS TO USE

To decrease skin inflammation:

- Aloe vera
- Boswellia serrata
- Mallow
- Niacinamide

- Arctium lappa (burdock root)
- Chamomile
- Cucumber
- Dexpanthenol (pro-vitamin B$_5$)
- Glycyrrhiza glabra (licorice extract)
- Licochalone
- Red algae
- Rose water
- Salicylic acid (beta hydroxy acid or BHA)
- Silymarin
- Sulphacetamide
- Sulphur
- Tea tree oil
- Zinc

To lessen acne:

- Azelaic acid
- Benzoyl peroxide (unless you experience facial redness)
- Resorcinol (dark-skinned OSPTs should use with caution)
- Retinol
- Salicylic acid (beta hydroxy acid or BHA)
- Tea tree oil (can cause allergy in some people)

To prevent pigment:

- Niacinamide

To reduce pigment:

Use when you have dark spots, melasma or undesirable pigmentation

- Arbutin
- Azelaic acid
- Bearberry extract
- Cucumber extract
- Epilobium angustifolium (willow herb)
- Kojic acid
- Glycyrrhiza glabra (licorice extract)
- Mulberry extract
- Resorcinol (dark-skinned OSPTs should use with caution)
- Salicylic acid (beta hydroxy acid or BHA)

Cleansing Ingredients to Avoid

- Avoid any products that have thick, 'vigorous' foam.

SKIN CARE INGREDIENTS TO AVOID

If acne prone:

- Butyl stearate
- Cinnamon oil
- Cocoa butter
- Cocos nucifera (coconut oil)
- Decyl oleate
- Isocetyl stearate
- Isopropyl isostearate
- Isopropyl myristate
- Isopropyl palmitate
- Isostearyl isostearate
- Isostearyl neopentanoate
- Jojoba oil
- Myristyl myristate
- Myristyl propionate
- Octyl palmitate
- Octyl stearate
- Peppermint oil

If you have skin allergies or rashes:

- Benzoyl peroxide
- Parabens
- Fragrances
- Lanolin
- Propylene glycol-2 (PPG-2)

Sun Protection for Your Skin

Often light-skinned OSPTs avoid the sun because they know that they will just burn and freckle. Thanks to the unique combination of oiliness and pigmentation, OSPTs with medium skin tone can achieve a glowing, gorgeous tan. However, medium- and dark-toned OSPTs should wear sunscreen to prevent the formation of dark spots, which are caused by UVB and UVA light. That's why a broad-spectrum sunscreen which blocks both UVA and UVB rays at all times is a must, regardless of your skin colour. Because OSPTs have oily skin, gels, light lotions and sprays will feel better than greasy creams and lotions. OSPT skin is sensitive, so physical barrier sunscreens that contain titanium dioxide and zinc oxide are better than chemical sunscreens that can sting and burn. You will notice you may still get a light tan, as no sunscreen blocks 100 percent of the sun's rays.

And remember, if you have an outbreak of melasma or acute sun spots, total sun avoidance is best. For extra 'security', choose a product that offers anti-inflammatory and skin-lightening ingredients as well as sun protection.

RECOMMENDED SUN PROTECTION PRODUCTS

£ Neutrogena Visibly Young Day Cream SPF 20

£ RoC Retinol Actif Pur Day Cream SPF 15

££ B. Kamins Sunbar Sunscreen SPF 30 Fragrance-Free

££ Dermalogica Solar Defense Booster SPF 30

££ Molton Brown Active Defence City-Day Hydrator

££ Origins Sunshine State SPF 30

££ Peter Thomas Roth Oil Free Sunblock SPF 30

££ SkinCeuticals Ultimate UV Defense SPF 30

£££ Philosophy A Pigment of Your Imagination SPF 18

£££ Prescriptives All You Need+ Broad Spectrum Oil Absorbing Lotion SPF 15

Baumann's Choice: Philosophy A Pigment of Your Imagination because it contains skin lighteners as well as sunscreen.

SUNSCREEN INGREDIENTS TO AVOID

Due to skin sensitivity, some OSPTs experience stinging, burning and redness in reaction to certain ingredients commonly used in sunscreens. If this occurs, stop using the offending product immediately and avoid these ingredients:

- Avobenzone
- Benzophenone
- Butyl methoxydibenzoyl methane
- Isopropyldibenzoylmethane
- Methylbenzylidene camphor
- Octyl methoxycinnamate
- Para-amniobenzoic acid (PABA)
- Phenylbenzimidazole sulphonic acid

Your Makeup

You can cover a pimple, dark spots, or redness with makeup that contains certain key ingredients that prevent these same problems. For acne control, look for products that contain salicylic acid which improves acne, increases skin exfoliation and decreases oiliness. To prevent dark spots, look for foundations that contain lightening ingredients like soy, such as Neutrogena Visibly Even Liquid Makeup. (This Neutrogena foundation is amazing, but is only found in the US. I'll try to make it available at www.Baumannstore.co.uk.) OSPTs should avoid heavier, oil-containing foundations, instead using oil-free ones. Most cosmetic lines contain three different foundation lines: one with oil; one without, and one with some added value, such as sunscreen. The oil-free version is best for you. Bypassing foundation altogether and instead using a powder with sunscreen is another good option.

Facial powders can temper your skin's shininess, if the recommended lotions and gels do not fully prevent it. As an added benefit, facial products that contain sunscreen will shield your skin from rays that stimulate pigmentation. Facial powders with sunscreen are more readily found in the USA, so stock up if you visit.The products I'll recommend can not only cover redness and dark spots, but absorb and camouflage skin oiliness while providing sun protection.

RECOMMENDED FACIAL POWDERS WITH SUNSCREEN

- £ Maybelline Pure Stay Powder SPF 15
- £ Neutrogena Healthy Defense Protective Powder SPF 30
- ££ Colorescience Foundation Powder SPF 20
- ££ Estée Lauder Amber Bronze Cool Bronze Loose Powder SPF 8
- ££ Jane Iredale's Amazing Base Loose Minerals SPF 20
- ££ Mirenesse Emulsion Pact with SPF 25
- ££ Philosophy The Supernatural Airbrushed Canvas Powder Foundation

Baumann's Choice: Colorescience Foundation Powder SPF 20. It comes in several shades.

RECOMMENDED FACIAL POWDERS WITH ACNE OR OIL CONTROL

- £ Avon Clear Finish Great Complexion Pressed Powder
- £ Maybelline Shine Free Oil Control Loose Powder
- ££ Bobbi Brown Sheer Finish Loose Powder
- ££ Clinique Stay-Matte Sheer Pressed Powder
- ££ Laura Mercier Translucent Pressed Setting Powder
- ££ Jane Iredale Pure Matte Finish Powder

££ Stila Loose Powder
£££ Lancôme Dual Finish Fragrance Free Powder
£££ Shu Uemura Face Powder Matte

Baumann's Choice: Lancôme Dual Finish Fragrance Free Powder is truly fragrance free and great for sensitive Skin Types.

RECOMMENDED FOUNDATIONS

£ CoverGirl Clean Oil-Control Makeup (for light coverage)
£ L'Oréal Air Wear Powder Foundation SPF 17
£ Maybelline Pure Stay Powder & Foundation SPF 15
£ Revlon Skin Perfecting Makeup for Oily Blemish Prone Skin
££ Acne Results Foundation by DermaBlend
££ Dermalogica Treatment Foundation
££ Fresh Face Luster Powder Foundation
££ Laura Mercier Oil Free Foundation
££ Mary Kay Dual-Coverage Powder Foundation
££ Philosophy The Supernatural Airbrushed Canvas Powder Foundation
£££ Chanel Double Perfection Fluide Matte Reflecting Makeup SPF 15

Baumann's Choice: Philosophy The Supernatural Airbrushed Canvas Powder Foundation

CONSULTING A DERMATOLOGIST

PRESCRIPTION SKIN CARE STRATEGIES

If after using your daily skin care recommendations and nonprescription treatments for two months, you find that you are still experiencing acute acne, the next step is to see a dermatologist. For acne, I would advise that you try a prescription antibiotic gel and retinoid first, and then consider oral antibiotics only if they fail to resolve the problem. Please follow my Stage Two Daily Skin Care Regimen below. If you take oral antibiotics long-term, I suggest that you take acidophilus along with them to maintain a healthy digestive tract.

Whether you suffer from acne, rosacea, or facial redness, this prescription regimen will help. Topical antibiotics have both anti-acne and anti-inflammatory properties.

DAILY SKIN CARE

STAGE TWO: PRESCRIPTION REGIMEN

To treat acne:

AM	PM
Step 1: Wash with cleanser	Step 1: Wash with cleanser
Step 2: Apply a toner (optional)	Step 2: Apply a toner (optional)
Step 3: Apply a skin lightener when you have dark spots (optional)	Step 3: If needed, apply skin lightener to dark spots (optional)
Step 4: Apply a prescription antibiotic gel	Step 4: Apply a prescription antibiotic gel
Step 5: Apply sunscreen (non-optional!)	Step 5: Apply a retinoid gel if you don't have dark spots, or a prescription skin lightener if you do have dark spots in place of lightener at Step 3
Step 6: Apply SPF-containing makeup	Step 6: Apply a moisturiser to dry areas if you have combination skin (optional)

In the morning, use a prescription cleanser to clean your face. Apply a toner if desired. Apply a prescription skin lightener to dark spots. Apply an antibiotic gel, such as Duac, to the entire face. If you currently have breakouts, you can also use an on-the-spot pimple treatment product (see recommendations in the nonprescription product lists) and take it with you to use if needed during the day as your final step before moving on with your morning.

Next, apply sunscreen and makeup if you desire.

In the evening, follow the same regimen, using a recommended retinoid, such as Differin. Since retinoids can be drying with combination skin (with an O/D score between 27 and 35), you can use a moisturiser as well.

RECOMMENDED PRESCRIPTION CLEANSERS

- Rosanil Cleanser
- Rosula Cleanser
- Triaz Cleanser
- Zoderm Cleanser

Baumann's Choice: Ask your dermatologist for cleansers containing benzoyl peroxide, salicylic acid, sulphur, sulphacetamide or zinc. The abovementioned product selections are available in the US.

RECOMMENDED PRESCRIPTION RETINOIDS TO TREAT WRINKLES, ACNE AND DARK SPOTS

- Aknemycin Plus (contains an antibiotic as well)
- Differin gel or cream
- Isotrex
- Isotrexin (contains an antibiotic as well)
- Retin-A gel, lotion or cream
- Retinova

PRESCRIPTION MEDICATION GELS FOR ACNE OR INFLAMMATION

- Aknemycin Plus (tretinoin and erythromycin)
- Benzamycin (benzoul peroxide and clindamycin)
- Dalacin T (clindamycin)
- Duac (Benzoyl peroxide and Clindamycin)
- Isotrexin (Isotretinoin and erythromycin)
- Stiemycin (erythromycin)
- Topicycline (tetracycline hydrochloride and 4-epitetracycline hydrochloride)
- Zindaclin (erythromycin and zinc)
- Zineryt (erythromycin and zinc)

Baumann's Choice: Ask your dermatologist to select a product right for you. There may be additional products not on this list.

If these treatments are not effective, the final option for acute acne is the prescription medication Accutane. Though highly effective, it can cause liver problems and birth defects, and thus should only be used in the most severe instances. Consult with your physician and be advised by his or her recommendations.

Treating Dark Spots

These prescription products contain hydroquinone, which inhibits the enzymes that produce colour, and thus helps to eliminate dark spots and other pigmented areas. Since hydroquinone is not available in the UK and many Asian countries, the list below contains prescription products available in the United States. Ask your dermatologist for substitutions, available in your country, that can be used for skin lightening in your Stage Two regimen.

RECOMMENDED PRESCRIPTION SKIN LIGHTENERS FOR DARK SPOTS

- Eldoquin Forte
- EpiQuin Micro
- Generic hydroquinones are also available
- Lustra-AF
- Solaquin Forte gel

Baumann's Choice: Ask your dermatologist to recommend similar products available in the UK.

PROCEDURES FOR YOUR SKIN TYPE

In most cases, OSPTs with dark skin get the best results with topical products, while most medical procedures are unnecessary, and sometimes harmful. However, you'll need patience because topicals require time to effect a change.

In general, dark-skin-toned OSPTs should avoid light therapy because it can lead to inflammation and worsening of dark spots. The sole exception is blue light therapy, which kills bacteria and helps with acne. Typically, you would go once to twice per week for six weeks. The cost is approximately £60–£80 per treatment.

On the other hand, if your skin tone is light to medium-light (ranging in skin tones from someone like Nicole Kidman on the light end to someone like Jennifer Lopez at the medium-light end) you have the option of Intense Pulsed Light treatments (IPL) performed by a dermatologist. Lighter-skinned OSPTs are less prone to inflammation than dark-skinned OSPTs and can benefit from IPL and other forms of light therapy to lighten dark spots more rapidly, in addition to blue light treatments for acne. Please see 'Further Help for Oily, Resistant Skin Types' for complete information.

Additional Options

People with darker skin tones, or those who do not want (or cannot afford) IPL, can benefit from chemical peels. Look for ones that contain salicylic acid (BHA) of 20 percent or 30 percent, which removes the top layers of the skin and triggers the cells to divide faster, thereby encouraging brown spots to depart through the natural process of cell renewal. Resorcinol can also effectively treat acne and dark spots in OSPTs. If you have darker skin, make certain that you go to a dermatologist who is skilled at treating people with darker skin, because dark spots can worsen if chemical peels are not done correctly. These peels range from £70 to £130 per peel and you will typically require a series of five to eight sessions.

ONGOING CARE FOR YOUR SKIN

Preventing the breakout–inflammation–brown spot cycle is the best strategy for OSPTs. To do that, follow the Daily Skin Care Regimen I've devised for you, and use my product recommendations. If you'd like, try a few simple procedures as well. Above all, make sure to avoid inflammation, eat the right foods, and de-stress whenever you can. By developing the right habits in youth, you can solve your skin problems. Managing this Skin Type definitely requires some effort, but over time, you'll come to appreciate your skin. In your later years, unlike some other Skin Types, you'll bypass costly antiaging routines and look good throughout life.

CHAPTER SIX

Oily, Sensitive, Non-Pigmented and Wrinkled: OSNW

THE LOBSTER SKIN TYPE

'After half an hour on the beach, I turn into a red lobster. I can't tan to save my life. But I'm not giving up yet . . .'

ABOUT YOUR SKIN

When the late English playwright Noel Coward wrote his famed and devastatingly witty song 'Mad Dogs and Englishmen (Go Out in the Midday Sun)', he undoubtedly had OSNWs in mind. As Coward reveals, the intrepid English with their insistence on sunning at noon, are indeed a nation of OSNWs, as are many people from English, Scottish, Irish, Australian, German and Scandinavian backgrounds. Fair skinned, with little pigment to handle sun exposure, what they lack in melanin, they make up for in dogged determination – they will produce a suntan where none is possible. This Skin Type also suffers from flushing and rosacea, but their wrinkling most commonly results from sun damage.

OSNW CELEBRITY

You could call Robert Redford an overachiever. Having risen to fame as an actor in such films as *Butch Cassidy and the Sundance Kid*, *The Sting*, *The Candidate*, and *All the President's Men*, Redford is also an Oscar-winning director, a longtime environmental activist, and the founder of the Sundance Film Institute. Since 1978, it's promoted the work of young and upcoming film directors, first bringing to popular attention such major talents as Kevin Smith, Quentin Tarantino and Jim Jarmusch.

Redford also owns a restaurant and a ski resort. Perhaps his passion for skiing led to the sun exposure that turned this handsome blond matinee idol into a wrinkled screen elder. The pale reddish skin, blond hair and blue eyes that typify his Irish ancestry reveal Redford as an N, while shiny photos and acne scars indicate that he is very likely an oily, sensitive type. A man's man and a woman's dream, Redford didn't protect his non-pigmented skin through either sun avoidance or sunscreen use, and now he has the wrinkles to show for it. He could be the poster child for sun abuse, but millions still find him handsome anyway, including me.

DON'T TAN, DON'T BURN

Back in the 1950s, there was a popular ad jingle for Coppertone suntan oil. Their slogan was, 'Tan, Don't Burn'. But, guess what, OSNW, they weren't talking about your type. You *always* burn in response to moderate to maximum sun exposure. The many OSNWs I see in my practice come to me with wrinkles, redness, and rosacea resulting from a bad mix of genetic predisposition and harmful behaviour. For you, sun avoidance is an absolute must.

Why?

As Coward accurately points out in his song, centuries of genetic adaptation did not prepare even pigmented types (like the Asians, Indians and Hispanics) for the tropical sun. That's why they wisely stay indoors during the heat of the day. Meanwhile, the foolhardy Brits (and other melanin-deprived OSNWs) are determined to brave it, to their detriment.

With less pigmentation to protect you, the results are disastrous. Although I don't recommend tanning for anyone, when pigmented types tan, at least they have a chance to work *with* the sun, by starting with short sun exposure at times of day when the rays are less harmful (such as before ten AM and after four PM). Then, as their pigment is activated, it provides some protection as they gradually increase exposure.

But most OSNWs lack both the genes to tan and the common sense as to how to go about it. After spending a year at a deskbound job, OSNWs will rush out to the beach, like lemmings to the sea, thinking to make up for the time spent indoors in one big blast. Instead, the pale, unprotected, unpigmented skin of the OSNW burns to a bright red. One or more burns over a lifetime will predispose skin to both non-melanoma skin cancers and the wrinkles that plague this type.

And when these lobsters show up in my office, with bright red necks, redder faces, and an array of other sun damage symptoms, they sheepishly confess, 'I overdid it at the beach.' No kidding!

Yet maddening as it is to see what you do to yourselves, I can't help forgiving and secretly admiring you intrepid OSNWs. Yours was the spirit that created the British Empire. But direct your determination at something other than getting a tan.

Escaping the rainy and cloudy weather, the British compulsion to get some sun is not entirely misguided since the sun *is* mood-enhancing, while depression is more prevalent in cloudier climes, like Alaska. Sunlight is actually a treatment for Seasonal Affective Disorder, in which feelings of depression and listlessness occur in grey, wintry weather when sunlight is scarce. Ultraviolet light helps increase the production of endorphins, the hormones that make you feel good. However, you can get these benefits from the sun even when wearing sunscreen and sun protective clothing.

Hannah and Joshua's Story

With their two-year-old son, Ryan, this attractive young couple took a holiday, and came to experience a real American Thanksgiving with Hannah's twin sister, Rebecca, who was living in Miami. Because it was November and the weather was overcast, they assumed that it would be all right for little Ryan to play out on the deck for forty-five minutes without any sunscreen. The next day they rushed him into my office, and I wished I'd been there to warn them. My heart sank when I saw that adorable little toddler with his cute carrot top and his beet-red burn. Poor baby! Fortunately, I was able to offer temporary relief via aloe vera gel and ibuprofen liquid. I also issued a stern warning to his parents. The sun can burn your skin even on grey, overcast days, so take heed and apply sunscreen no matter what the weather.

Some tan believing that sun is 'good for the skin' or improves acne. Not true. UV radiation was shown to cause changes in the skin's natural oils that led to an *increased* number of blackheads. And studies also report a higher incidence of acne in the summer months.

THE R-WORD, ROSACEA

Another prime reason to make sunscreen use a daily habit is that sun exposure causes breakage in blood vessels that can result in rosacea symptoms, such as flushing and facial redness. This occurs because sun exposure accelerates collagen loss, weakening the supportive structures around the blood vessels. In fact, a growing body of medical evidence indicates that in many instances rosacea is *caused* by sun damage.

OSNW skin is one of the types most prone to rosacea. If you've consulted a dermatologist, you may have received that diagnosis. Research shows that although fourteen million Americans suffer from rosacea, 78 percent of Americans are not aware of the disease – and many who have it do not realise that they do.

What Is Rosacea?

The four common symptoms of rosacea are:

1. Facial redness and flushing
2. Acne with pimples and papules
3. Visible facial blood vessels
4. Enlarged oil glands that cause the nose to redden and thicken

You can have one or more of these symptoms simultaneously, and each symptom requires a different treatment. But having one symptom does not necessarily mean that you will develop the others. If you experience any of these rosacea symptoms, seek help sooner rather than later because receiving treatment can prevent rosacea from developing to its later stages.

The later stages of the disease can and should be avoided. One of the most well-known rosacea sufferers was the American comedian W. C. Fields. The bulbous nose that contributed to his comic appearance is actually a telltale rosacea symptom, one that can be treated, if necessary, but is best prevented. The treatments I'll offer in this chapter will help do that.

Shannon's Story

A successful PA in a large firm, Shannon was a pale blonde, elegant in her understated blue and cream knit suit. After hearing an ad for one of my rosacea research projects, she came in to our clinic at the University of Miami.

Although she was not a candidate for the research project, Shannon's desperation became clear as we discussed her skin situation. At the comparatively young age of forty-two, Shannon had already consulted nine different dermatologists in an effort to master her skin care problems. Despite carefully following their advice, she had failed miserably, and that was something new to her, since she had experienced only success in her professional and personal life.

I was amazed and saddened to see a woman with a high-powered career, dressed impeccably in a St John's suit and Mikimoto pearls, break down in tears when she discussed her skin. 'It's not fair to have both pimples and wrinkles!' she wailed. For years, she lived with constant feelings of self-consciousness and shame about her skin, she confided.

As a teenager, she had acne and had taken several different kinds of antibiotics. Although she had never been treated with Accutane, a common medication for acute acne, she had regularly consulted a dermatologist. As she got older, along with her pimples, she now had symptoms of rosacea, including frequent flushing and broken blood vessels that appeared around her nose and then branched out onto her cheeks and chin. In the past she'd worn foundation to cover it. But now that she had passed her forty-second birthday, the foundation caked in the wrinkles that sprang up around her eyes and between her eyebrows. Shannon began a new campaign against those wrinkles with an arsenal of highly touted antiaging products. But they stung and turned her skin beet red. She felt so desperate that she responded to our ad for the rosacea study.

After hearing her story, I reassured Shannon that her skin issues were typical for her type and I had solutions. First, I put her on an anti-inflammatory, sensitive skin care regimen with antioxidants to prevent inflammation and combat aging. The products I recommended were inexpensive so that she could pay for procedures that would improve her skin's condition and enhance her appearance.

Shannon's rosacea cried out for prescription sulphur medication to calm the redness. In addition, I recommended a nonirritating, nonoily sunscreen specially made for sensitive skin. An Intense Pulsed Light Treatment erased her facial blood vessels and lessened the redness of her flushed cheeks.

Although these procedures were costly, taking into account the time she spent visiting dermatologists, searching for skin care products, and hiding out at home after harmful product choices, Shannon felt she came out ahead financially.

A CLOSE-UP LOOK AT YOUR SKIN

As Shannon experienced, it's stressful to have rosacea. Studies indicate that rosacea sufferers commonly experience low self-esteem. When rosacea acts up, people want to hide. But if you have it, it's better to face facts and get treatment.

Although not every OSNW has rosacea, if you are on the rosacea spectrum with any of the common OSNW symptoms, my treatment protocols will help.

If you, like Shannon, have OSNW skin and rosacea, you may experience any of the following:

- Facial redness and flushing
- Pink patches
- Difficulty tanning, frequent sunburns
- Pimples
- Facial oiliness
- Enlarged pores
- Facial rashes or pink scaling patches, especially around your nose
- Visible red or blue facial blood vessels
- Acne, burning, redness or stinging in response to many skin care products
- Yellow or skin-coloured bumps with a dent in the middle (These enlarged oil glands are called sebaceous hyperplasia.)
- Enlarged nose
- Wrinkles, frown lines, and crow's-feet
- Increased risk of non-melanoma skin cancer (basal cell carcinoma and squamous cell carcinoma)

Most OSNWs experience redness and flushing. 'My face looks red in photos' is a common complaint. You may also notice yellowish bumps on your face with central indentations. These are enlarged oil-producing glands that over time may cause your nose to appear enlarged. Sun exposure worsens rosacea and all the symptoms on the rosacea spectrum.

YOUR SKIN CARE HISTORY

Most OSNWs who come to my office have seen several dermatologists before finding their way to me, often suffering from decades of skin problems. Before the age of thirty, acne is an OSNW's biggest skin issue.

Long considered a teenager's condition that passes with time, many people find it endures. The thirties can be tough because that's when the sebaceous glands are at their largest, making even more oily sebum. Experimenting with products may make matters worse, because sensitive skin reacts to many skin care ingredients.

OSNWs over forty may still suffer from acne or rosacea. Plus, in your thirties and forties (and alas, sometimes even your twenties), wrinkles begin to appear as well. It can seem like the worst of all possible worlds. One positive note is that the oiliness causing acne tends to decrease in women in their forties and fifties due to menopause. (Sorry, men, your oil glands do not slow down until you are in your eighties.)

Hugh and Jean were a Scottish couple in their mid-sixties, who lived in a rural area of Scotland. Now retired, they both enjoyed their outdoor pursuits: for Hugh, it was golf, for Jean, gardening. They had friends who were my patients, and when Hugh and Jean flew into Key West for a visit, their friends insisted they come in for a checkup because Hugh had had a non-melanoma cancer removed from his face the previous year.

Both Hugh and Jean were sandy haired, blue eyed and ruddy faced. I enjoyed Hugh's self-deprecating sense of humour. Jean, a retired school-teacher, had the warm, no-nonsense personality that comes with teaching a couple of generations of kids their ABCs.

Both Hugh's skin and Jean's showed brown, flaky bumps on their arms and foreheads, signs of extreme sun damage. When I took their histories, I discovered why. Though regular sunscreen use would have protected their OSNW skin during Hugh's weekly midday golf game and Jean's vigorous gardening, that wasn't their worst problem. It was their annual vacation trip south. On August 1, like clockwork, the family motored down to the decaying Italian villa that had been in Hugh's family since the 1920s.

Although their OSNW skin lacked the melanin to cope with the Mediterranean sun, they did not realise it, and believing that tanning was healthy, they would expose their skin. They would burn and peel, burn and peel on every vacation. I shuddered to think of it.

Now they were paying the price. In inspecting their skin, I found actinic keratosis (precancerous lesion) on Hugh and a suspicious-looking dark mole on Jean. Fortunately, biopsies revealed neither to be malignant. I treated the precancerous lesion with Aldara, a prescription medication. Still, they would have to be checked regularly, as often as every year.

Their weather-lined faces were clearly the result of all that sun damage. Yet they carried it gracefully and with maturity.

Dr Baumann's Bottom Line: Following your Daily Skin Care Regimens and strict sun avoidance will help prevent your worst skin problems. Don't experiment with antiaging products. Follow my recommendations, find what works for you, and stop wasting money on expensive skin care products. Instead the right procedures will make the biggest difference.

EVERYDAY CARE FOR YOUR SKIN

What skin care products best serve your needs? Your primary concerns are oiliness and facial redness, along with the tendency to develop broken blood vessels on your face. You therefore need nonirritating products that will limit acne and redness. To find them, you may have tried products marketed for 'sensitive skin', but found them irritating or overly oily since many sensitive skin products are better suited for those with dry skin.

Whether you have active rosacea, acne or simply experience facial redness, breakouts, facial stinging or rashes, the regimens described in this section of the chapter will benefit you, and should be used on a daily basis.

All the products I'll recommend act to do one or more of the following:

- Prevent and treat redness
- Prevent and treat pimples
- Prevent and treat wrinkles

In addition, your daily regimen will also help to address your other skin concerns by:

- Helping to prevent non-melanoma skin cancer
- Helping to prevent skin fragility common for OSNW seniors

Anti-inflammatory and antioxidant products can help manage a wide range of typical OSNW symptoms, most of which are caused by inflammation, so I'll show you how to use them in your daily regimen. Please look over the two regimens I provide and determine which one is right for your needs. Next, you can choose the products you'll need from those I recommend in each category later in this chapter.

If after using either or both of these regimens for six weeks to two months, you find you need further help, consult a dermatologist, who can offer prescription cleansers, oral medications, and procedures that may make a huge difference for your Skin Type. If your symptoms are acute, you may wish to schedule an appointment at once, as there is often a waiting list.

DAILY SKIN CARE

STAGE ONE: NONPRESCRIPTION REGIMEN
For flushed skin:

AM	PM
Step 1: Wash with anti-inflammatory cleanser	Step 1: Wash with anti-inflammatory cleanser
Step 2: Apply antiaging serum	Step 2: Apply serum or moisturiser
Step 3: Apply moisturiser (optional)	Step 3: Apply retinol product
Step 4: Apply facial foundation with SPF or a gel sunscreen	

STAGE ONE: NONPRESCRIPTION REGIMEN
For acne:

AM	PM
Step 1: Wash with benzoyl peroxide cleanser	Step 1: Wash with benzoyl peroxide cleanser
Step 2: Apply spot treatment to pimples	Step 2: Apply serum or moisturiser with anti-inflammatory ingredients
Step 3: Apply antiaging serum	Step 3: Apply retinol product
Step 4: Apply moisturiser (optional)	
Step 5: Apply facial foundation with SPF product or a gel sunscreen	

Used morning and evening, a cleanser with anti-inflammatory ingredients will address acne by cutting down on skin surface oil. Those containing salicylic acid are a good option. If you have only slightly oily skin you may choose to apply a moisturiser. If so, choose one with anti-inflammatory ingredients. If you have a higher O/D score (35 or above) and shiny skin, skip this step.

In the evening, use a cleanser to gently remove makeup. Then apply a light nighttime serum or a mask, lotion or gel with anti-inflammatory ingredients.

Cleansing

I do not recommend toners for your type because they can increase flushing. However, if you have a medium S/R score (25–33) and acne is your main problem, you can use scrubs no more than two to three times a week. Make sure to apply gently to avoid provoking inflammation. I am not a big fan of scrubs for your Skin Type, so use them carefully. Do not use scrubs if your S/R score is higher than 33, or if you have redness and rosacea. You can use foaming cleansers, selecting one targeted to your main problem. For example, if you have acne, choose an acne wash, or if you have rosacea, look for cleansers that improve redness, such as RoC Calmance Soothing Cleansing Fluid.

RECOMMENDED CLEANSING PRODUCTS

- £ Eucerin Gentle Cleansing Milk
- £ Neutrogena Clear Pore Wipes
- £ Nivea Sensitive Balance Cleansing Milk
- £ PCA Skin pHaze 31 BPO 5% Cleanser
- ££ Clarins Purifying Cleansing Gel
- ££ Ella Baché Savon Adoucissant
- ££ Jurlique Cleansing Lotion
- ££ Kiehls Blue Herbal Gel Cleanser
- ££ Korres Hamamelis Cleansing Tonic Lotion
- ££ Lancôme Gel Contrôle Purifying Gel Cleanser
- ££ Laura Mercier Foaming One-Step Cleanser
- ££ Peter Thomas Roth Beta Hydroxy Acid 2% Acne Wash
- ££ Rodan & Fields Calm Wash Facial Cleanser
- £££ Darphin Intral Cleansing Milk
- £££ Darphin Purifying Foam Gel

Baumann's Choice: Korres Hamamelis Cleansing Tonic Lotion

RECOMMENDED SCRUBS

- £ Avon Clearskin Facial Cleansing Scrub
- £ Bioré Pore Perfect Pore Unclogging Scrub
- £ Clean & Clear Blackhead Clearing Scrub
- £ Clearasil Blackhead Clearing Scrub
- £ Nivea Facial Scrub for Men
- ££ Anthony Logistics for Men Facial Scrub
- ££ Peter Thomas Roth AHA/BHA Face & Body Polish

Baumann's Choice: Clearasil Blackhead Clearing Scrub is good if you have acne. However, scrubs can worsen acne in some people. If you have redness or rosacea, avoid scrubs.

Acne Control Products

You can use these products when you have active acne. While I don't recommend squeezing pimples, if you can't restrain yourself, please follow the guidelines in 'The Proper Way to Pop' in Chapter Five.

RECOMMENDED ACNE TREATMENT

- £ Neutrogena Oil-Free Acne Wash (Not in the UK but I love it.)
- £ Clearasil Complete Instant Effects Roller-ball Pen
- £ PanOxyl Acne Gel 5% or 10%
- ££ Avon Clearskin Overnight Blemish Treatment
- ££ Brevoxyl Cream
- ££ Jurlique Blemish Cream
- £££ Dermalogica Medicated Clearing Gel
- £££ Erno Laszlo Total Blemish Treatment

Baumann's Choice: PanOxyl Acne Gel 5% with benzoyl peroxide

Moisturisers

Moisturisers are unnecessary for most oily types. However, wrinkles and redness, prime concerns for OSNWs, are often addressed via moisturisers, so I'll make some recommendations while warning you away from products that could worsen your sensitive skin. If your skin is very oily (with an O/D score over 34), look for serums, fluids, or lotions.

Products with anti-inflammatory ingredients can be used both to treat active redness and to calm your skin to prevent flushing and skin sensitivity. Once redness calms, you can prevent wrinkles with the antioxidant moisturisers and serums.

To prevent wrinkles, many OSNWs experiment with antiaging products, but these may contain harsh ingredients, like fruit acids and other active ingredients, that can irritate OSNW skin, causing acne, facial burning or redness.

Instead use moisturisers and serums with antioxidants, which have been shown to prevent wrinkles and other signs of aging. In addition, I recommend that you increase antioxidant foods and even take an anti-oxidant supplement. I'll explain this in greater detail in 'Further Help for Oily, Sensitive Skin'.

Since you will not be using toner, serums (and if desired, certain moisturisers) are an ideal delivery system for OSNW skin because they often contain a higher percentage of the active ingredients which penetrate better to combat wrinkles. But beware of ingredients that cause inflammation. The trick is to combine the right cocktail of ingredients, including those strong enough to work tempered by others that soothe irritation.

Powerful and costly antioxidants, like green tea, are more concentrated in serums and also stay on your skin longer than when used in cleansers, which rinse off. Delivered via a dropper-style bottle, serums are thick in texture, so that a little goes a long way. Use only a few drops and spread over your face. When you get to Stage Two and incorporate prescription antiaging products, you will use the serum as a delivery system. This is a highly effective combination for wrinkled skin, much more so than many anti-wrinkle creams, which are often too oily and not effective to begin with.

Looking ahead, some moisturisers currently being developed will contain higher amounts of active ingredients; however, these may be pricey. While antioxidants help prevent wrinkles, those of you over thirty may choose retinol and prescription retinoids to help get rid of wrinkles that you already have.

RECOMMENDED ANTI-INFLAMMATION MOISTURISERS

£ Olay Regenerist Rehydrating Lotion SPF 15
££ Avène Eau Thermale Skin Recovery Cream

££ Clinique CX Soothing Moisturiser
££ La Roche-Posay Rosaliac Anti-Redness Moisturiser
££ Paula's Choice Skin Relief Treatment
£££ Dermalogica Barrier Repair Moisturiser
£££ Prescriptives Redness Relief Gel
£££ Ren Calendula Omega 3/7 Hydra-Calm Moisturiser (not for acne)

Baumann's Choice: La Roche-Posay Rosaliac Anti-Redness Moisturiser is my favourite.

RECOMMENDED SERUMS AND MOISTURISERS

£ Olay Regenerist Daily Regenerating Serum
£ Revlon Anti-Wrinkle Day Lotion
££ Aesop Oil Free Facial Hydrating Serum
££ Bobbi Brown Shine Control Face Gel with Seaweed Extract and Green Tea
££ Caudalie Face Lifting Serum with Grapevine Resveratrol
££ Clarins Skin Beauty Repair Concentrate
££ Elizabeth Arden Ceramide Advanced Time Capsules
££ Garnier Shine Control Moisturiser
££ Laura Mercier Multi Vitamin Serum
££ MD Skincare Antioxidant Firming Face Serum
££ Tolerance Extreme Crème by Avène
£££ Decléor Contour Firming Serum
£££ Jurlique Herbal Recovery Gel
£££ SkinCeuticals Serum 10

Baumann's Choice: Olay Regenerist Daily Regenerating Serum

RECOMMENDED WRINKLE TREATMENT PRODUCTS

£ Avon Anew Advanced All-In-One Max SPF 15
£ Roc Retin Ox Correxion Antiwrinkle Serum – soft
££ Philosophy Help Me
££ Sothy's Retinol 15
££ Topix Replenix Retinol Smoothing Serum
£££ Clarins Renew Plus Night Lotion
£££ Estée Lauder Diminish Anti-Wrinkle Retinal Treatment

£££ Jan Marini Factor A Plus Lotion
£££ Lancôme Resurface
£££ Prescriptives Skin Renewal Cream

Baumann's Choice: All products except the Avon product contain retinol. I prefer Philosophy Help Me and Topix Replenix Retinol Smoothing Serum because they are packaged in small-mouthed aluminium tubes that minimise air exposure.

Eye Creams

Eye creams are not always necessary. I personally choose to use a regular facial moisturiser around my eyes. However, if you prefer a separate eye cream you can look for these products and use them before your moisturiser.

RECOMMENDED EYE CREAMS

£ Derma E Pycnogenol Eye Gel with Green Tea Extract
£ Neutrogena Visibly Young Eye Cream
£ Nivea AntiWrinkle Q 10 plus eye cream
£ Olay Regenerist Eye Lifting Serum
££ Clarins Eye Contour Balm
££ Dermalogica Intensive Eye Repair
££ Jo Malone Green Tea and Honey Eye Cream
££ Laura Mercier Eyedration
££ Osmotics Antioxidant Eye Therapy
££ Philosophy Hope in a Tube for Eyes and Lips
££ SkinCeuticals Eye Balm
£££ Darphin Soothing Eye Mask
£££ Du Wop Igels (These are actually masks)

Baumann's Choice: Olay Regenerist Eye Lifting Serum because it contains niacinamide which helps soothe inflammation and prevent wrinkles.

Masks

Use masks when you're flared with acne or redness, or otherwise about once or twice a week.

RECOMMENDED MASKS

£ Montagne Jeunesse Cucumber Peel-Off Masque
£ Mudd Mask
£ Nivea Visage Active Purifying Mask
£ Paula's Choice Skin Balancing Carbon Mask
££ Aesop Chamomile Concentrate Anti-Blemish Masque
££ Dermalogica Skin Refining Mask
££ Kiehl's Soothing Gel Masque
££ Origins Out of Trouble Mask
££ Peter Thomas Roth Therapeutic Sulphur Masque Acne Treatment
£££ Laura Mercier Hydra Soothing Gel Mask
£££ Pevonia RS2 Rosacea Mask

Baumann's Choice: Peter Thomas Roth Therapeutic Sulphur Masque because the sulphur helps decrease redness.

SHOPPING FOR SKIN CARE

You can widen your choice of products by reading labels to determine product ingredients, so that you can select those that contain beneficial ingredients for you, while avoiding ones that may cause irritation, inflammation or oiliness. If you find products that you like that are not on my lists, please go to www.DrBaumann.co.uk and share your finds with other OSNWs.

SKIN CARE INGREDIENTS TO LOOK FOR

Antioxidants to prevent wrinkles:

- Basil
- Caffeine
- Camilla sinensis (green tea, white tea)
- Coenzyme Q_{10} (ubiquinone)
- Feverfew
- Genistein
- Ginger
- Ginseng
- Grape seed extract
- Idebenone
- Lutein
- Lycopene
- Pomegranate
- Pycnogenol (a pine bark extract)
- Silymarin
- Yucca

To decrease inflammation:

- Aloe vera
- Basil
- Boswellia serrata
- Arctium lappa (burdock root)
- Chamomile
- Dexpanthenol (also known as provitamin B$_5$)
- Epilobium angustfolium (willow herb)
- Feverfew
- Ginger
- Hamamelis
- Licochalone
- Mallow
- Niacinamide
- Red algae
- Salicylic acid (beta hydroxy acid or BHA)
- Sulphacetamide
- Sulphur
- Tea tree oil
- Zinc

To improve acne:

- Benzoyl peroxide (but see below)
- Retinol
- Salicylic acid (beta hydroxy acid or BHA)
- Tea tree oil

COMMON BEAUTY PRODUCT NO-NO'S

- Acetone
- Alcohol
- Benzoyl peroxide (see below)

A No-No for OSNWs: Benzoyl Peroxide

Benzoyl peroxide (BP) is one of the most commonly used topical preparations for acne. It helps fight bacteria and moderates oiliness. Although it
works, it may cause burning, stinging and redness in sensitive OSNW skin.
However, not all OSNWs will experience this problem, and many individuals who suffer from acne will benefit from its use. People with lower S/R
scores (from 30 to 34) may be able to use benzoyl peroxide. Also it may be
easier to tolerate a product that contains a lower concentration of BP (2.5
percent or less). Combining a benzoyl peroxide product with an anti-
inflammatory product, such as Paula's Choice Skin Relief Treatment, may
help you use benzoyl peroxide. Ask your pharmacist for help choosing a
benzoyl peroxide product.

SKIN CARE INGREDIENTS TO AVOID

Due to stinging and itching from skin care products:

- Acetic acid
- Balsam of Peru
- Benzoic acid
- Cinnamic acid
- Lactic acid
- Menthol
- Parabens
- Quaternium-15

To minimise pimples or blackheads:

- Butyl stearate
- Chemical additives such as decyl oleate, isocetyl stearate, isopropyl myristate, isostearyl neopentanoate, isopropyl isostearate, isopropyl palmitate, myristyl myristate, myristyl propionate, octyl palmitate, octyl stearate
- and propylene glycol-2 (PPG-2)
- Cinnamon oil
- Cocoa butter
- Cocos nucifera (coconut oil)
- Lanolin
- Peppermint oil

To minimise skin redness:

- Alpha hydroxy acids (lactic acid, glycolic acid)
- Alpha lipoic acid
- Benzoyl peroxide (for some people)
- Vitamin C

Sun Protection for Your Skin

Tanning is not for you. But so many forces in our society drive women to want to look like models, actresses or people they see on television. I believe in being yourself, and using the best of skin care to enhance who you are.

Kristen's Story

Kristen was nineteen years old, a beautiful girl, with fine facial features she'd inherited from her Norwegian-American mother. She'd also inherited pale blond hair, light blue eyes and flushed red skin from her Scandinavian ancestry. But no longer living in the land of the midnight sun that her forebears inhabited, Kristen was (like me) a Texas native, so from an early age, her fine Nordic skin was subjected to the harsh southern sun.

To make matters worse, Kristen was a cheerleader at her university, and, as she told me in her charming accent, 'Texas cheerleaders just have to be tay-an.' Believe me, I know all about it.

It turned out that Kristen and her cheerleading pals were emulating certain role models they saw on television, namely the bathing beauties on the hit show *Baywatch*. Darkly tanned in their bikini uniforms, the men and women of *Baywatch* set a trend, and Kristen followed along in its wake.

But her skin wasn't cooperating. When she tried to tan, over and over and over, her skin burned and then peeled; it was like a bucking bronco trying to throw its rider. If her skin could speak, it would have said, 'Don't tan me.'

But it couldn't, so I had to speak for it. 'Excess sun exposure is not good for anyone, but it's worst for pale-skinned OSNWs like you,' I told her. Kristen didn't want to believe me, but her very low N score of 14 told the story: OSNW.

'That means I can't safely tan. It's impossible?' she wondered.

'That's right, stay off the beach, and wear sunscreen every day of your life,' I advised her. I let Kristen in on a little secret I'd learned as well. Those gorgeous tans you see coming and going on that show don't come from hours on the beach, they come from a bottle. The *Baywatch* babes used self-tanners. They saved their skins, while encouraging millions of Americans to sacrifice their skin future to looking good today.

Kristen was first amazed, then angered, and finally motivated to follow my plan. But part of the problem, she admitted, was that many sunscreens irritated her skin, causing itching, stinging and burning. I pointed her towards an oil-free product ideal for sensitive skin and ended her tanning days, which were really just burning days, once and for all.

Like Kristen, sunscreen is an absolute must for you. You need to wear it at all times except at night. Use an SPF of 30 daily, and when outside, or in a sunny climate, use an SPF of 45–60. To get the most benefit from sunscreens apply them after cleansing to reduce surface skin oiliness. Lotion or gel sunscreens are better choices for you than cream sunscreens, because creams will make your skin look oilier. Powders that contain sunscreen are also a great option.

RECOMMENDED SUN PROTECTION PRODUCTS

£ Jack Black Oil-Free Sun Guard, SPF 20
£ L'Oréal Air Wear Powder Foundation SPF 17
£ Neutrogena Visibly Young Day Cream SPF 20
££ Dermalogica Waterproof Solar Spray SPF 25
££ Elizabeth Arden First Defence Anti-Oxidant Lotion SPF 15
££ Garnier Ambre Solaire Sheer Protect Shine Free SPF 30
££ Kiehls Ultra Protection Water-Based Sunscreen SPF 25
££ Origins Sunshine State SPF 20 Sunscreen
£££ Natura Bisse C+C Vitamin Fluid SPF 10
£££ Prada Hydrating Gel Tint SPF 15

Baumann's Choice: Neutrogena Visibly Young Day Cream SPF 20 because it contains copper peptide which may improve wrinkles. (10% of my patients do not like the smell, but others love it.)

How to Apply Sunscreen

Smooth a hands portion of product the size of a 10p coin over the entire face, neck, hands and chest every morning. If you are in the sun for longer than one hour, reapply sunscreen every hour.

SUNSCREEN INGREDIENT TO AVOID

If skin burns, itches or turns red
in response to sunscreen avoid:

- Avobenzone
- Benzophenone
- Octyl methoxycinnamate

Your Makeup

Since talc helps control oil, pressed powder, powdered eyeshadow and blusher will absorb oil and last longer. According to the National Rosacea Foundation, mineral makeup can help people with rosacea since it's nonirritating and naturally protective to the skin. Although some companies claim that their makeup offers sun protection as well, I recommend applying mineral makeup over your sunscreen to assure that you have the right degree of sun protection.

RECOMMENDED MAKEUP FOUNDATION

£ Avon Clear Finish Great Complexion Foundation
£ Maybelline Shine Free Oil Control Makeup
£ Revlon Skin Perfecting Make Up
£ Rimmel Stay Matte Compact Powder Foundation
££ Boots No7 Uplifting Foundation SPF 15
££ Bloom Compact Foundation
££ Dermablend Acne Results Foundation
££ Laura Mercier Oil Free Foundation
££ Mirenesse Matte Liquid Silk Foundation SPF 15
££ Nutrimetics Perfect Matte Oil Free Foundation
££ Philosophy The Supernatural Airbrushed Canvas Powder Foundation
£££ Nars Oil Free Foundation
£££ Prescriptives Traceless Skin Responsive Tint

Baumann's Choice: Philosophy The Supernatural Airbrushed Canvas Powder Foundation has an SPF of 15 and absorbs oil well.

RECOMMENDED POWDER

£ Avon Clear Finish Great Complexion Pressed Powder
£ Maybelline Shine Free Oil Control Pressed Powder
£ Rimmel Stay Matte Pressed Powder
££ Bloom Loose Powder
££ Garden Botanika Natural Finish Loose Powder
££ Laura Mercier Translucent Pressed Setting
££ Molton Brown Under Control Compact Loose Powder
££ Stila Illuminating Powder Compact

Baumann's Choice: Garden Botanika Natural Finish Loose Powder, because it has antioxidants and aloe. Increase your sun protection by dusting an SPF-containing powder over your sunscreen. This will help prevent shine from the sunscreen and give you some added protection.

RECOMMENDED FACIAL POWDER
WITH SUNSCREEN

£ l'Oréal Idéal Balance Pressed Powder for Combination Skin with
SPF 10 Sunscreen

£ Maybelline Pure Stay Powder SPF 15

££ Colorescience Foundation Powder

££ Estée Lauder Amber Bronze Cool Bronze Loose Powder SPF 8

££ Jane Iredale's Amazing Base Loose Minerals SPF 20

£££ U2B+ Sheer Finish Pact SPF 24

Baumann's Choice: They are all good. Jane Iredale's is available on-line at
www.Baumannstore.co.uk or from your dermatologist.

SKIN CARE INGREDIENTS TO AVOID

Foundation:

• Oil

Powder:

• Avoid pressed powders with
isopropyl myristate. Look for oil-
control products instead.

Blusher:

• Avoid D & C red dyes (xanthenes,
monoazoanilines, fluorans and
indigoids).
• Look for the natural red pigment
carmine instead.

CONSULTING A DERMATOLOGIST

PRESCRIPTION SKIN CARE STRATEGIES

As an OSNW, you may suffer from acne, flushing, redness and wrinkles, as
well as rosacea. That's why I've provided three Stage Two regimens that

incorporate prescription medications to treat each of your three main problems. Please consult your doctor and then select and follow for at least two months the regimen that addresses your main problem. You may need to follow it indefinitely. But make sure that you do not move up to address wrinkles until after you've cleared flushing, redness and rosacea using the regimens I recommend.

DAILY SKIN CARE

STAGE TWO: PRESCRIPTION REGIMEN

For acne:

AM	PM
Step 1: Wash with a prescription cleanser	Step 1: Wash with a prescription cleanser
Step 2: Apply an antibiotic gel	Step 2: Apply an antibiotic gel
Step 3: Apply a moisturiser (optional)	Step 3: Apply an anti-inflammatory moisturiser
Step 4: Apply an SPF-containing facial foundation or powder with anti-inflammatory ingredients, such as salicylic acid	Step 4: Apply a retinoid such as Isotrex

In the morning, wash with your prescribed cleanser and apply an antibiotic gel. If you have only slightly oily skin, you may choose to apply a moisturiser. If so, choose one with anti-inflammatory ingredients. Use makeup powder and foundation formulated to treat inflammation and protect from sun exposure.

In the evening, cleanse as in the morning, apply the antibiotic gel, and then the moisturiser. Wait a few moments to allow absorption of beneficial ingredients before applying retinoid. (Another option is Isotrexin, a product that combines both an antibiotic and a retinoid; if you use it, you can skip Step 2.)

In addition, if you wish to use a prescription mask when acne or redness is a concern, you can use it once or twice a week with any of the Stage Two regimens.

RECOMMENDED PRESCRIPTION CLEANSERS

Benoxyl-4 Creamy Wash
Rosanil Cleanser
Rosula Cleanser
Triaz Cleanser
Zoderm Cleanser

Baumann's Choice: Ask for cleansers containing benzoyl peroxide, sulphacetamide, sulphur, and zinc. The above-mentioned products are available in the US but your dermatologist can make recommendations of similar products for you.

RECOMMENDED ANTIBIOTIC GELS FOR ACNE

Aknemycin Plus (tretinoin and erythromycin)
Benzamycin (benzoyl peroxide and clindamycin)
Dalacin T (clindamycin)
Duac (Benzoyl peroxide and Clindamycin)
Isotrexin (Isotretinoin and erythromycin)
Stiemycin (erythromycin)
Topicycline (tetracycline hydrochloride and 4-epitetracycline hydrochloride)
Zindaclin (erythromycin and zinc)
Zineryt (erythromycin and zinc)

Baumann's Choice: Gel formulations work best for oily skin.

Treating Rosacea and Redness

OSNWs can find themselves at any point along the spectrum that leads to rosacea, so whether you have simple flushing or active rosacea, the prescription medications and procedures I'll recommend here will be very helpful. If you have any rosacea symptoms, I advise you to first use my anti-inflammatory regimens, and graduate to prescription meds and procedures if you need more help in addressing the problem.

STAGE TWO: PRESCRIPTION REGIMEN

For flushed skin, rosacea and redness:

AM	PM
Step 1: Wash with prescription cleanser	Step 1: Wash with prescription cleanser
Step 2: Apply a prescription gel to reduce redness	Step 2: Apply the same prescription gel used in the morning
Step 3: Apply an SPF-containing foundation or powder with anti-inflammatory ingredients	Step 3: Apply anti-inflammatory moisturiser

In the morning, wash with prescription cleanser, selecting from the product list earlier in this section of the chapter. Next, apply an antibiotic gel. If you have only slightly oily skin you may choose to apply a moisturiser. If so, choose one with anti-inflammatory ingredients. Use sunscreen, makeup powder and/or foundation to treat inflammation and protect from sun exposure, assuring a minimum SPF of 15.

In the evening, cleanse as in the morning, and apply the same prescription medication to soothe redness. Wait a few moments to allow absorption of beneficial ingredients before applying a moisturiser.

In addition, if you wish to use a prescription mask for redness, you can use it once or twice a week.

RECOMMENDED PRESCRIPTION MEDICATIONS FOR FACIAL REDNESS

- Avar gel (sodium sulphacetamide 10 percent and sulphur 5 percent)
- Klaron lotion (sodium sulphacetamide 10 percent)
- MetroGel (metronidazole 0.75 percent) is available in the UK
- Noritate emollient cream (metronidazole 1 percent)
- Plexion gel (sodium sulphacetamide 10 percent and sulphur 5 percent)
- Rosac Cream with Sunscreens (sodium sulphacetamide 10% and sulphur 5 percent)
- Rosanil Cleanser (sodium sulphacetamide 10 percent and sulphur 5 percent)
- Rosasol Cream (metronidazole 1 percent with SPF)
- Rosula Aqueous Gel (sodium sulphacetamide 10 percent and sulphur 5 percent)
- Sulfacet-R (sodium sulphacetamide 10 percent and sulphur 5 percent)

Baumann's Choice: Unless noted otherwise, these brands are available in the United States. Please ask your dermatologist to prescribe similar products available in your country.

Medications to Avoid

Topical steroid creams may temporarily improve facial flushing. However, long-term use can worsen facial redness, rosacea and acne because a rebound effect occurs. Steroids temporarily shrink the blood vessels, making the skin less red, but then the vessels rebound and dilate again. Eventually your blood vessels will dilate whenever you are not applying the steroid, creating a dependency on the medication. Steroids can result in visible blood vessels on the face in addition to worsening acne and redness.

Other medications can also worsen facial redness, so look out for niacin, minoxidil, nifedipine, amiodarone, cyclosporine, nitroglycerin and sildenafil. In addition, if you are on medications to address any other kind of health issue, please ask your physician about your medications to determine if any of them could be worsening facial redness.

Rosacea Treatment: A Varied Treatment Approach

Doctors believe that certain symptoms can lead to others. For example, frequent facial flushing can lead to broken blood vessels. Typically people who come for treatment complain that the broken blood vessels 'make me look like an alcoholic'. But don't worry: they can be eliminated permanently. First, try the prescription medications I recommend, as they can help prevent the problem and, in many cases, address it as well. If you find after eight to twelve weeks that they are not effective, you can ask your dermatologist about using advanced light technology (discussed in the next section). I've treated literally thousands of people, both men and women, for this problem, and usually one or the other treatment helps.

Medications for Wrinkles

As you get your redness, flushing or other rosacea symptoms under control, you can begin to prevent and treat wrinkles with prescription products. This Stage Two regimen adds retinoids to your basic daily regimen.

Don't step up to this particular regimen until after your flushing, redness and rosacea symptoms have cleared. Until then, retinoids will be too irritating to your skin. However, if acne is your main problem, you can get started with retinoids at once, since retinoids help acne as well as prevent wrinkles. In the 1970s many people first began to use Retin-A for acne. Years later, Dr Albert Kligman and Dr Jim Leyden of the University of Pennsylvania noticed that those on Retin-A for acne had fewer wrinkles. Voilà, a new wrinkle treatment was born.

STAGE TWO: PRESCRIPTION TREATMENT

To prevent wrinkles:

AM	PM
Step 1: Wash with prescription cleanser	Step 1: Wash with prescription cleanser
Step 2: Apply an antibiotic gel	Step 2: Apply an antibiotic gel
Step 3: Apply moisturiser (optional)	Step 3: Mix two drops of a serum containing antioxidant ingredients with a pea-size dollop of Differin cream
Step 4: Apply an SPF-containing facial foundation or powder with anti-inflammatory ingredients	Step 4: Apply moisturiser with antioxidant ingredients (optional)

In the morning, wash with a prescription cleanser and apply antibiotic gel. If desired, apply a moisturiser with antioxidants or anti-inflammatory ingredients. Use sunscreen, makeup powder and/or foundation to treat inflammation and protect from sun exposure assuring a minimum SPF of 15.

In the evening, cleanse as in the morning, and apply antibiotic gel. Mix two drops of serum with retinoid and apply to face, avoiding contact with the eye area. If you wish to moisturize, choose a nonprescription moisturiser with antioxidants and anti-inflammatory ingredients.

Another optional step is to use a prescription mask once or twice a week to calm acne or redness.

RECOMMENDED PRESCRIPTION
MEDICATIONS FOR WRINKLES

- Aknemycin Plus (contains an antibiotic as well)
- Differin gel or cream
- Isotrex
- Isotrexin (contains an antibiotic as well)
- Retin-A gel, lotion or cream
- Retinova

Baumann's Choice: Differin gel (adapalene) is my favourite for OSNWs' sensitive skin because it seems to be less irritating than other retinoids. Avage and Tazorac are only available in the US. Your dermatologist can recommend comparable brands.

PROCEDURES FOR YOUR SKIN

As an OSNW, you have three main problems – facial redness, overactive oil glands and wrinkles – and my procedure recommendations will help treat all three. In your type, after your blood vessels dilate, they do not constrict properly as they do in other types.

Intense Pulsed Light Treatments (IPL) may help decrease wrinkles long-term by stimulating fibroblasts, the skin cells in the dermis that make collagen. Short-term, IPL causes slight swelling that puffs out your fine wrinkles and smoothes your skin's texture. Although future research will evaluate whether this treatment has any long-term antiwrinkling effect, its benefits for the treatment of facial flushing and visible blood vessels are well established.

However, please note that the rosacea and aging process will most likely continue despite these treatments, necessitating future treatments and current prevention strategies. Although capable of thwarting the progression of aging and rosacea, the procedures I recommend will not end it permanently.

IPL and Vascular Lasers

A highly effective treatment for flushing, redness, visible blood vessels and other symptoms on the rosacea spectrum combines Intense Pulsed Light (IPL) with various vascular lasers. They work synergistically to reduce blood vessels and facial flushing symptomatic of rosacea. For more information about these treatments, please consult 'Further Help for Oily, Sensitive Skin'.

Treating Advanced Rosacea

Most of the recommended procedures also work for dilated blood vessels. They cost between £75 and £200 per session. Although it may require between two to five treatments for the vessels to disappear, once vessels disappear, they are usually gone permanently. An annual maintenance treatment can treat any new ones that appear.

There are several different options for treating the enlarged nose that may occur with more advanced rosacea, including surgery, dermabrasion and CO_2 laser. All these procedures remove enlarged oil glands on the nose. Although each procedure is done by a different instrument, the action performed is virtually the same. The doctor removes the top and middle layers of the skin. Naturally, this can be uncomfortable, and the total downtime is about ten days. The wound remains bandaged for four days, while ten days after surgery, the skin will be healed. The nose will remain pink for six months, and it can be covered with makeup. This is the last stage of rosacea, and frankly, I don't see it much. Taking antibiotics can prevent it.

Other Treatment Options

For more advanced options to remove wrinkles, you can consider cosmetic procedures, such as the use of Botox, Reloxin, and dermal fillers. However, make sure that you have substantially reduced your rosacea and flushing first. As a precaution, be aware that you will be more likely than other types to experience redness due to the rubbing and the use of ice and anaesthetic creams that occurs during the procedures. However, the redness usually resolves in about twenty minutes. For more information about these treatments, please consult 'Further Help for Oily, Sensitive Skin'.

ONGOING CARE FOR YOUR SKIN

Coming in from the midday sun (or indeed, any sun) is absolutely critical for your sensitive, redness-prone skin. Wear sunscreen regularly, and adhere to your daily regimen to address your skin care problems. Anti-inflammatory and antioxidant foods and ingredients in skin care products can help tremendously. Don't experiment with antiaging products. The right procedures (Botox, dermal fillers, and Intense Pulsed Light) will help resolve your type's most persistent issues.

CHAPTER SEVEN

Oily, Sensitive, Non-Pigmented and Tight: OSNT

THE FLUSHED SKIN TYPE

'I'm in my thirties, but I still get adolescent acne and blush bright red like a little kid! It's so-o-o embarrassing. Hello! I'm a grown-up! When will my skin mature?'

ABOUT YOUR SKIN

As an OSNT, your biggest problem is facial flushing, which never fails to give you away in social situations. No one wants the world to know their secrets, but OSNTs are walking lie-detector tests, as their face reveals everything they feel.

Tense at the meeting? It shows on your face. Attracted to that new acquaintance? It's hard to hide. If you need a cool head or an impassive look, you'd better forget about it. Your face will always give you away, and you just have to learn to deal with it by relaxing, doing things you find calming, and avoiding ingredients, products, and (when possible) life situations that are inflammatory. Don't worry, it's not that you're thin-skinned. You may suffer from rosacea, a dermatological condition, common among OSNTs, that affects fourteen million Americans and millions of others.

OSNT CELEBRITY

Wearing her feelings on her sleeve is actress Renee Zellweger's forte. In *Jerry Maguire* when she told Tom Cruise, 'You had me at hello,' her candour, vulnerability, and sensitivity won Cruise's heart – and the audience's. She continues to win us over through displaying those same traits, most recently as Bridget Jones, a screen character with whom many women identify. Key to Zellweger's skill at revealing feeling is the actress's flawless, near transparent skin. She is able to take the responsiveness of OSNT skin and use it in her art.

With her pale, slightly pink complexion, Zellweger has the colouring common to rosacea sufferers and so-called flushers, people who flush bright red in response to various stimuli. She appears to blush easily and may perhaps have a mild tendency to rosacea, which is prevalent in the countries of her ancestors, Norway and Switzerland. Since we're both from Texas, I wonder if Tex-Mex food (one of my favourites) causes her to flush?

Her face appears shiny in photos, hinting that she is indeed an oily type, and although she has the delicate, unpigmented, Caucasian skin most prone to wrinkling, her skin is wrinkle free. I have no doubt that Zellweger carefully protects her skin from sun exposure. Although she was willing to gain weight to portray the pleasantly plump, Bridget Jones in *Bridget Jones' Diary* and *Bridget Jones: The Edge of Reason*, Zellweger has not succumbed to the pressure to tan. I've never seen a photo of her tanned, and the white shoulders and legs she bares in fabulous designer gowns on the red carpet reveal the glamour of flawless white skin.

She is one of a new breed of actresses (women like Cate Blanchett, Uma Thurman, Nicole Kidman and Julianne Moore) who'd rather go pale than risk the premature wrinkling and skin cancers that result from sun exposure. And I say, Bravo! Their delicate fair skin is wrinkle prone by genetics, but good habits (such as sun and cigarette avoidance) should keep their beauty shining for decades to come.

THE R-WORD

OSNT skin is a perfect setup for rosacea, pronounced rose-AY-sha. Despite the scientific terminology, rosacea is really a collection of symptoms that you may know well. It's vital to recognise and treat it early to slow the disease process. By identifying which symptoms trouble you, you can manage them or, in some cases, eliminate them and thereby prevent later-stage symptoms.

How does flushing occur? First, blood vessels dilate more in sensitive types due to heightened sensitivity to neurotransmitters (similar to hormones). Second, like Bill Clinton, many OSNTs have light skin, which reveals the redness of dilated blood vessels more readily than dark skin. Over time, blood vessels lose their ability to contract back to their normal size, so they remain dilated. These visible red or blue blood vessels look like spider veins. Many people of Irish and Scottish descent have the OSNT type, as do members of my own family. To find out if you have rosacea, please consult Chapter Six, 'The R-Word, Rosacea'.

Doctors believe that certain symptoms can lead to others. For example, frequent facial flushing can lead to broken blood vessels, in turn leading sufferers to complain that that they 'make me look like an alcoholic'. But don't worry; they can be eliminated permanently using Intense Pulsed Light technology. I've treated literally thousands of people, both men and women, for this problem.

If you are an OSNT with darker-toned skin who experiences the same burning and stinging but without the visible flushing and dilated blood vessels, you'll find my daily regimens, product recommendations, and lifestyle guidelines helpful. The procedures for treating more intensive rosacea symptoms are not necessary.

If you're Asian and your test results indicated that you are an OSNT, you should double-check your answers because a special trait common to Asians could produce misleading scores. Many Asians lack an enzyme that processes alcohol, causing flushing when they drink. So if you're Asian and you flush only when you drink, you're probably not a true OSNT. Most Asians fall into the pigmented category, and worry more about dark spots than wrinkles.

Isabella's Story

A lively and attractive blue-eyed blonde, Isabella was a quick-witted woman who loved to play poker. Six months prior to the World Series of Poker in Las Vegas, she came to see me, worried that if she had a good hand, her face would flush red. With that dead giveaway, her competitors would know what Isabella was up to. To win, she needed to have a classic poker face.

Despite much research, there's no permanent cure for facial flushing, but I offered practical suggestions to minimise it. First, I recommended a makeup brand appropriate for sensitive skin to conceal the redness. Foundations and powders with yellow undertones hide redness better than pink ones. 'Skip the blusher,' I also told Isabella.

For more permanent help, relaxation techniques, anti-inflammatory topical agents, and nutritional approaches each played a part in decreasing stress and inflammation. Isabella's husband, Alfredo, a charming, and mild-mannered Argentinian attorney, was delighted that she was finally making an effort to relax. 'He thinks I need to calm down, I don't know why!' she confided. I advised Isabella to bypass the salsa, a favourite condiment she'd learned to make from her mother-in-law.. She also agreed to avoid vessel-dilating alcohol, even the great wines of Argentina.

In addition, to decrease redness and oil, I gave her an anti-inflammatory skin care regimen that she used every day. Isabella was intent on going the course to control this problem, so I offered an advanced procedure, Intense Pulsed Light (IPL) treatment, which is highly effective in zapping hyper-active blood vessels.

After following my skin care regimen, dietary changes, and going for six light treatments, Isabella's blushing lessened. Still when she played poker, she wore a yellow-based foundation – just to be sure. After she returned from Las Vegas, she called me in triumph. She had made it to one of the final tables in the tournament and was set up to compete internationally.

If, like Isabella, you don't want an opponent to guess your moves, wear a thick layer of foundation or else use a medication to control facial flushing. Make sure to follow my recommendations for products designed for sensitive skin, to avoid causing further irritation, stinging and redness. As for blushing, some men find it charming, so with courage, you can make your flaw your asset.

With an S/R score of 34 or higher, you may experience one (or more) inflammatory skin problems: rosacea, acne, skin allergies, and burning in response to some skin care ingredients. Whatever the cause, my recommendations will help you.

If you have severe acne, excess hair on your face and irregular menstrual periods, it could also indicate an underlying medical condition known as polycystic ovarian syndrome. If you've had trouble treating acne and suffer from these other symptoms, please consult a gynaecologist.

A CLOSE-UP LOOK AT YOUR SKIN

With OSNT skin, you may experience any of the following:

- Facial redness and flushing
- Pimples
- Facial oiliness
- Pink patches
- Yellow or skin-coloured bumps with a dent in the middle. (These enlarged oil glands are called sebaceous hyperplasia.)

- Acne, burning, redness or stinging in response to many skin care products
- Facial rashes or pink scaling patches, especially around your nose
- Difficulty tanning, frequent sunburns
- Visible red or blue facial blood vessels

Although rosacea and rosacea-like symptoms can be uncomfortable and embarrassing, they occur within an overall pattern of skin oiliness and sensitivity that you can treat and prevent. Also, facial redness is not always due to rosacea.

Twenty-two-year-old Bonnie, a DJ of Norwegian ancestry, had pale blonde hair, pale skin, and large pale, blue eyes. Although she was very nearsighted, she hated to wear glasses. 'They make me look like a geek!' Instead, at her first appointment she wore purple contact lenses, silver stiletto heels, and metallic blue nail polish. Definitely funky. Her complaint? The skin around her eyes was red and inflamed.

A year earlier, friends suggested that her facial redness was due to rosacea, so Bonnie tried to address it. She quit using her usual skin care line, switching to one for sensitive skin. But it didn't help. Then she consulted a doctor and tried rosacea medication, to no effect. She changed her diet and cut out alcohol. No change. She began cleansing with Cetaphil, designed for sensitive skin, but it made no difference. Puzzled, Bonnie consulted a second dermatologist, who performed patch tests to determine if allergies were the cause. But they were not.

At last, she came to see me. I decided to retest Bonnie for allergies, but she was not allergic to any common allergens. Looking further, I tested her for rarer allergic triggers. Sure enough, she *was* allergic – to an ingredient in her blue nail polish, which caused irritation whenever her hands came into contact with her eye area. This occurred every day when Bonnie applied makeup or put in her contact lenses. No wonder her eye area was red and inflamed! When I advised Bonnie to stop using that brand of nail polish, she moaned, 'But I feel naked without it.' Fortunately, she decided to take my advice, and within a month her problem resolved. I'd recommended a brand of hypoallergenic nail polish, but its colour choices were 'too junior prom for me', Bonnie told me. Nevertheless, it's a good option for people who are sensitive to the chemicals in nail polish, unless, like Bonnie, it's metallic blue or nothing.

It's not uncommon for sensitive types to react to harsh chemicals like those found in nail polish. Some people are also allergic to nickel in the little ball, which helps mix the polish when you shake the bottle. The new euro coin also has a high nickel content, and when people with nickel allergies handle these coins and then touch their faces, redness and irritation can result.

All by themselves my daily regimens will help many OSNTs, but keep in mind that people with highly reactive skin often have specific allergies beyond those mentioned. If you follow my guidelines, and notice no change in your skin reactivity, you may want to consult an allergist to identify allergies to specific foods, products or environmental factors.

OSNTS AND AGING

Hormones regulate the production of your skin's oil, or sebum. In the human life cycle, birth is an initial high point in oil production, with a second taking place between the ages of nine and seventeen – the acne years. Thereafter, oil production normalises at adult levels. In women, sebum levels begin to fall during menopause. In men, this decrease is deferred until their eighties. In other words, the oiliness of OSNT skin improves with time (and women improve sooner than men). As you age, the acne caused by overactive oil production usually lessens. Finally, a benefit to going through menopause! However, women aren't out of the woods, since the hot flushes that some women experience can result in increased facial flushing – your biggest complaint.

To prevent or reduce the signs of aging, many people use antiaging skin creams, but OSNTs should stay away from them. You don't need them and their fruit acids and other ingredients can irritate your skin. Their exfoliation action is good for others, but not for you. Your best age prevention technique is the regular use of sunscreen and anti-inflammatories in your skin care and diet.

Believe it or not, the OSNT Skin Type is a great one to have. Younger OSNTs may not believe me, but all I can say is: Wait until you're forty.

When other types are scrambling to minimise the signs of aging, you'll look in the mirror with gratitude for your youthful looks. Believe me, a lot of people would trade places with you! One of the great assets of this type is that you rarely wrinkle. What's more, your skin is free of the dark spots and blotches that mar so many people's complexions.

OSNTs will save a fortune because aging will not bring the wrinkles and sags that drive others to costly procedures like Botox, collagen injections, face lifts, and microdermabrasion. If you read other chapters of this book, you'll see that I don't hesitate to advise antiaging treatments when necessary. But I have a different message for OSNTs: Don't waste your time or money on those costly procedures. You don't need them. You can skip facials, facial steaming, chemical peels and microdermabrasion. Are any advanced skin care options right for your Skin Type? Yes, and in the procedure section of this chapter, you'll find effective interventions for your main problems – redness, flushing and acne.

NON-MELANOMA CANCER

Light-skinned OSNTs with a history of excess sun exposure are at risk for non-melanoma skin cancer. Even though you're less likely to wrinkle or get dark spots, you should always wear sunscreen to prevent skin cancer. One study has shown that the incidence of basal cell carcinoma (BCC), the most common type of non-melanoma skin cancer, may be inversely proportional to the amount of wrinkling present. In other words, the more wrinkles you have, the less BCC you will develop. So, if you get a significant amount of sun exposure but do not have the genetic tendency to wrinkle, you may develop skin cancers instead.

How to Recognise a Non-Melanoma Skin Cancer

There are two types of non-melanoma skin cancer, so make sure to check yourself for both kinds regularly.

1. Squamous cell carcinoma (SCC): SCC commonly appears as a red, scaling patch that scabs in sun-exposed areas, such as the face, ears, chest, arms, legs and back. Although they resemble scabs, unlike scabs, they do not heal. An SCC may also be covered by a hard white scale that resembles a wart. Consult a dermatologist if you have a spot that fits this description and persists for three months or more.
2. Basal cell carcinoma (BCC): BCCs are bumps that look white, shiny and luminous like a pearl. They usually appear with a central raised ridge. Another variation is tiny blood vessels which appear around their borders. BCCs may also resemble a crater that shows up suddenly and resembles a scar, though no trauma or injury has caused it. Sometimes the border is 'ruffled', or heaped up around the central crater.

While avoiding skin cancer is vital, increased sun exposure also causes blood vessel breakage that can produce unsightly spider veins, flushing and facial redness. Sun exposure accelerates collagen loss, weakening the supportive structures around the blood vessels. In fact, a growing body of medical evidence indicates that in many instances rosacea is caused by sun damage.

Dr Baumann's Bottom Line: Save money on skin products, and instead go for relaxation therapies, like massage or yoga, or visits to a dermatologist. Remember, if you spend a lot of time outside, the increased risks of developing rosacea and skin cancer give you two good reasons to use generous amounts of sunscreen to protect your skin at all times.

EVERYDAY CARE FOR YOUR SKIN

What skin care products best serve your needs? Your primary concerns are oiliness and facial redness, along with the tendency to develop broken blood vessels. You therefore need nonirritating products that will limit acne and redness. If you've tried products marketed for 'sensitive skin', you may have found them irritating or overly oily since these products are usually formulated for dry skin. All the products I'll recommend act to do one or more of the following:

- Prevent and treat rosacea
- Prevent and treat oily skin

In addition, your daily regimen will also help to address your other skin concerns by:

- Preventing and treating inflammation

I've provided three different nonprescription regimens. If you experience facial redness, breakouts, facial stinging, rashes or active rosacea, use the first one daily. Use the second regimen if you have active acne. Use the maintenance regimen when your problems have cleared. Next, you can choose the products you'll need from those I recommend in each category later in this chapter.

If after following these regimens for six weeks, you find you need further help, consult a dermatologist, who can prescribe the prescription cleansers and oral medications I'll recommend later in this chapter.

DAILY SKIN CARE

STAGE ONE: NONPRESCRIPTION REGIMEN

For rosacea and redness:

AM	PM
Step 1: Wash with cleanser	Step 1: Wash with cleanser
Step 2: Apply an anti-inflammatory gel or lotion	Step 2: Apply an anti-inflammatory product
Step 3: Apply an oil control product (optional)	
Step 4: Apply sunscreen	
Step 5: Apply oil-free foundation or powder with sunscreen	

In the morning, wash with cleanser and apply an anti-inflammatory gel or lotion. If you have a high O/D score (above 35), you can apply an oil-control product before putting on sunscreen and makeup. Always use a sunscreen, even if you spend the day indoors.

In the evening, cleanse to gently remove makeup. Then apply a light nighttime lotion or gel with anti-inflammatory ingredients. Use masks or peels when skin is flared with acne or redness, and lotions and gels for maintenance when skin is calm. If your skin is less oily (with an O/D score of 27–35), choose lotions over gels. OSNTs with a higher score (above 35) may prefer gels.

STAGE ONE: NONPRESCRIPTION REGIMEN

For acne:

AM	PM
Step 1: Wash with cleanser	Step 1: Wash with cleanser
Step 2: Apply spot treatment for pimples	Step 2: Apply anti-inflammatory gel

Step 3: Apply oil-control product   Step 3: Apply a retinol product

Step 4: Apply oil-free foundation   Step 4: Apply moisturiser (optional
    or powder with sunscreen   if skin feels dry)

In the morning, wash with cleanser and use spot treatment for pimples, if needed. Then apply an oil-control product before putting on sunscreen and makeup. Always use a sunscreen.

In the evening, use a cleanser to gently remove makeup. Then apply a light nighttime mask, lotion, or gel with anti-inflammatory ingredients. Use masks when skin is flared with acne or redness, or serums for maintenance when skin is calm. If you scored between 27 and 35, your skin is slightly more combination, and serums are a better choice, as the recommended masks may be too drying. OSNTs with higher O/D scores (above 35) can benefit from both serums and masks.

STAGE ONE: NONPRESCRIPTION REGIMEN

For maintenance when acne and redness are under control:

AM   PM

Step 1: Wash with cleanser   Step 1: Wash with cleanser

Step 2: Apply oil-control product   Step 2: Apply anti-inflammatory
                                                   gel
Step 3: Apply oil-free foundation
    or powder with sunscreen   Step 3: Apply a retinol product

                                               Step 4: If skin feels dry, apply
                                               moisturiser

In the morning, wash with cleanser and apply an oil-control product before putting on sunscreen and makeup.

In the evening, use a cleanser to gently remove makeup. Then apply a light nighttime mask, lotion or gel with anti-inflammatory ingredients. Wait three to five minutes, and then follow with a retinol-containing product. Next, you can use a moisturiser if your skin feels dry or if you scored between 27 and 35 on the O/D questions.

Cleansers

My recommended cleansers contain anti-inflammatory ingredients that cut down on skin surface oil. Those with salicylic acid, sulphacetamide or sulphur are a good option.

RECOMMENDED CLEANSING PRODUCTS

- £ Eucerin Gentle Cleansing Milk
- £ Neutrogena Clear Pore Wash (if you have acne)
- £ Nivea Sensitive Balance Cleansing Milk
- £ Olay Total Effects Cleansing Cloths
- £ PanOxyl Bar 5% by Stiefel
- £ Paula's Choice One Step Face Cleanser
- £ Stiefel Acne-Aid Cleansing Bar
- £ Clean & Clear Blackhead Clearing Cleanser
- ££ DDF Salicylic Wash 2%
- ££ La Roche-Posay Effaclar Purifying Foaming Gel
- ££ Laura Mercier Foaming One-Step Cleanser
- ££ Philosophy On a Clear Day Super Wash for Oily Skin
- ££ Quintessence Skin Science Purifying Cleanser
- ££ Vichy Normaderm Deep Cleansing Gel
- £££ Darphin Intral Cleansing Milk
- £££ Guerlain Pure Dew Cleansing Foaming Gel
- £££ PCA Skin pHaze 31 BPO 5% Cleanser

Baumann's Choice: Olay Total Effects Cleansing Cloths

Toners

Most OSNTs won't need toners, which can worsen the flushing and redness you experience, because they often contain ingredients (like menthol) that can trigger flushing. People with severe rosacea should totally avoid toners.

However, if you like toners, choose ones with anti-inflammatory ingredients, like witch hazel. If cosmetic products often cause redness or stinging, pick a toner designed for sensitive skin.

Acne-Prone OSNTs

With acne but only minimal facial flushing and redness, you can use products containing benzoyl peroxide. The popular Proactiv system, composed of various benzoyl peroxide treatments, is geared towards this type. Any of their products can be substituted or combined with the other recommendations in this chapter. However, you can't buy the treatments individually; you must buy the entire kit, and it's not cheap. Many similar products containing benzoyl peroxide are available by prescription, which could save you money.

RECOMMENDED ACNE PRODUCTS

- £ Brevoxyl Cream
- £ Clean & Clear Quick Clear Treatment Gel
- £ PanOxyl Acne Gel 5% or 10% by Stiefel
- £ Panoxyl Wash
- ££ Biotherm Acnopur Emergency Anti-Acne Treatment for Blemish Prone Skin
- ££ DDF Benzoyl Peroxide Gel 10% & Sulphur 3%
- ££ Eve Lom Dynaspot
- ££ Kiehl's Blue Herbal Spot Treatment
- £££ Murad Exfoliating Blemish Gel
- ££ Peter Thomas Roth AHA/BHA Acne Clearing Gel
- ££ Philosophy On a Clear Day Acne Blemish Serum
- £££ Proactiv Repairing Lotion

Baumann's Choice: PanOxyl Acne Gel 5% with benzoyl peroxide. It's only sold at pharmacies.

Flushing- and Redness-Prone OSNTs

OSNTs with flushing and redness may not tolerate high-strength benzoyl peroxide products and the other acne treatments mentioned above. Instead, look for products with licochalone, feverfew, and other anti-inflammatory ingredients.

RECOMMENDED ANTI-INFLAMMATORY PRODUCTS

£ Olay Regenerist Regenerating Serum Fragrance Free
££ Avène Anti-Redness Light Moisturising Cream (It is green)
££ Clinique CX Redness Relief Cream
££ La Roche-Posay Rosaliac Hydrante Perfecteur
££ Mary Kay Calming Influence
££ Prescriptives Redness Relief Gel

Baumann's Choice: Rosaliac Hydrante Perfecteur by La Roche-Posay, because it contains thermal water with selenium and niacinamide, both of which are good anti-inflammatory ingredients.

Moisturisers

Due to your skin's naturally occurring oil, moisturisers may clog your pores and increase oiliness. However, if you have an O/D score of 27–35, you may use a light moisturiser that also contains ingredients that minimise inflammation and acne. But make sure to apply it to the dry areas only.

RECOMMENDED MOISTURISERS FOR COMBINATION SKIN

£ L'Oréal Pure Zone Skin Relief Oil-Free Moisturiser
£ Nivea Anti-Wrinkle Q_{10} Plus Day Cream
£ RoC Calmance Intolerance Repair Cream
££ Biotherm Biopur Melting Moisturising Matifying Fluid
££ Elizabeth Arden Sensitive Skin Calming Moisture Lotion
££ Paula's Choice Skin Balancing Moisture Gel
£££ Dior Energy-Move Skin Illuminating Moisturiser Crème

Baumann's Choice: Nivea Anti-Wrinkle Q_{10} Plus Day Cream

Peels

Discuss with your dermatologist or aesthetician whether or not you should use peels. If recommended, ask for peels with anti-inflammatory ingredients such as sulphur and salicylic acid.

Masks

Masks are helpful when your skin is especially oily. You can use a mask prior to an important event or even daily – there's no harm done with frequent application.

RECOMMENDED MASK PRODUCTS

££ Astara Blue Flame Purification Mask
££ DDF Sulphur Therapeutic Mask
££ Jurlique Moor Purifying Mask
££ Laura Mercier Deep Cleansing Clay Mask
££ Paula's Choice Oil Absorbing Facial Mask
££ SkinCeuticals Clarifying Clay Masque

Baumann's Choice: DDF Sulphur Therapeutic Mask

Skin Exfoliation

I recommend skin exfoliation only for certain types, and OSNTs should definitely avoid it because vigorous exfoliation can lead to inflammation. Always treat your skin as gently as possible, using only soft washcloths to wash your face. Avoid any harsh facial cleansing products, such as disposable facial cleansing cloths and cleansing pillows. These products are designed to be slightly abrasive and are not for you.

Tara, a thirty-nine-year-old mother of two, came to see me after consulting three other dermatologists. She'd received multiple treatments, but her acne was as bad as ever. As we chatted, Tara told me about her daily skin routine. She used a facial sponge to wash her face – the same sponge for *three years*. Once she threw it away and replaced it with a new one, her acne vastly improved. Sponges like the one Tara used can harbour bacteria that may cause acne and folliculitis. Anyone using a sponge should replace it every four to six weeks, as there's no point in using antibacterial and antibiotic treatments and then reinfecting your face with a skuzzy old sponge. However, OSNTs should use washcloths in any case.

SHOPPING FOR PRODUCTS

Your recommended skin care products contain anti-inflammatory ingredients to calm your skin's redness. Widen your selection by reading ingredient labels to include additional products with beneficial components. Always avoid products with ingredients that could cause irritation, inflammation or oiliness. If you find products that you like that are not on my product lists, please go to www.DrBaumann.co.uk and tell me what treasures you have found.

SKIN CARE INGREDIENTS TO USE

- Aloe vera
- Chamomile
- Cucumber
- Dexpanthenol (pro-vitamin B_5)
- Feverfew
- Glycyrrhiza glabra (licorice extract)
- Licochalone
- Niacinamide
- Salicylic acid (beta hydroxy acid or BHA)
- Tea tree oil
- Zinc

SKIN CARE INGREDIENTS TO AVOID

- Acetic acid
- Allantoin
- Alpha lipoic acid
- Balsam of Peru
- Benzoic acid
- Camphor
- Cinnamic acid
- Cinnamon oil
- Cocoa butter
- Cocos nucifera (coconut oil)
- DMAE
- Isopropyl isostearate
- Isopropyl myristate
- Lactic acid
- Menthol
- Parabens
- Peppermint oil
- Quaternium-15

Sun Protection for Your Skin

To get the most benefit from sunscreens, apply after cleansing to reduce surface skin oiliness. Lotions or gels are better for you than cream sunscreens.

Apply additional sunscreen even if using an SPF makeup (foundation or powder). Smooth a 10p-size portion of product over your entire face, neck, hands and chest. Reapply after six hours or every hour if you are out in direct sun. For complete instructions on sunscreen use, please reread Chapter Two.

RECOMMENDED SUN PROTECTION PRODUCTS

- £ Eucerin Q10 Active Anti-Wrinkle Fluid SPF 15
- £ L'Oréal Dermo-Expertise Future Moisturiser for Normal to Oily Skin with SPF 15
- £ Neutrogena Visibly Young Day Cream SPF 20
- £ Nivea Men Moisturising Lotion SPF 15
- £ Nivea Sun Age Defence Moisturising Facial Sunscreen SPF 30
- £ Paula's Choice Essential Non-Greasy Sunscreen SPF 15
- ££ Biotherm Biosensitive Soothing Anti-Shine Oil-Free Fluid Moisturiser SPF 15
- ££ Garnier Ambre Solaire Sheer Protect Shine Free SPF 30
- ££ Laura Mercier Tinted Moisturiser with SPF 20
- ££ Philosophy The Supernatural Airbrushed Canvas Powder Foundation
- ££ Prescriptives Daily Protection SPF 30 for Face
- £££ Chanel Précision Skin Conscience Total Health Oil Free Moisture Fluid SPF 15

Baumann's Choice: Garnier Ambre Solaire Sheer Protect Shine Free SPF 30

SUNSCREEN INGREDIENTS TO AVOID

If you have sunscreen sensitivity

- Avobenzone
- Benzophenone
- Butyl methoxydibenzoylmethane
- Isopropyldibenzoylmethane
- Octyl methoxycinnamate
- Methylbenzylidene camphor
- Para-amenobenzoic acid (PABA)
- Phenylbenzimidazole sulphonic acid

Your Makeup

OSNTs benefit from makeup with ingredients to minimise, treat, or conceal skin problems. Depending on which problems are paramount, you can select from various options.

For redness around the eye area, use an under-eye concealer with anti-inflammatory ingredients such as Beta Alisine Age Delete I-Zone Gel. People with a high O/D score (over 34) may prefer powders to foundations, while those with scores lower than 34 may like the coverage of a foundation. For acne or rosacea, look for foundations and powders with salicylic acid.

In general, OSNTs benefit from using medicated facial powders, especially if you have acne. But if you need to cover flushing or blemishes, choose an oil-free, yellow-tinted foundation that helps mask the redness, such as Giorgio Armani Fluid Sheer Foundation No6 formula. Or else apply a tinted makeup primer, such as Biotherm's Pure Bright Moisturising Makeup Base with a purple tint to cover redness. With an SPF of 25, this product can take the place of sunscreen. O/D scores over 34 may find this product too oily, but if you've scored in the 27–33 range, you may enjoy its coverage.

If eyelid redness is a problem, avoid shiny, frosted or iridescent eyeshadows. The rough edges of the ingredients used to give the product shimmer may cause skin irritation. Powder eyeshadows and blushers are recommended rather than cream products, because creams may streak on oily skin.

RECOMMENDED FOUNDATIONS

£ Almay Clear Complexion Blemish Healing Makeup
££ Boots No7 UpLifting Foundation SPF 15
££ Bloom Liquid Foundation
££ Laura Mercier Oil Free Foundation
££ MAC Studio Fix Powder Plus Foundation
£££ Giorgio Armani Fluid Sheer

Baumann's Choice: Almay Clear Complexion Blemish Healing Makeup, because it contains salicylic acid to clear pimples, is anti-inflammatory, and has aloe and chamomile – all at a great price.

RECOMMENDED POWDERS

£ Bonne Bell No Shine Pressed Powder (with tea tree oil)
£ Revlon Skinlights Face Illuminator Loose Powder
££ Avon Clear Finish Great Complexion Pressed Powder
££ Bloom Loose Powder
££ Laura Mercier Foundation Powder
£££ Lancôme Matte Finish Shine Control Sheer Pressed Powder

Baumann's Choice: Avon Clear Finish Great Complexion Pressed Powder, because it contains anti-inflammatory ingredients and oil control, comes in many colours, and has a great price.

CONSULTING A DERMATOLOGIST

PRESCRIPTION SKIN CARE STRATEGIES

Many OSNTs are on a spectrum that leads to rosacea; the daily regimen, prescription medications, and procedures in this section of this chapter will help, wherever you happen to be on that spectrum.

Sulphur or sulphacetamide cleansers will reduce inflammation and prevent both acne and rosacea breakouts, while antibiotic gels or lotions will reduce the skin bacteria, which can lead to inflammation. Avoid creams, as they're too oily for you. You can use these products even if you only experience a little facial redness, and they will be equally effective if you've been diagnosed with rosacea. I provide two regimens, the first for redness, the second for acne. I'll show you how to combine the prescription meds with some of the over-the-counter products recommended earlier in this chapter.

DAILY SKIN CARE

STAGE TWO: PRESCRIPTION REGIMEN

For rosacea and inflammation:

AM	PM
Step 1: Wash with prescription cleanser	Step 1: Wash with prescription cleanser
Step 2: Apply prescription antibiotic gel or lotion	Step 2: Apply prescription antibiotic gel or lotion
Step 3: Apply powder foundation with sunscreen	Step 3: Apply anti-inflammatory moisturiser

In the morning, use a cleanser followed by an antibiotic gel to help lessen inflammation. Next, you can apply a powder foundation with SPF. Assure you have a minimum SPF coverage of 15.

Wash again with the cleanser in the evening. Then apply the antibiotic, which will help the rosacea, and lastly, the anti-inflammatory moisturiser.

Once a week, use a prescription mask with anti-inflammatory action such as Plexion mask by Medicis.

RECOMMENDED PRESCRIPTION CLEANSERS TO COMBAT INFLAMMATION

Plexion Cleanser (sodium sulphacetamide 10% and sulphur 5%)
Rosanil Cleanser (sodium sulphacetamide 10% and sulphur 5%)
Rosula Aqueous Cleanser (sodium sulphacetamide 10% and sulphur 5%)
Zoderm Cleanser (8.5% benzoyl peroxide)

Baumann's Choice: They're all good. Please ask your dermatologist to recommend products comparable to these US brand name products.

Recommended Prescription
Anti-Inflammatory and Antibiotic
Lotions and Gels

Aknemycin Plus (tretinoin and erythromycin)*
AVAR gel (sulphacetamide and sulphur)
AVAR Green gel (sulphacetamide and sulphur)
Azelex cream (azelaic acid)
Benzamycin (benzoul peroxide and clindamycin)*
Clindagel (Clindamycin)
Clindets (Clindamycin)
Dalacin T (clindamycin)*
Duac (benzoyl peroxide and clindamycin)*
Finacea gel (azelaic acid)
Isotrexin (Isotretinoin and erythromycin)*
MetroGel (Metronidazole)*
Nicosyn (sulphacetamide and sulphur)
Noritate cream (Metronidazole)
Nocacet (sulphacetamide and sulphur)
Plexion SCT cream
Stiemycin (erythromycin)*
Sulfacet-R, available tinted and non-tinted, (sulphacetamide and sulphur)
Rosanil (sulphacetamide and sulphur)
Rosula Aqueous Gel (sulphacetamide and sulphur)
Topicycline (tetracycline hydrochloride and 4-epitetracycline hydrochloride)*
Zindaclin (erythromycin and zinc)*
Zineryt (erythromycin and zinc)*

Baumann's Choice: Ask your dermatologist which is right for you. Since many of these are US brand name products, he or she can identify similar ones that will work for you. Those marked with an * are available in the UK.

If these topical medications are not sufficiently effective, consider getting a prescription for oral antibiotics such as minocycline, doxycycline or tetracycline to control inflammation. Although highly effective, they do have some potential downsides: in some cases, they can inactivate oral contraceptives, cause yeast infections, or make you more sun sensitive. To obtain a full list of your oral antibiotic options, please consult your dermatologist or physician.

Periostat, a new medication that is a form of doxycycline, can be helpful in treating rosacea, recent studies show. Since it's given in very low doses, it does not lead to the above complications and can be used for longer periods of time.

STAGE TWO: PRESCRIPTION REGIMEN

For acne:

AM	PM
Step 1: Wash with prescription cleanser	Step 1: Wash with prescription cleanser
Step 2: Apply nonprescription spot treatment to pimples if needed	Step 2: Apply antibiotic gel and wait five to ten minutes
Step 3: Apply antibiotic gel to entire face	Step 3: Apply a retinoid
Step 4: Apply sunscreen and foundation assuring an SPF of 15.	Step 4: Optional moisturiser
Step 5: Apply powder with oil control	

In the morning, use a medicated cleanser followed by a nonprescription pimple treatment product. Next, apply the antibiotic gel. Finally, you can use foundation and powder with oil control.

Wash again with the cleanser in the evening. Then apply the antibiotic gel to treat acne, and after waiting for five to ten minutes, use a retinoid as directed. If skin feels dry or if you have combination skin, you can also use a moisturiser.

Once a week see your dermatologist or spa for a beta hydroxy acid (salicylic acid) peel.

RECOMMENDED PRESCRIPTION CLEANSERS

Brevoxyl-4 Creamy Wash (cleanser with benzoyl peroxide 4% for acne)
Plexion (cleansing pads with sulphacetamide and sulphur)
Triaz Cleanser (benzoyl peroxide, glycolic acid, zinc)

Baumann's Choice: The above-mentioned products are available in the US. Ask your dermatologist to identify comparable ones that are right for you.

RECOMMENDED PRESCRIPTION
ANTIBIOTIC GELS AND LOTIONS

Aknemycin Plus (tretinoin and erythromycin)
Benzamycin (benzoyl peroxide and clindamycin)
Dalacin T (clindamycin)
Duac (benzoyl peroxide and Clindamycin)
Isotrexin (isotretinoin and erythromycin)
Stiemycin (erythromycin)
Topicycline (tetracycline hydrochloride and 4-epitetracycline hydrochloride)
Zindaclin (erythromycin and zinc)
Zineryt (erythromycin and zinc)

Baumann's Choice: OSNTs with very sensitive skin and redness may prefer products, that do not contain benzoyl peroxide. Your dermatologist can recommend similar products that are available in your country.

Retinoid Use

If you suffer from both skin redness and acne, you may have trouble tolerating the retinoid. For complete instructions, please consult 'Further Care for Oily, Sensitive Skin'.

RECOMMENDED RETINOID
PRODUCTS FOR ACNE

Aknemycin Plus (contains an antibiotic as well)
Differin gel or cream
Isotrex
Isotrexin (contains an antiobiotic as well)
Retin-A gel, lotion, or cream
Retinova

Baumann's Choice: Isotrexin or Aknemycin Plus.

PROCEDURES FOR YOUR SKIN TYPE

All of the sulphur, sulphacetamide, and antibiotic-containing skin care products as well as the oral medications can help treat the flushing and acne forms of rosacea. Blue or red light therapy can also help reduce acne. The light therapy works by killing facial bacteria that causes acne. You can schedule treatments every two weeks for a series of ten to twelve treatments.

At this time, no topical or oral product is available to successfully treat the two other symptoms of rosacea: the dilated blood vessels (spider veins) and the yellowish, enlarged nose with large pores. A number of dermatological office procedures are effective in treating the dilated blood vessels, including the electric needle, an injection of saline solution, a laser, or a light device such as Intense Pulsed Light, IPL.

Most of the recommended procedures for dilated blood vessels cost between £150 and £250. It typically takes from two to five treatments for the vessels to disappear. But rest assured that these treatments are worth it, because once vessels disappear, they are gone permanently, and an annual maintenance treatment can handle any new ones that appear.

Brian was a clergyman who participated in a clinical trial I conducted for a medication that we hoped would prove effective in treating spider veins. After the trial had concluded, the trial physicians offered light treatments to the participants in thanks for their participation. Brian hadn't responded to the experimental medication so I treated him with a combination of IPL and Metvix, erasing the tiny spider veins that covered his cheeks. He was very grateful because this rid him of an embarrassing problem that had troubled him throughout his adult life. Parishioners saw his red face and whispered that he was an alcoholic. When highway cops pulled him over for driving a tad above the speed limit (which often occurred when he was on his way to counsel the dying), they would see his red face and conclude that he had been drinking, Brian confided. After the treatments, Brian reported that his former symptoms were gone, and with them the unfounded suspicion that he drank.

IPL and Metvix

My preferred procedure for rosacea spectrum is using IPL and Metvix together. They work synergistically to reduce the oil, blood vessels, and yellow papules that are symptomatic of rosacea. Your skin's oil-producing glands and red blood vessels absorb Metvix, which makes them more sensitive to light. Then, when the IPL is flashed on the skin, it shrinks and partially destroys them. The end result is that oil glands are less able to produce oil. This helps to eliminate yellow papules, the enlarged oil glands that so many OSNTs complain about. In addition, the IPL erases many of the visible facial blood vessels and improves red cheeks. This occurs because the enlarged blood vessels take up the heat of the light and it destroys them, leaving normal skin untouched. For more information on this treatment, please see 'Further Help for Oily, Sensitive Skin'.

Treating Advanced Rosacea

There are several different options for treating the enlarged nose that may occur with more advanced rosacea, including surgery, dermabrasion and laser. All these procedures remove enlarged oil glands on the nose. Although each procedure is done by a different instrument, the action performed is virtually the same. The doctor removes the top and middle layers of the skin. Naturally, this can be uncomfortable, and the total downtime is about ten days. The wound remains bandaged for four days; ten days after surgery, the skin should be healed. Pinkness, which persists for about six months, can be covered with makeup. An enlarged nose is the last stage of rosacea, and frankly, I don't see it much. Taking antibiotics at the first signs of a worsening rosacea condition can prevent it.

Cosmetic Procedures to Avoid

Although you may be tempted by a variety of services and products promising to help you address skin care problems, most of the following are a waste of time and money:

- Microdermabrasion is too harsh for your sensitive skin.
- Facials are too heating and inflammatory for your redness-prone skin.
- Non-ablative lasers, except those designed to improve rosacea and get rid of blood vessels, are more geared to wrinkles; you don't need them.

In addition, you probably do not need either Botox or fillers such as collagen and hyaluronic acid because you don't have wrinkles. However, they can be used to change eyebrow shape or make the lips bigger if desired.

ONGOING CARE FOR YOUR SKIN

Since the OSNT Skin Type is on the rosacea spectrum, your skin will never be as trouble free as other types. However, if you follow my programme and treat problems early, in most cases, you will be able to avoid the more advanced stages of rosacea. I see many OSNTs (both men and women) since what I offer is the most effective approach. So feel confident in following my recommendations. And as I've mentioned, if you begin taking good care of your skin now, you have something you can look forward to. Your skin will improve with age.

Further Help for Oily, Sensitive Skin

In this section, you'll find follow-up information, instructions on product use, and procedures for Oily, Sensitive Skin Types, as well as diet and lifestyle recommendations, and supplements that can help your skin.

USING RETINOIDS

Derived from vitamin A but with a different chemical structure, retinoids may limit oil production, reduce skin oiliness, and prevent acne and pigmentation. In addition, retinoids improve visible wrinkles for wrinkled types and dark spots for pigmented types, and can even act to prevent future outbreaks in oily types. I recommend that you start retinoid use slowly, using the lowest strength available sparingly, especially if you have rosacea, acne, or skin redness. It will take weeks of use before you can tolerate them without experiencing redness and flaking; however, the long-term benefits are worth it. If you experience excess irritation and redness, you can either stop, try another brand, or reduce the amount. If no excessive redness occurs after two weeks, you can begin using it every other night as per these instructions. Your skin will slowly become accustomed to the retinoid, so don't give up. In six months you will wonder how you lived without it.

RETINOID USE

1. In your hand, mix together a pea-size portion of retinoid with a couple of drops of serum. If you have pigmented skin, use serums recommended in Chapter Four. For non-pigmented skin, use serums in Chapter Six.
2. Apply to face and neck using upward strokes, and wipe a touch on the backs of your hands. With only a trace of product on your hands, place

your fingertips gently on the skin area under the eye (never on top of the eyelid or elsewhere around the eye), being careful not to get too close to the eye.

3. Use once every three days for two weeks or until no redness or dryness is visible.

4. At the end of two weeks, begin applying the mixture every other night for another two weeks.

5. After those two weeks are up, use nightly and indefinitely.

IPL and Vascular Lasers

Dermatologists use Intense Pulsed Light, or IPL (a combination of different colours of light), to remove the dark spots, blood vessels, and enlarged oil glands that produce excess oil and cause acne. There are various types of IPL devices, but I prefer the Quantum from Lumenis because it is much more powerful than the types used by salons. IPL can also be used in combination with a topical medication called Metvix that makes the skin sensitive to light and intensifies the light's effect. When used in combination with Metvix, the light therapy is called Photodynamic Therapy, or PDT.

This treatment is effective for the dark spots and oiliness of OSPTs and OSPWs. It's also a highly effective treatment for flushing, redness, visible blood vessels, and other symptoms on the rosacea spectrum experienced by OSNTs and OSNWs. IPL can also be combined with various vascular lasers. The red blood vessels absorb the light produced by the vascular laser or the Intense Pulsed Light. The blood vessels then heat up and burst, leaving the skin untouched. My favourite vascular laser is the Dornier 940nm laser. Its energy is absorbed by deoxyhaemoglobin, a component in the blood. As a result, this laser does not produce bruising after the procedure, as do many vascular lasers. It can also be used on people with dark skin. Usually, the IPL treatment is administered first to the entire face, followed by the Dornier laser directed to large blood vessels only.

Preparing for Light or Laser Treatment:

You can reduce the number of IPL treatments needed to treat dark spots by regular retinoid use for a month or more in advance. Differin gel is ideal.

On the day of your treatment, do not wear sunscreen, makeup or moisturiser. When you arrive, the doctor or nurse will clean your face to remove any oils. Some doctors like to perform microdermabrasion in advance to smooth the skin's surface and enhance the procedure's effects, but this is optional.

What to Expect:

In advance of the light therapy, Metvix gel is spread on your face for thirty minutes or more and then removed. Your doctor can then perform an IPL or other light treatment. It generally takes ten minutes, and you will notice a mild feeling of warmth; but don't worry, it's rarely painful. Since the Metvix sensitises the skin to light, you will need to use sunblock for thirty-six hours after treatment.

Following Treatment:

You'll notice that your skin retains light sensitivity, which can result in sunburn if you're not protected by a broad-spectrum sunblock of SPF 45–60. Apply sunblock immediately and avoid sun exposure for two days. After the IPL treatment your cheeks may be slightly pink for a few days, like after a hot shower. However, other than avoiding the sun, you can go about your usual daily activities.

After Photodynamic Therapy:

Your skin may look red, peeling or crusted for three to seven days after the PTD procedure.

After blue light treatment for acne:

There is no downtime from this procedure.

After vascular laser treatment for blood vessels:

Some vascular lasers cause intense bruising, so be sure to discuss this with your dermatologist prior to treatment so you will know what to expect. The Dornier 940nm laser, which I use in my office, does not result in downtime, bruising or sun sensitivity, so you can return to your regular activities right away.

After Care:

For all of these light and laser procedures, continue your skin care regimen.

Your Treatment Results:

After several treatments, you'll notice that brown spots fade and flake off, but resist the temptation to peel them off yourself.

In treating redness, enlarged blood vessels, and other rosacea symptoms, after several treatments you will notice a distinct change in your skin texture and colour. Your skin's redness will be diminished, the blood vessels will disappear or become less visible, and your skin will feel smoother.

This procedure's cost varies between £100 and £400 for different light sources. How many treatments will you need? The severity of your skin problem will dictate the type of light used and the number of treatments recommended by your doctor. Four to ten treatments is the average amount people require, with annual treatments for maintenance.

Metvix combined with light treatments (either blue light or IPL) is also helpful in knocking out early skin cancers. Although it does not get rid of melanoma, it can sometimes address early non-melanoma skin cancers.

TREATING WRINKLES WITH BOTOX AND RELOXIN

Wrinkles are born of squinting, smiling, frowning – any facial movement – as well as time and aging. If your wrinkles are getting you down and you don't mind injections, you might consider botulinum toxin treatments. In this procedure, botulinum toxins are injected into facial muscles to relax and improve wrinkles. At this time, Botox is the only FDA-approved treatment in the US for this indication, and it has been safely used for facial wrinkles since the very early 1980s. Reloxin (also called Dysport) is available in Australia as well. Studies assessing Reloxin are expected to result in its FDA approval in the US in the next few years. In addition, there is a product called Myobloc on the market. Myobloc injections only last about six weeks, which makes them a good option if you aren't ready to commit to the longer-term results of Botox and Reloxin (which last up to about four to six months) and want to 'try it out'.

BOTOX/RELOXIN TREATMENT

In Preparation:

For ten days prior to your appointment, avoid supplements or medications that make you bruise, such as medications that reduce inflammation (ibuprofen products like Advil and Nurofen), as well as aspirin, green tea, vitamin E, *Ginkgo biloba,* and Saint-John's-Wort. However, you may take Tylenol, which does not affect blood platelet function like these others do. Purchase a product containing arnica or vitamin K, and/or retinol, which can be applied after the procedure to prevent and treat bruises.

On the day of your treatment, try to be as relaxed as you can – remember, this really is easy. If your doctor hasn't applied a topical anaesthetic cream to the area being treated, usually the forehead, between the brows, or the crow's-feet at the outside corners of the eyes, be sure to request it about twenty minutes before the treatment begins. Or you can buy this cream (called LMX or EMLA) behind the pharmacist's counter without a prescription and apply it (with your doctor's approval) twenty minutes prior to your treatment.

What to Expect:

The treatment involves injections via a tiny needle, which is smaller than the size of a pinhead. Since a topical anaesthetic is always used in my practice, most people don't feel anything. Frown lines usually require three injections, crow's-feet receive three injections per side, and lines in the forehead usually get five to eight injections. Following treatment, your skin will have a few raised bumps in the area of injection that look like insect bites. These typically last about thirty minutes. Bruising can also occur (though this is more likely in redheads), so remember to apply the arnica or vitamin K and retinol at the first sign of bruising.

Follow-Up Care for Botox/Reloxin:

Your doctor will ask you to move the muscles in the treated area off and on for ten minutes. In other words, if you had frown lines treated, she will ask you to frown and relax, frown and relax. Patients can immediately resume all skin care and makeup use after the treatment.

What to Expect After Botox/Reloxin:

After three days you will notice decreased movement in the treated area. It takes ten days for the full effects to be seen. Return to your doctor in two weeks if you are not happy with the results. If you can make the treated area move by flexing the muscles, or if you notice any asymmetry – uneven results on one side or the ability to move only on one side – the treatment hasn't worked as it should.

If this is the case, see your doctor immediately so that he or she can give you more Botox to treat the asymmetry.

Your Treatment Results:

Your wrinkles themselves may not completely disappear but the muscles underneath them should quit moving. It may take four to eight months without movement before the wrinkles begin to smooth out, which they will do especially if you are following the recommended skin care regimen at the same time. With continuous treatment, wrinkles smooth out; however, if treatment is discontinued, they will return.

Botox and Reloxin injections vary between £150 and £250 per treated area. Frown lines, crow's-feet, and forehead lines would be considered three separate areas. Expect to return for follow-up treatments every three to six months.

DERMAL FILLERS

Dermal fillers, including collagen products (like Zyplast and CosmoPlast), and hyaluronic acid products (Restylane, Hylaform, Captique, and Juvéderm) do exactly as the name implies: help skin fill gaps in wrinkles via injections of collagen and hyaluronic acid, two biochemicals present in the skin that decrease with aging.

In Preparation:

I recommend the same preparation for dermal fillers as I do for Botox. Most doctors like to use several different types of fillers. Be sure they discuss with you what types are available and which they think are best for your needs.

What to Expect:

In advance of the treatment, some doctors will do a dental block anaesthetic injection, similar to those dentists perform, to numb the entire area between the nose and mouth. This makes the treatment injections painless but the anaesthetic can last about an hour or more after treatment. You can elect instead to numb the area with a topical cream. This does not result in a numb mouth and is more convenient if you plan to return to work that day. Most of my patients prefer it. You can expect to feel slight pain with each treatment injection, even with the numbing cream. The hyaluronic acid (HA) fillers such as Hylaform, Restylane, and Juvéderm are more painful than collagen injections such as CosmoPlast, because the collagen-containing fillers have the anaesthetic lidocaine. Each wrinkle will require about three to five injections to treat.

Following treatment, your skin will be slightly red and swollen around the injected area. This improves in twenty minutes and usually resolves completely by the next day. The amount of swelling varies depending on what filler is used. Collagen fillers tend to have less swelling than HA fillers. Injecting first with collagen and then following it with a hyaluronic acid filler will often reduce swelling and decrease the risk of bruising as well as providing the benefits of both types of fillers. Collagen gives structure, while hyaluronic acid provides volume by drawing water into the area.

Follow-Up Care for Dermal Fillers:

Applying ice immediately following treatment is recommended. The only other aftercare necessary is using the above-mentioned vitamin K/retinol cream or arnica if you experience bruising. Patients can immediately resume all skin care and makeup use after dermal fillers.

What to Expect After Dermal Fillers:

If you've decided to pursue a course of treatments because your wrinkles bother you, the disappearance of unwanted lines and wrinkles is immediately gratifying.

Your Treatment Results:

While the results from this treatment are quite good, there is a chance that your deeper wrinkles may not disappear completely. Your doctor will discuss this with you prior to treatment.

This procedure costs between £150 and £750, or even more, depending on the amount of wrinkles you need to treat. With most fillers, you'll need to re-treat yourself once every four to six months. Sculptra, a new product on the market, may yield results that last for as long as two years. It is injected every month for three to five months until the desired result is achieved. This product is ideal for the treatment of multiple or very deep wrinkles, and can be used in combination with botulinum toxin and other fillers as well.

LIFESTYLE RECOMMENDATIONS FOR OILY, SENSITIVE TYPES

Avoiding sun exposure is particularly important for types at an increased risk of skin cancer and for those who suffer from rosacea. One study showed that sunlight exposure caused a rosacea flare in 81 percent of the one thousand patients surveyed. To prevent what are known as deep 'smoker's wrinkles', I also strongly advise you to quit smoking. Many people I know have used smoking cessation patches successfully. And remember, if at first you don't succeed, try, try again.

Sensitive, Non-Pigmented Skin Types need to prevent rosacea and redness through lessening skin sensitivity. To do that, avoid all ingredients, conditions, and actions (both internal and external) that might provoke an inflammatory reaction. Exercising in a cool environment is best, if possible. Swimming is an ideal exercise, if you do not react to chlorine.

Overall, you should avoid heated, humid environments (such as steam rooms) whenever possible. The combination of heat and humidity causes the skin to swell, which can lead to clogged pores and acne.

Avoid abrupt changes in environmental temperature, which lead to facial redness and irritation. The hearty Scandinavians used to go from a hot sauna outdoors to roll around in the snow. Not that you'd be tempted, but this kind of radical change in climate would play havoc with your skin. Excessive cold during downhill skiing and many winter sports should be avoided. Sensitive types are susceptible to windburn, so use a heavy facial moisturiser to protect your skin. Protective facial clothing and scarves should be used in extremely cold temperatures.

Going back and forth between air-conditioning and a hot summer day is not ideal. Try to arrange your life so that you can avoid or minimise such changes wherever possible. Don't sit by the fire and then head directly outdoors. Plan your moves so you give your skin's internal thermostat time to adjust gradually.

Avoid external heat or irritating conditions. Hot tub use can exacerbate rosacea due to heat and the chemicals used to keep it clean. Chlorine in swimming pools can worsen skin problems. Avoid touching your face if you come in contact with inks, carbon, grease or other chemicals. Perfumes, cleansing products, even room fresheners can contain ingredients that cause a reaction.

Keep hot drinks to a minimum, and allow them to cool before drinking, to avoid stimulating vascular dilation. Enjoy cool water and iced herbal teas, such as green or peppermint tea. In hot weather or when working in a hot environment, chew on ice chips to keep your body temperature down. Or drape a cool towel across the back of your neck. Wear clothes that breathe. Some people find that all-cotton clothing is more cooling than clothes made with synthetic fabrics.

Facial steaming can increase oiliness, while antiaging ingredients can irritate sensitive skin, causing both acne and redness.

Friction against your skin can also lead to acne, especially in acne-prone areas. For example, male oily, sensitive types often complain that their neck breaks out after wearing a shirt with a tie, due to the friction of the collar against their skin. Buying shirts one-half inch larger in neck size can help.

Oily types need to reduce stress, which can increase oil secretion, worsen acne, and increase the production of the skin pigment melanin, studies show. In fact, one study of twenty-two university students showed that acne worsened during exam time. Stress can also impair the skin's protective barrier, making it more susceptible to skin allergies.

Stress reduction is a habit you can cultivate. If you catch yourself stressing, interrupt the stress pattern as you go about your day. At times, when you feel tense or pressured, take a few deep breaths, concentrating on exhaling fully. Catch yourself when you react with anxiety or anger: practise taking a step back and letting it go. Make sure to make 'unwinding' activities, like walking, playing with a pet, chatting with a friend, or anything else you find relaxing, a regular part of your day. Treat yourself well, and address stress so that you lessen your skin's tendency to act like a barometer of your emotions.

Marguerite, a concert violinist with pale skin and flaming red hair, had an artistic temperament. Her face instantly flushed bright red whenever the conductor snapped at her impatiently in rehearsal. The next day, without fail, Marguerite's chin would be dotted with acne, which she tried unsuccessfully to camouflage with a creamy foundation. But it only further irritated her sensitive skin.

I put Marguerite on an anti-inflammatory daily skin care regimen and urged her to avoid alcohol (which dilates blood vessels) on days leading up to performances. Seeking ways to de-stress, Marguerite found she enjoyed silent meditation, as a respite from a world filled with sound. After a few weeks on this new treatment, Marguerite felt calmer, reacted less to the conductor's outbursts, and was able to control her skin symptoms.

Still, she was relieved when the temperamental conductor accepted a new appointment in a distant city. It turned out that her orchestra's new conductor was a Frenchman with a great appreciation for fine red wine and artistic redheads.

To make stress management a part of *your* weekly routine, here are a few options:

- Getting a relaxing massage
- Doing restful, restorative yoga
- Walking in nature
- Meditating in a peaceful place
- Applying calming essential oils
- Listening to serene and soothing music
- Playing with a beloved pet
- In Miami Beach I like to go watch the ocean waves. It works for me every time!

BODY TREATMENTS

Skin problems are not confined to your face, since you can also get acne (and dark spots) on all parts of your body. That's why I want to offer you a few treatment suggestions that may help. Spas and resorts offer therapeutic baths of mineral waters that contain a high concentration of the mineral sulphur, which is beneficial for acne-plagued skin. In baths, sulphur functions in the same way for your body as it does for your face in the sulphur-based facial products I've recommended earlier. Bath has been famous for its Roman baths and natural springs, which are rich with healing minerals, and have been a pilgrimage site since Roman times.

Balneotherapy

Balneotherapy, which means bathing in mineral water baths and pools, evolved as a core offering of spas in the 1800s, first in Europe and then in the United States.

The active ingredient in these baths is the mineral sulphur, which prevents inflammation, scarring and infection, as well as reducing the formation of skin outbreaks, itching and rashes. In dermatology research, sulphur has been shown to be especially helpful in the treatment of rosacea and acne, but beyond these conditions, it seems to have an overall benefit to the skin.

Diet

All OS types need to prevent inflammation and breakouts. Studies show that some foods can increase acne, while other foods help prevent outbreaks. So here are some dos and don'ts to help manage oil production.

Eating a diet rich in high glycaemic foods can lead to acne, while eating a low carb diet can help curb outbreaks. Here's why: high glycaemic foods (such as sweets, sweetened jams and jellies, certain fruits, and foods with refined grain products, like bread, pastry, cake, scones, and cold cereals) cause a rapid rise in blood glucose levels. Blood glucose stimulates the release of insulin, and excess insulin production can contribute to acne. Obesity itself may also be linked with acne. That's why you'll get a double benefit by controlling your weight, your insulin production, and your acne via a low carb diet. Dairy products are known to stimulate insulin production and should also be avoided. However, chocolate, long considered a no-no for acne sufferers, is no longer believed to cause instant breakouts. Vitamin A has also been shown to be associated with decreased oil secretion. Vitamin A-rich foods include liver, shellfish, and cod liver oil (taken as liquid or capsules). Although vegetables do not contain vitamin A, many provide beta-carotene, a related nutrient. Some foods are also vitamin A fortified. Beta-carotene can be found in sweet potatoes, mangoes, spinach, cantaloupe, kale, dried apricots, egg yolks and red peppers.

The mineral iodine, in high dietary levels, can contribute to acne by causing pores to swell, leading to acne breakouts. To reduce your iodine levels, avoid iodised salt, shrimp, and sea vegetables. Instead, use Celtic Sea Salt (available from http://www.celtic-seasalt.com), which contains no added iodine.

Avoiding beer may also be prudent for OSPTs and OSPWs since hops, the ingredient that gives beer its aroma and flavour, acts in an oestrogen-like way to increase dark spots and melasma. Hops can also cause acne, and it was discovered that hop pickers had increased acne due to their exposure.

For OSNTs and OSNWs who suffer from rosacea-type symptoms such as facial flushing, certain foods can contribute to your condition. Alcohol, especially red wine, can aggravate rosacea and facial flushing. Avoid stimulants like caffeine that act as vascular dilators. Vinegar, hot spices, spicy seasonings, hot sauces, peppers (including black pepper), and meat marinades may also dilate blood vessels. Any of these can worsen facial redness. Look out for fermented foods like some cheeses and the nitrates in cured meats, sausages or hotdogs, which can also worsen your symptoms.

While overall avoidance of alcohol, hot foods (temperature), and spicy foods is recommended, to identify your specific triggers, it can be helpful to keep a diary of what you eat, and then note when you later develop symptoms. That way you can make sure to avoid them.

The ideal diet for OSNs should accent foods that decrease inflammation, such as eggs, fish, and cool salads. The omega-3 fatty acids may have anti-inflammatory effects. Omega-3 fats can be found in wild Pacific salmon, flax seeds, omega-3 enriched eggs, wild game, grass-fed meats, wild plants, and cod liver oil supplements, such as Carlson's Brand Cod Liver Oil or Nordic Naturals Arctic Cod Liver Oil (available in gel caps or liquid form). In supplementing with cod liver oil to decrease inflammation, make sure to use a product like these two, which have been processed to remove both mercury contamination and the 'fishy' taste that so many find disagreeable. Although tuna is another omega-3 rich fish, mercury contamination is an issue, especially for pregnant and nursing women and those planning to become pregnant. The National Center for Policy Research for Women and Families advises that the above-mentioned categories of women limit fish consumption to twelve ounces per week and limit tuna consumption to six ounces of 'light' canned tuna per week. Salmon is low in mercury contamination while still rich in omega-3 fatty acids.

Vegetarians (and vegans who do not eat fish or eggs) will have more difficulty finding a source of omega-3 fatty acids. Although flaxseed and flaxseed oil are well-known vegetarian sources, for many people, the fat component they carry is not well converted into the more essential forms, DHA and EPA, which are found only in animal products. However, one vegan source of DHA alone is O-Mega-Zen3, derived from marine microalgae and encapsulated in vegicaps (available from www.nutru.com).

OSNTs are at an increased risk of developing non-melanoma skin cancer (basal cell or squamous cell carcinoma). That's why I recommend that you consume foods and supplements that contain antioxidants to decrease your skin cancer risk. Antioxidants act by lowering the activity of free radicals and destructive enzymes that lead to skin cancer. Fruits, especially pomegranate and berries of all kinds, contain them and should be a regular part of your diet. In addition, foods containing beta-carotene, as recommended previously, also show a protective effect against certain types of cancers.

Other plant phytonutrients have been shown to offer some protection against skin cancer: spinach, kale and broccoli contain the phytonutrient lutein, while tomatoes contain another cancer-fighting phytonutrient, lycopene. For OSNWs and OSPWs, antioxidant foods and supplements can help prevent wrinkles. Antioxidants help defuse free radicals, renegade oxygen molecules that, when out of balance in the body, can cause cells to break down and age more rapidly. Most vegetables and many fruits contain antioxidants, particularly berries, cherries, kiwis, and even artichokes. Green tea is a powerful antioxidant, which is why I recommend both topical skin care products that contain it and oral supplements. In addition, you should drink the tea itself regularly. Apple peels have also been shown to contain higher amounts of antioxidants, so eat your apples with the peels on!

While an Australian study showed that blueberries are the number-one source of antioxidants, they are also found in such foods as cranberries and pomegranates. Out of season, you can obtain the benefits of these fruits via unsweetened juice concentrates. A tablespoon or two can be mixed with water and sipped, to deliver both hydration and antioxidant benefits. Make sure to obtain unsweetened brands, as excess sugars have been shown to contribute to acne. Other sources of antioxidants are tomatoes (which also contain lycopene, a pigment shown to have anticancer benefits) and basil (which can be enjoyed in salad and pasta).

Antioxidants are also amply present in vegetables such as spinach, kale, collard greens, turnips, romaine lettuce, broccoli, leeks, corn, red peppers, peas, and mustard greens. Egg yolks and oranges contain the antioxidant lutein. While obtaining your antioxidants from whole foods is advisable since the body is designed to recognise and process these and other beneficial nutrients from food sources, you can also use supplements, if wished. Grapes and grape seed extract also rate high in antioxidants. Grape seed extract can be obtained via supplements.

SUPPLEMENTS

On a recent trip to the UK, I discovered that supplements are not widely available. What's more, the few supplements that are readily available usually contain only a low concentration of active ingredients. Since supplements are very popular in France, Australia and Germany, you may want to pick some up on one of your trips there. Zinc has been shown to help acne sufferers at a recommended dose of 100mg per day. Or if you prefer, you can eat zinc-rich foods such as oysters and beef or lamb kidneys and liver. Vitamin A supplements are also an option for this type to decrease oil production. However it is important not to take too much vitamin A, so please consult your physician first. Avon's VitAdvance Acne Clarifying Complex with vitamins A, C and E, as well as zinc, selenium and alpha lipoic acid is a good option, as is Murad Pure Skin Clarifying Supplement.

Those of you who are 'W' types should look for supplements with antioxidants such as vitamin C, vitamin E, green tea, Coenzyme Q10, lutein, lycopene and pycnogenol. Heliocare, an oral supplement, contains PL extract from ferns, which has been shown to be a powerful antioxidant.

PART THREE

Skin Care for Oily, Resistant Skin

CHAPTER EIGHT

Oily, Resistant, Pigmented and Wrinkled: ORPW

THE TEFLON SKIN TYPE

'Will every decade bring some new skin problem? Each morning, I look in the magnifying mirror and I don't like what I see: enlarged pores, blackheads, wrinkles, brown spots. Skin care products? You name it, I've tried it. But nothing seems to work.'

ABOUT YOUR SKIN

Put down that magnifying mirror! It will only reveal what you already know. If your questionnaire results showed that you have ORPW skin, it's no surprise that you have ongoing skin care challenges. There is hardly any skin issue from which you are exempt (except for skin sensitivity), and picking at your face will not solve the problem.

I can't guarantee that the oiliness, enlarged pores, and dark spots that have marred your complexion since adolescence can be cured in an instant, nor will your skin problems disappear with age. However, for ORPW women, skin oiliness *will* lessen in midlife, although it can leave enlarged pores and acne scars in its wake. What's more, the aging process will result in wrinkling. Yes, ORPWs, you get a hit on both sides of the youth-age spectrum.

ORPW CELEBRITY

No one reveals the up- and downsides of ORPW skin better than the original blonde bombshell, Brigitte Bardot. Her signature long blonde tresses, voluptuous body, pouty mouth, and uninhibited carnality made her the incarnation of desire during her heyday. As a sex symbol, she was the French counterpart to Marilyn Monroe.

From her dark eyes and ease in tanning, I surmise that BB is an Oily, Pigmented Skin Type. I've never seen pictures of her with acne so I'm guessing that she had resistant skin. Her ability to tan could have protected her from skin cancer that might have ravaged the skin of a blonde, blue-eyed beauty with the same habits. Although she tanned well and looked great with a tan, as do many ORPWs, she definitely paid the price for it later in life.

Unlike Marilyn Monroe, who avoided the sun to protect her creamy, pale skin, Bardot bared all – or nearly all – to the camera and to the sun. In the 1950s, when Bardot ruled, tanning first came to be considered appealing. In Europe, for many centuries before the mid-twentieth, tanned skin had been viewed as unattractive, unfashionable, and low class, because the hard-working people who performed the labour that sustained society had to endure sun exposure, while the ruling class, living in thick-walled palaces, did not. But in the post-World War II era, the French Riviera became popular with rich society folk, as did tanning. Beauty pioneer Helena Rubinstein was part of this crowd, but she took care to wear sunscreen and sit under an umbrella to protect her skin. The new appeal of tanning spread to the masses via movies and tanned starlets like Bardot. People discovered the sun, and tanned skin came to be seen as healthy, sexy and fun. It is that perception that drives people to tan today.

From her late fifties on, Bardot is practically unrecognisable in photos that reveal the deeply lined face and leathery skin resulting from excess tanning. By then, Bardot was rich and retired, and probably couldn't care less. Perhaps her deeply lined face permits her to go to a shop or museum without being mobbed. But since you don't have that problem, learn from her mistakes, and protect yourself from premature aging with sunblock. For those of you born after Bardot's era, look to Donatella Versace as a contemporary blonde with a tan and an attitude. Sexy Sir Sean Connery also most likely has this Skin Type.

FREE TO EXPERIMENT

All ORPWs are at risk for wrinkles. But if you quit smoking and sunning, the right skin care products can help alleviate your skin problems. But be warned: most over-the-counter products will not be sufficiently concentrated for your tough all-weather skin!

Resistant skin has one significant upside: it's nonreactive. That means you can experiment with different products without negative responses. For you, no rashes, no burning or stinging – all hallmarks of skin sensitivity. Sensitive types get paranoid about products, afraid to try new things. But you can freely sample different products at department store cosmetic counters. You can wash your face with any soap that's handy. When visiting relatives or staying in a hotel, you can use the shampoo without experiencing dryness or irritation.

Your Skin Type proves why 'one size fits all' skin care can never work. While sensitive types need to calm skin reactivity, you need products and ingredients that turn up the juice. While in their respective chapters, I warn sensitive types *away* from products that are too intense for them, in this chapter, I'll point ORPWs *towards* powerhouse concentrations of active ingredients that your hardy skin calls for.

Ian's Story

I an, a handsome executive in his early forties, retired to Bermuda, where he lived the good life. He first came to see me with the complaint of dark spots on his cheeks when he and his current girlfriend were on vacation in Miami. Developing gradually over the last few years, these dark spots had worsened lately. Although he wasn't worried that they were dangerous or cancerous, he didn't like the way they looked.

What's more, he was embarrassed to admit that they bothered him because he believed that guys shouldn't care about their skin's appearance. He'd been given gift certificates for facials at a skin care salon in Bermuda. He was way too embarrassed to even consider receiving a beauty treatment.

So there he was, treating his dark spots in my Miami office, where no one would discover his secret. I was glad that he'd overcome his reservations and placed his trust in me.

During our consultation, Ian was surprised to learn that facials would not have helped since aestheticians can't use ingredients strong enough for his resistant skin. Nor could they prescribe a strong retinoid such as Retin-A gel or Tazorac gel, which is what he really needed. As I wrote a prescription, Ian sat up and took notice.

'All I have to do is fill this prescription? Now, that's more like it,' Ian said with relief. Also, because Differin, the prescription I recommended, has a medical-sounding name, Ian no longer feared that someone might see it in his bathroom cabinet. Although prescribed for his brown spots, Differin will help prevent wrinkles as well. Even if he wouldn't have wanted to admit it to his golfing buddies, Ian was receiving antiaging treatment.

A CLOSE-UP LOOK AT YOUR SKIN

Like Ian, with ORPW skin, you may experience any of the following:

- Large pores
- Shiny, oily skin
- Trouble finding sunscreen that doesn't make your skin oilier
- Dark spots in sun-exposed areas
- Wrinkles
- Occasional acne breakouts
- Easy use of most skin care and cosmetic products
- Increased risk of skin cancer if you have light skin

I recommend sunscreen for all types, but since you are prone to oiliness, it's essential to find a product that does not increase it. Later in this chapter, I'll offer daily skin care regimens using both nonprescription and prescription products. While prescription medications are always more active and therefore most effective, they are particularly important for you because you won't see results with less active products.

HOW YOUR SKIN AGES

ORPW skin changes over time. Younger ORPWs have problems with oil, while older ORPWs lose their oiliness and develop wrinkles. In your fifties your skin may even change to a DRPW Skin Type. That's why using prescription retinoids in your younger years is paramount. These products possess a dual action ideal for you: they help decrease oil secretion *and* prevent wrinkles.

Aging improves oiliness while reducing new dark spots. As your hormone levels drop, so does your production of pigment, causing melasma and dark spots to lessen. However, taking hormone replacement reverses that effect. This is a double bind for ORPWs, since hormone replacement, while worsening pigmentation, helps prevent further wrinkling. I recommend that you consult your gynaecologist to make your decision, taking into account both personal and family history.

To prevent and treat both wrinkles and dark spots, I recommend sun avoidance, daily skin care, retinoid use, and other suggestions offered in the procedures section of this chapter. If desired, use self-tanners, which do not worsen dark spots, as some pigmented types fear. Tanners temporarily dye the surface layer of dead skin cells, but don't activate the skin pigments that cause dark spots. To learn more about their use, please see Chapter Ten, 'Self-Tanners'.

WHAT PRODUCTS DO I NEED?

In search of a solution for wrinkles, ORPWs easily fall victim to marketing ploys, purchasing antiwrinkle creams geared for dry skin. When I gave my Skin Type questionnaire to four hundred patients, I discovered that most oily types use moisturiser. Smearing on a heavy night cream increases oiliness and blackheads and is definitely contraindicated for you. Yet most Americans have been fooled into believing that everyone needs moisturiser. Not true!

Increasing skin hydration will not reduce wrinkle formation, although it may cause tiny, dry lines to puff up temporarily. Nor does moisturiser help prevent wrinkles unless it contains ingredients like antioxidants and retinoids. Although dry types need moisturizing, you definitely do not (unless you tested nearer the combination range of 27–35 on the oily/dry spectrum of the questionnaire).

AN UNDERSERVED SKIN TYPE

For the most part, product researchers and developers fail to formulate products for your special needs. Cosmetic shelves overflow with products for sensitive skin, but none for resistant skin. It's perceived by the industry to be 'easy', but with multiple skin problems, yours is not the easiest Resistant Skin Type. Both resistant and oily, your skin's strong barrier keeps out irritating ingredients. The downside is it keeps out *all* ingredients, even beneficial ones your skin needs. That's why it's tough to find nonprescription-strength products that work. Have you ever seen skin care products designed for 'tough skin'?

Companies can't regulate who purchases their over-the-counter products. They therefore produce products of lower strength that a sensitive type can safely use because they want to avoid the negative publicity that could result from consumers reacting adversely to their products.

As Skin Typing becomes well known and people learn their Skin Type, I hope that manufacturers will be able to offer products specifically geared towards the different types. If that occurs, ORPWs will no longer be underserved.

Until that time, a prescription retinoid is most valuable for ORPW skin because it may decrease oil production and prevent, or even help to eliminate, dark spots and wrinkles. For more information on retinoids and their use, please see 'Further Help for Oily, Resistant Skin'. Buy the cheapest cleansers and sunscreens because your resistant skin does not require babying.

Save your money for prescription medications that really do the job.

Amanda was a throaty-voiced museum curator whom I met at a cocktail party. Once she heard I was a dermatologist, she stubbed out her cigarette and perched near me, ready with a litany of skin care problems. 'As a teenager, my skin was oily,' she explained. 'By my twenties, my cheeks looked like a combat zone, with enlarged pores and visible oil glands that gave my skin a pebbly appearance. In my thirties, dark spots accumulated on my cheeks and upper lip,' she enumerated. 'Now that I am past forty, hello, wrinkles.' I shook my head sympathetically as Amanda lit another cigarette and confided, 'I feel like an old bag. Now, you're a dermatologist. Just tell me what I'm supposed to do. I mean, most of these so-called products are worse than useless.' I handed her my card. She peered at it. 'You're the director, really?' she declaimed doubtfully. 'Huh, hard to believe, you look so young.'

I'd had enough. After all, secondhand smoke is harmful to my skin too. I urged her to call and assured her that I would be happy to refer her to an older associate if need be. Then I headed out to the deck.

No, I wasn't trying to drum up business. For ORPWs like Amanda, it's definitely worth the expense of an office visit to a dermatologist, who can recommend the powerful prescription medications and medical procedures that will really make a difference. It may very well save you hundreds of pounds that you might have spent on useless skin care products, facials, facial exercising machines, and other minimally effective treatments.

The recommendations I'll offer you will definitely help, but there is no quick fix. Over a lifetime, to help your skin look its best will require dedication, along with the use of retinoids, sunscreen, antioxidants, and the right diet. Your skin's future is up to you.

Dr Baumann's Bottom Line: Go for it! You can use the strongest products. And don't forget to prevent wrinkles by smoking cessation, sun avoidance, and a healthy diet with ample fruits and vegetables.

EVERYDAY CARE FOR YOUR SKIN TYPE

The goal of your skin care routine is to address dark spots with products that deliver depigmenting ingredients such as kojic acid, arbutin and vitamin C, and to address wrinkles with products containing retinoids and antioxidants. All the products I'll recommend act to do one or more of the following:

- Prevent and treat dark spots
- Prevent and treat wrinkles

In addition, your daily regimen will help address your other skin concerns by:

- Treating oiliness
- Addressing blackheads and enlarged pores

ORPWs who are under thirty will have more problems with oily skin; for those who are older, oil production will have leveled off, but you'll be seeing increased wrinkles. For younger ORPWs, therefore, your goal is to address oiliness and to prevent wrinkles with appropriate skin care. For older ORPWs, wrinkle prevention and treatment is paramount.

I'll provide you with a two-stage regimen, including both nonprescription and prescription recommendations. In my opinion, no amount of over-the-counter (OTC) skin care will get rid of wrinkles – you need retinoids or a procedure such as Botox or Juvéderm injections. If you choose to follow the prescription recommendations and procedures, then use the nonprescription protocol to care for your skin for eight weeks or until your dermatology appointment. Since often you may have to wait a few months to see a dermatologist, I suggest you go ahead and make the appointment right away if you think you might need it. You can always cancel it.

If you choose to forego the prescription route, you can follow the nonprescription regimen indefinitely. In that case, look for toners, sunscreens, facial foundations, and evening treatment lotions or gels that contain retinol, a related but less powerful ingredient. Most retinol products only contain a low amount, so you can safely use several different kinds of skin care products with retinol to increase the results.

DAILY SKIN CARE

STAGE ONE: NONPRESCRIPTION REGIMEN

AM	PM
Step 1: Wash with oil-control cleanser	Step 1: Wash with glycolic acid or salicylic cleanser
Step 2: Use toner (optional)	Step 2: Apply skin lightening serum to entire face
Step 3: Apply skin lightener to spots	Step 3: Apply retinol or antioxidant skin serum
Step 4: Apply an oil-control product (optional)	Step 4: Apply moisturiser (optional)
Step 5: Apply moisturiser (optional)	
Step 6: Apply sunscreen	
Step 7: Apply powder with SPF or oil-absorption qualities	

In the morning, wash your face with an oil-control cleanser, then use a toner if you choose. Then apply a skin lightener to dark spots that you wish to treat. Next, you may choose to apply an oil-control product if you have an O/D score over 33. Or if instead you have combination skin (O/D score of 27–33), you can choose to apply a moisturiser in the dry areas (avoid the T-zone). Also, for combination skin, if your face feels slightly dry overall, you can apply moisturiser to your entire face. Then apply a sunscreen. Finally, apply either a powder with SPF or an oil-absorbing powder.

In the evening, wash with a cleanser containing glycolic or salicylic acid. Apply a skin lightening serum to your entire face to help prevent dark spots, then your choice of retinol product or antioxidant serum to help prevent wrinkles. Finally, apply moisturiser if you are using one.

You can also increase exfoliation by using facial scrubs directly after cleansing at night. See the products I recommend later in this section.

Cleansers

To control oil and prevent enlarged pores, keep your skin clean by using cleansers both morning and evening. ORPWs should stay away from cream cleansers or cold creams. Choose a gel cleanser or a foaming cleanser. Oil-control cleansers and those with glycolic acid and salicylic acid are also good for you. Glycolic acid cleansers are easier to find in the US than in the UK. When travelling or shopping at www.Baumannstore.co.uk, look for ones by Neostrada and MD Formulations that you don't have in the UK.

RECOMMENDED CLEANSERS

- £ Botanics Skin Brightening Deep Clean Gel
- £ Neutrogena Visibly Refined Facial Wash
- £ Time Dimensions Clarifying Facial Exfoliator
- ££ Biotherm Biopur Pore Refining Exfoliating Gel – Exfoliator for Oily Skin
- ££ Exuviance Purifying Cleansing Gel
- ££ Laura Mercier Oil Free Gel Cleanser
- ££ PCA Skin pHaze 13 Pigment Bar
- ££ Paula's Choice One Step Facial Cleanser for Oily Skin
- ££ Philosophy On a Clear Day Super Wash for Oily Skin
- £££ Cellex-C Betaplex Gentle Foaming Cleanser
- £££ Dermatologica Dermal Clay Cleanser
- £££ Jurlique Foaming Facial Cleanser
- £££ Lancôme Ablutia Fraîcheur Purifying Foaming Cleanser
- £££ N.V. Perricone M.D. Pore Refining Cleanser

Baumann's Choice: PCA Skin pHaze 13 Pigment Bar contains lighteners like kojic acid and niacinamide.

Toner Use

Look for toners with oil-control, depigmenting, and antioxidant ingredients. If using a prescription retinoid, use a toner with alpha hydroxy or beta hydroxy acids. Otherwise, look for a toner with retinol. Those with O/D scores above 33 will probably want to use only a toner and skip the moisturizing step altogether.

RECOMMENDED TONERS

£ Dove Essential Nutrients Toner
£ Johnson & Johnson Clean & Clear Black Head Clear Toner
£ Neutrogena Visibly Refined Facial Toner
£ Nivea Visage Gentle Refreshing Toner
£ Time Dimensions Refining Toning Water
££ Dr Hauschka Clarifying Toner
££ Natura Bisse Oily Skin Toner
££ Ole Henriksen Pick-Me-Up Face Tonic
££ SkinCeuticals' Equalizing Toner
££ YonKa Lotion PNG for Normal to Oily Skin
£££ Cellex-C Betaplex Fresh Complexion Mist
£££ N.V. Perricone M.D. Firming Facial Toner

Baumann's Choice: Time Dimensions Refining Toning Water because it has alpha hydroxy acid.

Oil-Control Products

You can use an oil-control product in addition to or instead of toners if you have an O/D score of 33 or more. You can also choose oil-control foundations and powders. Blotting tissues are helpful in absorbing oil throughout the day. Many oily types like to keep them handy.

RECOMMENDED OIL-CONTROL PRODUCTS

£ Crabtree and Evelyn Facial Blotting Tissues
£ Seban liquid
£ Simple Oil Control Facial Wipes
££ Ferndale O.C. Eight Oil Control Gel
££ Mary Kay Beauty Blotters Oil-Absorbing Tissues
££ Paula's Choice 1% Beta Hydroxy Acid Gel
£££ Clarins Mat Express Instant Shine Control Gel
£££ Dermatologica Oil Control Lotion
£££ Gatineau Purifying Regulating Serum
£££ Korres Lemon Anti-Shine Gel
£££ Molton Brown Instant Matte Shine Control SPF 15

£££ Ole Henriksen Grease Relief Face Tonic
£££ Thalgo Intense Regulating Serum

Baumann's Choice: Molton Brown Instant Matte Shine Control because it has sunscreen.

Treating Dark Spots

For dark spots, use skin lightening products after cleansing and toning, but before other products. Apply at the first sign of a dark spot, and continue until the spot has disappeared completely. To both treat and prevent dark spots, use products containing retinol and other ingredients that increase cell turnover, such as alpha hydroxy and beta hydroxy acids. Niacinamide and soy help prevent the formation of brown spots. Look for soy products that have had the oestrogenic components removed like the ones from Neutrogena that contain 'active soy'. If you find that these nonprescription skin lighteners do not produce results in eight weeks, a dermatologist can prescribe a prescription lightener. Hydroquinone, which is commonly found in skin lighteners in the US, is not available in the UK and many Asian countries.

RECOMMENDED PRODUCTS FOR TREATING DARK SPOTS

£ Neutrogena Ultimate Moisture Day Cream
£ Olay Regenerist Daily Regenerating Serum
££ La Roche-Posay Active C Light
£££ DDF Intensive Holistic Corrector Swabs
£££ Estée Lauder Re-Nutriv Intensive Lifting Serum
£££ Prescriptives Skin Tone Correcting Serum
£££ Rodan & Fields Radiant 3 Treat
£££ SkinCeuticals Phyto + Corrective Gel

Baumann's Choice: SkinCeuticals Phyto + Corrective Gel. (The US has many more choices in this category. See www.Baumannstore.co.uk)

Wrinkle Prevention

Although retinoids are the only effective products for treating wrinkles that have already developed, many OTC products can help *prevent* wrinkles.

RECOMMENDED ANTIOXIDANT SERUMS TO PREVENT WRINKLES

£ Roc Retin Ox Anti-Wrinkle Serum Max (with retinol)
££ Dr Andrew Weil for Origins Plantidote Mega-Mushroom Face Serum
££ La Roche-Posay Active C Light
££ Laura Mercier Multi Vitamin Serum
££ Origins A Perfect World White Tea Skin Guardian
££ Pure Simplicity White Tea Line Prevention Serum
££ SkinCeuticals C E Ferulic
££ SkinCeuticals Serum 20
£££ Allergan Prevage MD Anti-Aging Treatment
£££ Elizabeth Arden Prevage Anti-Aging Treatment
£££ Estée Lauder Re-Nutriv Intensive Lifting Serum
£££ MD Formulations Moisture Defence Antioxidant Serum
£££ Organic Pharmacy Antioxidant Serum
£££ Prada Hydrating Gel Matte (with lightening ingredients)
£££ Ultraceuticals Antioxidant Serum

Baumann's Choice: SkinCeuticals C E Ferulic to prevent aging. Use Skinceuticals Serum 20 to prevent aging and improve dark spots. The research behind these is brilliant!

Moisturisers

If your O/D score is high (above 35), you probably won't need a moisturiser. With scores of 34 to 44, you may opt to use moisturiser on the dry areas only. If so, look for products formulated for oily skin with oil-control ingredients.

For daytime use, pick a moisturiser with sunscreen. In night creams, search out products with retinol. If you choose to use a moisturiser all over your face – something I recommend only for those with scores between 27 and 33 – look for products with lightening ingredients or antioxidants.

RECOMMENDED DAYTIME MOISTURISERS

- £ Roc Retin Ox Anti-Wrinkle Serum Max (with retinol)
- £ Eucerin Q10 Active Anti-Wrinkle Fluid SPF 15
- £ Nivea Anti-wrinkle Q10 Plus Day Cream
- £ Paula's Choice Skin Balancing Moisture Gel
- ££ Skinceuticals Renew Overnight Oily
- ££ SkinMedica Ultra Sheer Moisturiser
- ££ YonKa CremePG
- ££ Jurlique Day Care Face Lotion
- £££ Caudalie Day Fluid SPF12 with Resveratrol
- £££ pH Advantage Control Regimen AM Facial Multi-Complex SPF 20

Baumann's Choice: For AM, Eucerin Q10 Active Anti-Wrinkle Fluid SPF 15. For PM, Roc Retin Ox Anti-Wrinkle Serum- Max.

Masks

Masks, used once or twice a week, are another good way to give your skin the strong ingredients it needs. I personally think you'd do better going to a spa, salon, or a dermatologist for a chemical peel or microdermabrasion, which can help improve fine lines and dark spots, but if you don't have the time or the money, try a mask. They improve skin oiliness only temporarily, but that can be useful before special occasions, when you want to look your best.

RECOMMENDED MASKS

- £ Ahava Advanced Mud Masque for Oily Skin
- £ Bioré Pore Perfect Self-Heating Mask
- £ Palmers Skin Success Even Tone Brightening Facial Mask
- £ Montagne Jeunesse Cucumber Peel-Off Masque
- ££ DDF Clay Mint Mask
- ££ Decléor Clay and Herbal Cleansing Mask
- ££ Elizabeth Arden Deep Cleansing Mask
- ££ Jurlique Moor Purifying Mask
- ££ Laura Mercier Deep Cleansing Clay Mask
- ££ True Blue Spa All in a Clay's Work Detoxifying Facial Mask
- £££ Chanel Précision Masque Pureté Express Instant Purifying Mask
- £££ Dr Brandt Poreless Purifying Mask

Baumann's Choice: True Blue Spa All in a Clay's Work Detoxifying Facial Mask has clay to absorb oil and licorice root extract to decrease pigment.

Exfoliation

Cleopatra, famous for her gorgeous skin, was very likely this type. She was known to use sour milk on her face. Without knowing it, she was giving herself a lactic acid–alpha hydroxy acid peel, which speeds the removal of dark spots.

Scrubs and microdermabrasion kits can remove the top, dead layer of the skin to allow better penetration of the active ingredients in toners and moisturisers. If your daily routine includes a prescription retinoid, retinol, alpha hydroxy acid, or beta hydroxy acid product, any form of scrub or exfoliation should only be done twice a week. If you are not using any of these products, you can use your choice of exfoliation product every other day, so long as you don't experience redness or soreness.

Do not use both scrubs and peels; pick one or the other. Too much exfoliation can cause redness and skin sensitivity, making you feel like an OSPW. If you choose peels, however, I advise that you go to a salon or spa, since they are licensed to offer stronger peels than those available in kits for at-home use, which have a much lower concentration of active ingredients. (Of course, dermatologists can give you the most potent peels.) Note: the Obagi system, recommended below, has six steps, including one using prescription Retin-A, but you can go ahead and get started without it.

RECOMMENDED SCRUBS

£ Benefit Pineapple Facial Polish
£ Fresh Sugar Face Polish
£ L'Oréal Refinish Micro-Dermabrasion Kit
££ Decléor Micro-Exfoliating Gel
££ Laura Mercier Face Polish
££ Rodan & Fields Reverse Exfoliate
££ Dr Brandt Microdermabrasion In A Jar
£££ La Prairie Cellular Microdermabrasion Cream
£££ Prescriptives Dermapolish System

Baumann's Choice: L'Oreal Refinish Micro-Dermabrasion Kit

RECOMMENDED AT-HOME PEEL PRODUCTS

£ L'Oreal ReNoviste Home Peel Kit

££ Dermalogica Daily Microfoliant

££ Elizabeth Arden Peel & Reveal Revitalising Treatment

££ MD Skincare Alpha Beta Daily Face Peel

£££ Lancôme Resurface Peel

£££ Natura Bisse Glyco Peeling 50% Pump

Baumann's Choice: Alpha Beta Daily Face Peel by MD Skincare, which combines AHA and BHA.

RECOMMENDED KITS

££ M.D. Forté Normal/Combination Skin Introductory Set

££ Philosophy Microdelivery Peel

££ DDF Holistic Lightening Protocol

££ DDF Potent Lightening Protocol

££ Dermalogica Skin Brightening System

£££ Dr Michelle Copeland Anti-Aging Kit

£££ Obagi System

£££ Rodan & Fields Reverse Regimen

£££ Vichy Microabrasion Peel Kit

Baumann's Choice: Rodan & Fields Reverse Regimen is expensive, but I like the ingredients and it's perfect for your type. If you want to, this is a recommended way to splurge. It's not in the UK yet but you can find it at www.Baumannstore.co.uk.

SHOPPING FOR PRODUCTS

To widen your choice of products, read product labels and choose those that contain beneficial ingredients for the particular problem you want to address, as listed below.

There are also ingredients you need to avoid. Some products contain ingredients that can increase oiliness. Others may make your skin more sensitive to sunlight, causing more tanning and dark spots in localised areas. For example, perfumes containing oil of bergamot (also found in Earl Grey tea) can create darkening on the neck. Also, if you drink margaritas while out in the sun, you may notice increased tanning around your mouth or in other areas that come into contact with lime juice.

RECOMMENDED INGREDIENTS

For wrinkle prevention:

- ALA
- Caffeine
- Coenzyme Q_{10} (Ubiquinone)
- Copper peptide
- Ginseng
- Grape seed extract
- Green tea
- Idebenone
- Lutein
- Lycopene
- Moringa
- Pinus pinaster (Pine bark)
- Pomegranate
- Resveratrol
- Rosemary
- Vitamin C
- Vitamin E

For wrinkle treatment:

- Alpha lipoic acid
- Copper peptide
- DMAE
- Glycolic acid (alpha hydroxy acid or AHA)
- Lactic acid
- Phytic acid
- Retinol
- Salicylic acid (beta hydroxy acid or BHA)
- TGF-Beta

To prevent dark spots:

- Cocos nucifera (coconut fruit juice)
- Niacinamide

To hasten removal of dark spots:

- Arbutin
- Bearberry
- Cucumber extract
- Epilobium angustifolium (willow herb)
- Gallic acid
- Glycyrrhiza glabra (licorice extract)
- Kojic acid
- Mulberry
- Pycnogenol (a pine bark extract)
- Resorcinol
- Retinol
- Salicylic acid (beta hydroxy acid)
- Saxifraga sarmentosa extract (strawberry begonia)
- Vitamin C (ascorbic acid)

SKIN CARE INGREDIENTS TO AVOID

Due to excess oiliness:

- Mineral oil
- Other oils such as coconut oil
- Petrolatum

Due to hormonal activity that increases pigmentation and dark spots:

Topical oestrogen and estradiol are oestrogens present in hormone replacement treatments and some topical creams; these can increase pigmentation. Phyto-oestrogens, compounds found in plants, also produce similar effects. These include:

- Cimicifuga racemosa (black cohosh)
- Vitex agnus-castus (chasteberry)
- Humulus lupulus (hops)
- Trifolium pretense (red clover)
- Soy (except in Roc, Aveeno and Neutrogena products, where the oestrogenic ingredient has been removed)
- Wild yams

Due to skin darkening effects:

- Extracts of celery, limes, parsley, figs and carrots
- Oil of bergamot

Sun Protection for Your Skin

Most sunscreens are formulated in an oil base because their active ingredients are usually oil soluble. Oily sunscreens can make your skin look shiny, so use gels or sprays. Powders with SPF are another excellent option. One of my new favourites is a powder foundation with sunscreen (SPF 15) made by Philosophy that's called The Supernatural. Formulated for oily skin, it comes in two shades to match different skin tones.

Avobenzone is one superior UVA sunscreen that comes in gel forms. You can also decrease sunscreen oiliness by mixing and applying sunscreen together with O.C. Eight Oil Control Gel by Ferndale.

My favourite sunscreen, Anthelios by La Roche Posay, contains a UVA blocker called Mexoryl that's superior to those available in the US or the

UK, but you can always stock up if you take a holiday in France or Ireland. (Buy the Anthelios Fluid Extreme; it's best for oily skin.)

RECOMMENDED SUN PROTECTION PRODUCTS

- £ Eucerin Q$_{10}$ Active Anti-Wrinkle Fluid SPF 15
- £ Neutrogena Visibly Refined Moisturiser SPF15
- ££ Boscia Oil-Free Daily Hydration SPF 15
- ££ Clarins Sun Control Stick SPF 30
- ££ Clinique Super City Block Oil-Free Daily Face Protector SPF 25
- ££ Estée Lauder Multi-Protection Sun Spray (Oil-Free) SPF 15
- ££ Exuviance Fundamental Multi-Protective Day Fluid SPF 15
- ££ Exuviance Multi-Defence Day Fluid SPF 15 with AHAs
- ££ Garnier Ambre Solaire Sheer Protect Shine Free SPF 30
- ££ La Roche-Posay Anthelios XL SPF 60 Fluide Extreme
- ££ NeoStrada Oil-Free Lotion SPF 15
- ££ Philosophy A Pigment of Your Imagination SPF 18 (not in the UK)
- £££ La Mer SPF 18 Fluid

Baumann's Choice: Neutrogena Visibly Refined Moisturiser SPF15 because it contains alpha hydroxy acid. If you shop online, look for Philosophy A Pigment of Your Imagination SPF 18. It contains skin lightening ingredients as well as sunscreen.

Your Makeup

ORPWs may have trouble choosing makeup foundations. To cover dark spots, you need a heavier foundation, which may streak. If you're over forty, heavier makeup products can run into wrinkles, making them more noticeable.

If pigment is not a problem, choose a sheerer foundation and cover it with a powder. If pigment is a problem, choose a heavier foundation that hides dark spots and also works well for oily skin.

Since you can never get enough sunscreen, use makeup products containing SPF whenever you can. Also listed below are a concealer and lip colour that both have sunscreen.

RECOMMENDED FOUNDATIONS

£ Avon Beyond Colour Perfecting Foundation with Natural Match Technology SPF 12

£ Boots No7 Uplifting Foundation SPF 15

££ Bobbi Brown Oil-Free Even Finish Foundation SPF 15

££ Exuviance CoverBlend Concealing Treatment Makeup SPF 20

££ FACE Stockholm Powder Foundation

££ Laura Mercier Oil-Free Foundation

£££ DiorSkin Compact with SPF 20

£££ Lancôme Maquicontrôle Oil-Free Liquid Makeup

Baumann's Choice: Boots No7 Uplifting Foundation SPF 15

RECOMMENDED POWDERS

£ L'Oréal Air Wear Powder Foundation SPF 17

£ Maybelline Pure Stay Powder & Foundation SPF 15

£ Paula's Select Healthy Finish Pressed Powder with SPF 15

££ Bare Escentuals i.d. bareMinerals SPF 15 Foundation

££ Bloom Pressed Powder

££ Laura Mercier Translucent Pressed Setting Powder

££ Philosophy The Supernatural Airbrushed Canvas

£££ Lancôme Star Bronzer Bronzing Powder Compact SPF 8 for Face and Body

Baumann's Choice: Maybelline Pure Stay Powder & Foundation SPF 15

RECOMMENDED CONCEALER

£ Avon Beyond Colour Line Diminishing Concealer SPF 15

££ Bloom Concealer

££ Cover Blend Multi Function Concealer

££ Laura Mercier Undercover

££ Paul and Joe Stick Concealer SPF 15

££ Philosophy Supernatural Airbrushed Colour Corrector

££ MAKE Under Eye Transformer

£££ Sisley Phytocernes Botanical Concealer

Baumann's choice: Philosophy Supernatural Airbrushed Colour Corrector because it has several shades.

RECOMMENDED LIP COLOURS

£ Avon Beyond Colour Plumping Lipcolour with Retinol SPF 15
££ Bloom Lip Tint SPF 8
££ Elizabeth Arden Eight Hour Cream Lip Protectant Stick Sheer Tint SPF 15
££ Laura Mercier Lip Kisses with SPF 15
£££ Ole Henriksen Fresh Lips SPF 15

Baumann's Choice: Any of the above because they have sunscreen.

You can make your makeup needs work for you. Look for a powder compact that can also be a fashion statement. I have dry skin and do not use much facial powder; however, I have a passion for collecting powder compacts. I have vintage ones, gorgeous new ones by Jay Strongwater and look forward every Christmas to the new compacts by Estée Lauder. I have to admit that I'm addicted to shopping for powder compacts on eBay. For those of you with oily skin, carry one of the gorgeous compacts with you and touch up your makeup every few hours or before a photograph to prevent the telltale signs of oily skin.

CONSULTING A DERMATOLOGIST

PRESCRIPTION SKIN CARE STRATEGIES

I'll offer two Stage Two prescription regimens; the first is for treating dark spots when you have them, and it will treat wrinkles as well. The second is a maintenance regimen that treats wrinkles once the dark spots have cleared. Both feature retinoids, which address all your skin problems: wrinkles, oiliness, and dark spots. With a high O/D score (35 or above), your best retinoids are gel forms. If you have a middle or low O/D score (27–34), you can tolerate creams without feeling too greasy. For more information about retinoids and how to use them in this regimen, please consult 'Further Help for Oily, Resistant Skin'.

DAILY SKIN CARE

STAGE TWO: PRESCRIPTION REGIMEN

For treating dark spots:

AM	PM
Step 1: Wash with a cleanser	Step 1: Wash with a glycolic acid cleanser
Step 2: Apply a prescription skin lightener to spots	Step 2: Apply a prescription skin lightener to spots
Step 3: With higher O/D score, apply oil-control gel; with lower O/D score, apply a moisturiser	Step 3: Apply a retinoid or an antioxidant serum
Step 4: Apply sunscreen	Step 4: Apply moisturiser (optional)
Step 5: Apply powder with SPF	

In the morning, wash with a cleanser containing glycolic acid. Then apply a prescription skin lightener to the spots. Depending on your O/D score, you'll next apply either a nonprescription oil-control product for O/D scores of 35 and above, or moisturiser with SPF for O/D scores of 27–34. Next apply the sunscreen. (You can mix the oil-control product with the sunscreen, if wished.) Last, apply powder containing SPF.

In the evening, wash with the same cleanser. Next, apply a prescription skin lightener followed by a retinoid. Apply a moisturiser as the last step, if your O/D score is in the range indicated.

You can stay on this regimen until dark spots improve (approximately eight weeks) and then switch to the maintenance regimen.

STAGE TWO: MAINTENANCE REGIMEN

To treat and prevent wrinkles:

AM	PM
Step 1: Wash with a cleanser	Step 1: Wash with a glycolic acid cleanser
Step 2: Apply oil-control gel or a moisturiser depending on your O/D score	Step 2: Apply a prescription retinoid or antioxidant serum
Step 3: Apply sunscreen	Step 3: Apply moisturiser (optional)
Step 4: Apply powder with SPF	

In the morning, wash with a cleanser. Depending on your O/D score, apply either nonprescription oil-control product, for scores of 35 and above or moisturiser with SPF, for scores of 27–34. Next, apply sunscreen. Last, apply powder containing SPF.

In the evening, wash with a cleanser containing glycolic acid. Next, apply a prescription retinoid or a nonprescription antioxidant serum. Apply a moisturiser as the last step, if you choose.

RECOMMENDED PRESCRIPTION PRODUCTS

To treat dark spots:

- Claripel (lightener cream with SPF)
- Eldoquin Forte
- EpiQuin Micro
- Lustra-AF (with SPF)
- Solaquin Forte (with SPF)
- Tri-Luma

Baumann's Choice: These products contain hydroquinone so they are not available in the UK. Please ask your dermatologist for a comparable product.

To combat wrinkles and dark spots:

- Aknemycin Plus (contains an antibiotic as well)
- Differin gel or cream
- Isotrex
- Isotrexin (contains an antiobiotic as well)
- Retin-A gel, lotion, or cream
- Retinova

Baumann's Choice: Use the highest strength that you can tolerate.

PROCEDURES FOR YOUR SKIN TYPE

Procedures like lasers and light treatments can't be used on dark skin. Instead, ORPWs with dark skin tones can use topical products to decrease oiliness and dark spots. Resistant types have an advantage over sensitive types, because you can use stronger ingredients without fear of sensitivity, so you may see results faster. Expect to wait about four to eight weeks to see the dark spots improve. Dark-skinned ORPWs may also benefit from chemical peels containing salicylic acid (BHA) 20 percent or 30 percent or combinations of glycolic acid and other depigmenting ingredients. Retinoids used in your skin care regimen will enhance the penetration of the peel and will help you heal faster afterwards by stepping up cell division.

If you have darker skin, choose a dermatologist who is skilled at treating dark-skinned people, because dark spots can worsen if chemical peels are not done correctly. These peels range from £50 to £100 per peel and a series of five to eight is normal.

To Reduce Pores

Skin care procedures such as facials and microdermabrasion don't really decrease pore size. However, you can obtain temporary pore reduction by using products containing AHAs, BHA, and vitamin C as recommended in the nonprescription product section.

To Reduce Oiliness

For those with light skin, light procedures, such as IPL procedures with Metvix, may decrease oil secretion by shrinking the oil-producing glands (for details see the section on light treatments, in 'Further Help for Oily, Resistant Skin Types').

Procedures to Treat Wrinkles

A number of procedures are available to treat wrinkles. They include injections of botulinum toxin (Botox) and dermal fillers. For more information, see the sections on Botox and dermal fillers in 'Further Help for Oily, Resistant Skin Types'. Lasers and other forms of light treatment for wrinkles show promise for the future, but they are not yet undisputedly effective. In addition, there is a new technique called Thermage. ORPWs are ideal candidates for it. Please see the section on Thermage in 'Further Help for Oily, Resistant Skin Types'.

ONGOING CARE FOR YOUR SKIN

Avoid the sun and stop smoking to preserve your skin. Plus, use retinols and retinoids to reverse sun damage and the signs of aging. Eat an anti-oxidant-rich diet. If your wallet will permit, go for procedures that will bring real results. Your resistant, non-pigmented skin will help protect you from the side effects that other types develop after these procedures. The latest technology is there for you!

CHAPTER NINE

Oily, Resistant, Pigmented and Tight: ORPT

THE GLOWING SKIN TYPE

'I have some skin problems, but nothing that hard to handle. Except for some dark spots and a little acne, I'm pretty happy with my skin. Is there something else I should be doing to go from good skin to great skin?'

ABOUT YOUR SKIN

Yours is definitely one of the easier Skin Types, since your type's strengths far outweigh its deficits. Oily, resistant and tight skin looks great and ages well. Yes, you may get acne (especially in youth) and some dark spots, but your easy care skin has a vibrancy and glow that many ORPTs take for granted.

Luckily, you rarely develop the stinging, redness or product allergies often experienced by more sensitive types. Oily skin is troublesome in youth but, for women, will often improve with menopause. The dark spots, which are your nemesis, do have an upside: the pigmentation that causes them also protects you from skin cancer. Finally, tight skin helps you retain your youthful appearance when other types are hunting down antiaging remedies. Your skin is to be coveted and also protected with regular sunscreen use (even if you have dark-toned skin) as well as a diet high in antioxidant-rich fruits and vegetables.

ORPT skin is quite common among people with a darker skin colour like the many Caribbean-Americans I see in my Florida practise. Lighter-skin-toned people from other ethnic backgrounds, like the Irish, English, Australians, Germans, and others, can also be ORPTs. A redhead with freckles, which are a form of pigmentation, is a classic ORPT type. With smooth, resilient, and tight skin, English actress, Kate Beckinsale, is very likely an ORPT. She has a few freckles, and is able to tan even though her skin usually looks smooth, pale and unblemished. As you can see, there's a lot of variety among people of this type, so if the questionnaire revealed that you're an ORPT, but you don't experience all the symptoms I'll cover, you shouldn't worry that your result is wrong. All ORPTs share a number of common problems, but there are some significant differences, so throughout this chapter, I'll discuss the range of symptoms and tendencies, as well as the various treatment options, available to dark-, medium and light-toned ORPTs.

ORPT CELEBRITY

Oprah Winfrey most likely has ORPT skin, a common Skin Type for people of colour. It's obvious that she has pigmented skin, as most African-Americans do. It's equally obvious that she has well-tended, tight skin, because she appears virtually ageless. If you compare photos of her now and when she was much, much younger, there's hardly any change. That's tight skin. Lucky Oprah! From one of my close colleagues, a female dermatologist who never misses Oprah's show, I understand that Oprah most likely has oily, rather than dry, skin. As to the sensitive vs. resistant factor, my educated guess points towards resistant skin. Why? Because Oprah has never hesitated to share all her personal struggles and triumphs with her legions of fans. If she had sensitive skin, I'm betting we would have heard about it. (OK, so I'm a fan too.)

As an ORPT, pigmentation and oil are most likely Oprah's chief skin issues, and she has them under control. And that's a good thing because a number of on-the-job factors could potentially worsen her skin's condition. Constant makeup touch-ups can increase oiliness and breakouts, while bright television lighting can reveal troublesome, hard-to-hide dark spots. On-the-job stress is another concern, which may be why Oprah has been a pioneer in finding ways to relax, de-stress, treat, and, most of all, be true to oneself. That special glow that emanates from Oprah and that magnetises people comes from her heart. But it doesn't hurt to having glowing ORPT skin as well!

SKIN COLOUR AND THE ORPT

The recommendations in this chapter will help your skin glow more vibrantly, whether you are a dark-skinned ORPT or a light-skinned one. While anyone can have this Skin Type, a high proportion of ORPTs are Africans, African-Americans, Latin-Americans, Middle-Easterners, Indians, Mediterraneans and Asians. By the way, even though Asian skin may look light, it often reacts similarly to darker skin. If you have Asian ancestry, consider yourself in the dark-skinned ORPT group, which will affect the skin recommendations you follow later in this chapter.

I've found that light-toned ORPTs generally have both good genes and healthy skin habits that protect them from the ravages of aging. They often eat lots of fruits and vegetables, do not smoke, and do not intentionally seek sun exposure. I say: good for you, as this combination helps to prevent wrinkles. For others reading this chapter, if you'd like to prevent wrinkles too, remember, genes tell only part of the story, and lifestyle factors can make a big difference!

Julia, a psychotherapist, practised in a small New England town. In her late forties, she had dark blonde hair sprinkled with plenty of grey, while her pale face was sprinkled with freckles. While visiting family in Florida, she came in to have her freckles checked for skin cancer. Melanoma is more prevalent in fair-skinned, freckled ORPTs like Julia.

Fortunately, there was no problem, though I urged her to follow up with regular dermatology checkups. Still, I couldn't help noticing the youthfulness of her skin. Although Julia had passed through menopause, she looked great, with few wrinkles and little sagging. She could have easily been in her late thirties. Curious, I asked about her lifestyle.

Julia was married to her college sweetheart and lived in a charming rural town. Her kids were healthy, and she loved her work, which she considered to be nothing fancier than 'helping people'. Julia and her family had been 'organic' for over ten years and ate a lot of health-protective fruits and vegetables. Every day, during her break, Julia walked around her village to get some exercise. And lo and behold, here was someone who didn't require my sunscreen lecture. To avoid freckling, Julia had been a regular sunscreen user since her teens. She'd learned it from her blonde mother, a sun protection fanatic, who'd coated Julia and her brothers with the 'white stuff' from the time they were tiny tots.

Finally, Julia's levelheadedness and humour protected her soul from life's vicissitudes, just as the sunscreen protected her skin. The balance that she found in her life was reflected in her smooth, unlined face. And the sunscreen didn't hurt either!

Over the years, I've seen a number of light-skinned ORPTs like Julia, who somehow manage to do it all – or most of it – right. It's one reason that I emphasise that though genes may be one part of your destiny, the other part of your destiny is what you do with those genes.

On the other hand, for darker-skinned ORPTs, the most common problem is that your skin is easy, leading many to take their skin for granted and subject it to unnecessarily harsh treatment. Stunning supermodel Naomi Campbell has that ORPT glow, along with the ageless quality that tight skin confers. Even though Campbell has been said to smoke, which ages the skin and can lead to wrinkling, her pigmented, tight skin may protect her from smoking's ravages during her middle years. However, light-skinned ORPTs can tip the balance and wind up as wrinkled ORPWs if they follow Campbell's lead.

YOUR SKIN ISSUES

Dark-skinned ORPTs like Campbell and light-skinned ones like Julia will have slightly different skin issues and treatment options, which I'll discuss separately throughout this chapter.

All dark-skinned ORPTs readily develop dark spots, triggered by any form of skin injury or inflammation, including cuts, burns, bruises and scrapes. Allergic reactions are less common for you than for sensitive types. In most cases, stronger topical products can easily prevent or lighten them, so thank your resistant skin that you can use them while sensitive types cannot. Ingrown hairs can cause dark spots, and dark-skinned male ORPTs experience this in the beard area, especially if they shave.

Women may have excessive facial hair above the lip, on the cheeks, or elsewhere. Darker-skin-toned ORPTs have darker-coloured hair, making unwanted hair growth more noticeable. However, hair removal can create further problems: waxing and chemical depilatories can irritate your skin and leave dark spots in their wake. Plucking hairs can lead to tweezer injury, subsequently leaving dark spots.

Your second major issue is acne and facial shine. You may battle with oily skin, struggle with troublesome breakouts, despair that your face always looks shiny in photos, and avoid wearing necessary sun protection because you can't stand its greasy feel. The trick is to find a sunscreen and other products that don't add to your skin's innate oiliness.

Dina, a beautiful oval-faced Lebanese woman, was a recent graduate of a hotel management programme in Miami. She came to see me, frustrated with what she called her 'all oily, all the time' skin, particularly her shiny forehead and jawline. 'Even my neck feels greasy,' she moaned. As an intern, she had once manned the reception desk of a prestigious hotel, and after a brief power blackout occurred, hotel guests 'told me they could find their way through the darkened lobby by the reflected light on my face. I thought I'd die of embarrassment!' she complained. Together we went over her morning and evening skin care regimen and I made a couple of cleanser and toner recommendations. But two weeks later, there was no improvement. Puzzled, I dug further. When I asked about other aspects of her personal care, I learned that Dina washed and conditioned her medium-length raven black hair daily with products suited for dry hair. Aha! I knew we had identified one of the culprits.

In order to smooth and soften, products like conditioners often include ingredients that remain after washing. They're good for your hair, but a big problem for your skin. Always wash your face after washing and conditioning your hair to remove all product residue. You should also be cautious with bug sprays, sunscreens, hair gels, leave-in conditioners, hand lotions, and other products that may come into contact with your face, as they can contribute to greasiness.

Finding products that fight oil and inflammation without adding oil, or triggering brown spots, is essential. Certain ingredients widely included in skin care stimulate hormones like oestrogen that activate pigmentation, thereby contributing to the formation of brown spots. That's where my ingredient lists will help. I'll offer you my recommendations for a daily routine with a selection of products most effective for ORPT skin. If you're inclined to shop and experiment, check ingredients, and make sure to avoid those that are 'oestrogenic', like the ones I detail in the 'Shopping for Products' section of this chapter.

In the past, some products may have backfired because of the combination of issues you must address. Others may not have been effective enough to help your sturdy and resistant skin. It's a matter of finding the right balance.

Selena's Story

When Selena, a thirty-five-year-old tax and estate attorney, strode into my office I saw a tall, striking, and impeccable woman in a tailored grey pinstripe suit and a crisp white shirt that contrasted smartly with her rich, medium-toned black skin. The reason for her visit was dark patches over her cheeks. She got them every winter.

In looking for lifestyle factors that could have triggered the problem, I learned that she was a single woman and a self-confessed workaholic, who devoted long hours to her full caseload, typically working twelve-hour days, seven days a week. When these dark patches sprang up, she couldn't understand why.

Since sun exposure stimulates pigmentation, I asked about sunscreen use and she confessed that she never would have dreamed of using any. 'I'm not one to laze around in the sun, so why bother?' she replied. She rarely went out in the sun and never went to the beach. On a typical day, Selena would arise; jog on the treadmill in her deluxe condo; bathe, drink a protein drink; and then, at 6:15 sharp, drive in her silver Lexus with tinted windows straight to the parking lot of the office building where she worked. Seven days a week. Her office was windowed. Only rarely did she take a lunch break. Sun exposure? Forget about it.

As I probed to discover the source of her skin complaint, I was frankly mystified.

'I've wondered if maybe I have an allergy,' she suggested.

While I was prepared to test for that, I was doubtful, since allergies are far more common in Sensitive Skin Types.

'And what do you do for fun?' I pursued further.

'Maybe once a month go out at night with friends to hear music,' she replied. 'And of course, I keep up with my skiing every winter.'

'How often?'

'Well, this old friend of mine from law school has a little place in Vail, and I can drop in whenever I want,' she reported.

When I heard that, I knew that I'd found the cause of and the solution to her skin problem.

I explained to her that without some type of barrier to keep the elements at bay (such as a scarf or mask or a heavy moisturiser), the winter weather would cause inflammation even on resistant skin like hers. Although inflammation is not as visible on dark skin as it is on lighter skin, where redness is apparent, for people with darker skin tones it can result in dark spots, a condition dermatologists call post-inflammatory hyperpigmentation. Despite her minimal skin problems, exposure to insults such as hotel soap (which weakens the skin barrier), air travel, cold air, wind, and low humidity were taking their toll, leaving her with those dark patches on her cheeks. I taught her to use protective moisturiser and a scarf when skiing. I urged her to avoid those harsh hotel soaps. The following year I received a Christmas card from her showing a photo of her on the slopes with a scarf. 'It worked!' she wrote.

A CLOSE-UP LOOK AT YOUR SKIN

Like Selena, ORPTs typically have minimal skin problems, but they may still find themselves in her ski boots if they use poor products or, worse, think their skin can take care of itself in all situations.

With either dark, medium or light ORPT skin, you may experience any of the following:

- Face looks shiny, especially in photographs
- Facial foundation streaks
- Sunscreens feel oily
- Dark spots develop on face
- Skin tans easily
- Minimal facial wrinkles
- Occasional acne breakouts

Whatever your skin colour, I don't recommend tanning or excess sun exposure and I do recommend regular sunscreen use for all ORPTs. Like Catherine Zeta-Jones, most ORPTs tan well. And a home on the beautiful island of Bermuda, like the one she shares with her husband, Michael Douglas, certainly offers much tanning temptation. But even though, like Zeta-Jones, you probably look gorgeous tanned, resist the urge, and use self-tanners. You'll thank me later! (For instructions on their use, please refer to 'Self-Tanners' in Chapter Ten.)

DARK-SKINNED ORPTS

When I surveyed my black patients, I found that few wore sunscreen, assuming that they did not need it. People with darker skin tones do have some built-in protection from the sun, but dark pigmentation alone won't prevent dark spots. I see proof of that every day, as many of my patients are people of colour, and the most common reason they come to see me is for help in treating their dark spots.

Beyond its role in activating the pigment production that triggers dark spots, excess sun exposure can also have other harmful effects. When you get too much sun, your body temporarily suppresses your immune system's response mechanisms for anywhere from a day to three days. As a result, for a few days following sun exposure, you may be more vulnerable to colds and flu, which is why some people get summer colds. (Obviously, winter colds in colder climes are due to other factors.) Viral infections, like herpes, may also occur more easily due to this temporary immunosuppression.

The bottom line is that sun protection should be a priority for everyone, regardless of skin colour or tone. And sunscreen should be used on a daily – not a sporadic – basis.

Finding the right colour of sunscreen, facial powder, and foundation can be a problem for darker-skin-toned people. For example, there are over two hundred different shades of Asian skin, but as far as I know, no company offers two hundred shades of makeup foundation! While often oily types dislike the greasy feel of sun products, many dark-skinned people find that creamy white products turn their skin a violet or whitish colour. Finding the right moisturiser is also key. Luckily, several tinted moisturisers are now available as companies recognise the need to develop skin care products geared to dark-skinned people.

With dark ORPT skin, you may experience any of the following:

- Dark spots in areas of previous irritation
- Shiny face, especially with sunscreen use
- White or purple skin hues when using sunscreens
- Difficulty finding the right colour of facial foundation
- Streaking of facial foundations
- Ingrown hairs with resulting dark spots
- Dark circles under the eyes

LIGHT-SKINNED ORPTS

Like dark-skinned ORPTs, light-skinned ORPTs will tend to develop dark spots. But in your case, they will most likely be freckles. As a consequence, you may have learned to avoid the sun. Remember in *Gone with the Wind* when Scarlett O'Hara was applying buttermilk to her shoulders to get rid of freckles from the sun? She was probably a light-skinned ORPT! (Do you think the real-life Southern belles knew that buttermilk contains lactic acid, an alpha hydroxy acid that helps remove dark spots by increasing exfoliation?)

ORPTs with light skin have it easier than those with dark skin for several reasons. Your freckles and sun spots can be greatly improved by laser and light treatments. Dark-skinned people's higher levels of melanin absorb too much of the laser or light energy, which damages the normal skin in the area.

If you have light ORPT skin, you may experience:

- Shiny face, especially with sunscreen use
- Freckling on face and body
- Sun spots on hands, arms and legs
- Increased risk for melanoma skin cancer, especially if you have red hair

THE DOWNSIDE OF TIGHT SKIN

Those of you with the ORPT Type may have genes on your side, but that doesn't make you immune to bad skin care habits. For example, let's take two people with similar but slightly different types, such as an ORPT (like you) and an ORPW. While excess sun and smoking will not cause wrinkles as much for your T skin, they will increase the likelihood of skin cancer, especially in light-skinned ORPTs, who are already at risk. Also, bad skin habits can cause you to revert to a W type. This is one skin factor that you can significantly control, so good habits are important. (See Chapter Two for more on tightness vs. wrinkling.)

Since light-skinned ORPTs are at higher risk of melanoma skin cancer, it's essential to wear sunscreen consistently, especially when out in the sun. This type of skin cancer is the most deadly kind, and that's why I urge all Pigmented, Tight Skin Types to make certain to check on anything suspicious. If you have fair skin, red hair, and freckles, please get annual skin exams to search for melanoma, which is completely curable when caught early.

Nicole was an attractive, fashionable, fifty-year-old redhead who came to our office for a liposuction consult. Revealing that she had never before been to a dermatologist's office, she proudly confessed that she had never had 'anything done' to her face. Her skin seemed to need no help whatsoever. It was naturally smooth, clear, unlined and glowing. Lucky Nicole!

During the routine skin exam I conduct in advance of scheduling liposuction, I noticed a dark mole on her back that was an irregular shape. As an Australian, Nicole was in a high-risk group for melanoma. Although her history did not reveal excessive sun exposure, melanoma can often occur without it, even on covered areas such as the back. In fact, redheads like Nicole are at a higher risk due to their genes. A biopsy of the mole showed that it was indeed an early melanoma.

Ironically, Nicole's decision to get liposuction inadvertently saved her life. Her good skin would likely have kept her out of a dermatologist's office, leaving the melanoma undiscovered until it might have been too late.

If you're an ORPT, it's vital that you learn to recognise the early warning signs of melanoma so that you can act promptly. Dermatologists take all melanomas very seriously, and we're trained to recognise them. While I recommend a regular, thorough, professional exam, you should also pay attention to and regularly inspect any and all moles.

The A, B, C and D of Melanoma

Four things to look out for include:

1. Asymmetry: one side of the mole is not a mirror image of the other side.
2. Borders: the borders are not distinct. It is hard to tell where the mole starts and stops.
3. Colour: the presence of more than one colour, or black, white, red and yellow hues
4. Diameter: greater than or equal to the size of a pencil eraser

If you have moles with any of these characteristics, see a dermatologist immediately. If you or your family have a history of melanoma, make an appointment with your GP for a routine skin exam every six months. If you are redheaded, Australian, or have a history of many sunburns, you are also at an increased risk of developing melanoma.

THE WRINKLE–SKIN CANCER SPECTRUM

Wrinkling and skin cancer may be on the far ends of the same continuum. Some people tend to wrinkle, while others tend to develop skin cancer. There is much that we don't know about skin aging and genetics. What we do know is that one study showed that skin with one particular kind of non-melanoma skin cancer tends to have less wrinkles than skin that did not have skin cancer. Whatever combination of good genes and good skin care gave you your youthful line-free skin, help out nature and prevent skin cancer through good skin care and avoiding excess sun exposure.

AGING AND THE ORPT

As you get older, your skin problems will likely decrease. The exception is that you may develop more sun spots if you have light skin and are prone to them. Most ORPTs enjoy their skin during their fifties and sixties, the decades of life when other types are reaching for wrinkle creams or are running for plastic surgery.

You're lucky for several reasons. First, as you go through menopause, oil secretion tends to decrease. Second, oestrogen levels (contributing to dark spots and melasma) will decline with age, causing those problems to improve. Hormonal fluctuations caused by pregnancy, birth control pill use, and perimenopause stabilise. Of course, if you opt to take hormone replacement therapy, you may continue to suffer from dark spots. People with dry, wrinkled skin may experience some improvement on hormone replacement therapy (HRT), but neither of these is a problem for you. Deciding for or against HRT is a decision to be made in consultation with your gynaecologist, along with an assessment of family history and other risk factors. But overall, ORPT skin has no compelling need for it.

Dr Baumann's Bottom Line: Enjoy your glowing skin, but don't take it for granted! Following my Daily Skin Care Regimen and other recommendations will help assure that your ORPT skin remains low maintenance and problem free. The right habits, like sunscreen use, smoking cessation, and getting plenty of antioxidants, will assure you youthful skin for a lifetime. Protect your skin and it will protect you.

EVERYDAY CARE FOR YOUR SKIN TYPE

The goal of your skin care routine is to address oiliness and brown spots, with oil-control products, bleaching ingredients, and ingredients that help prevent dark spots. All the products I'll recommend act to do either or both of the following:

- Prevent and treat dark spots
- Treat oiliness

Your skin can handle strong bleaching agents. I'll be recommending products that are strong enough to be effective yet are not heavy or greasy, so they don't make your skin look oilier.

Dark spots are your number one skin problem. Although some ORPTs are not bothered by oily skin, others are. I'll provide a two-stage regimen for you. The first stage is a nonprescription protocol in two parts: one part to get rid of the dark spots and freckles, and one for maintenance, to prevent them from coming back. The second stage is a two-part prescription protocol: the first part is for treatment and the second is for maintenance. Please look over your choice of regimen and then you can select each of the products you'll need from those I recommend in each category later in this chapter.

You can choose to see your dermatologist right away and jump straight into the prescription protocol or to try the over-the-counter protocol first for eight weeks, and then, if it does not work, see your dermatologist. (Make your appointment right away as it may take as long as two months for an opening.) While nonprescription products are not quite as strong as prescription ones, they can sometimes be effective in lightening dark spots, and they often contain additional ingredients that help improve acne. However, since your resistant skin can handle the high percentages of active ingredients in the prescription medications, I suggest you go for it – use the prescription meds.

DAILY SKIN CARE

STAGE ONE: NONPRESCRIPTION REGIMEN

For getting rid of dark spots and freckles:

AM	PM
Step 1: Wash with cleanser	Step 1: Wash with same cleanser as in AM
Step 2: Apply a glycolic acid product, such as toner or at-home peel	Step 2: Apply a skin lightener to spots
Step 3: Apply sunscreen	Step 3: Apply retinol-containing product
Step 4: Apply oil-absorbing powder or powder with SPF	

In the morning, use a cleanser to clean your face, then apply a glycolic acid face toner or peel. Next, apply sunscreen. Last, apply a powder, if desired. Many companies are now launching cosmetics with a range of colours suited to both light- and dark-skinned ORPTs.

In the evening, wash with the same cleanser that you used in the morning, then apply a skin lightener to dark spots. Last, apply a moisturiser containing retinol. This will help to control oil and prevent future brown spots, while also providing basic wrinkle prevention. Eye creams and serums, which are optional for your type, can be applied prior to sunscreen application in your morning protocol, and prior to moisturiser application in your evening protocol.

If you choose to try this regimen, continue it for eight weeks. If you find that it successfully eliminates the dark spots on your skin, move to the nonprescription maintenance regimen below to prevent new dark spots from occurring.

If this regimen does not successfully get rid of your dark spots and/or freckles after eight weeks, it's time to see your dermatologist and begin the prescription protocol I provide later in this chapter.

STAGE ONE: NONPRESCRIPTION REGIMEN

For preventing dark spots:

AM	PM
Step 1: Wash with cleanser	Step 1: Wash with same cleanser as in AM
Step 2: Apply glycolic acid toner or peel product	Step 2: Apply a retinol-containing product
Step 3: Apply sunscreen	

In the morning, wash your face with a cleanser, then use a facial peel, or toner if preferred. Next, apply sunscreen. If skin feels oily, you can also opt to use a facial powder that contains SPF.

In the evening, clean your face with the same cleanser that you used in the morning, then apply a retinol product for ongoing oil control, wrinkle and dark-spot prevention.

Eye creams and serums, which are optional for your type, can be applied prior to sunscreen application in your morning protocol, and prior to moisturiser application in your evening protocol.

RECOMMENDED CLEANSING PRODUCTS

£ Neutrogena Deep Clean Facial Wipes
££ Avon Clearskin Purifying Gel Cleanser
££ Ella Baché Pureté Demaquillant
££ La Roche-Posay Effaclar Foaming Purifying Gel
££ Laura Mercier Foaming One-Step Cleanser
££ MD Formulations Facial Cleanser
££ MD Forté Facial Cleanser II
££ Philosophy Purity Made Simple Facial Cleanser
££ Prescriptives All Clean Sparkling Gel Cleanser for Oilier Skin
££ SkinCeuticals Simply Clean Pore-Refining Cleanser
£££ Clarins Purifying Cleansing Gel
£££ Clinique Acne Solutions Cleansing Foam
£££ Estée Lauder Sparkling Clean Oil-Control Foaming Gel Cleanser

Baumann's Choice: Philosophy Purity Made Simple Facial Cleanser

Toner Use

You can use toners that contain ingredients that control oil production, absorb oil, exfoliate, or lighten dark spots.

RECOMMENDED TONER PRODUCTS

£ Avon Clearskin Purifying Astringent
£ Dove Essential Nutrients Toner
£ Johnson & Johnson Clean & Clear Black Head Clear Toner
£ Neutrogena Visibly Refined Pore Refining Mattifier
£ The Body Shop Soy & Calendula Gentle Toner
£ Time Dimensions Refining Toning Water
££ Bloom Soothing Rosewater Toner
££ Gly Derm Solution 5% (contains glycolic acid)
£££ Lancôme Tonique Contrôle (helps absorb facial oil)

Baumann's Choice: Avon Clearskin Purifying Astringent because salicylic acid will help unclog pores as well as remove dark spots

Oil-Control Products

These products offer options for on-the-spot oil control that you can use on an as-needed basis at any time.

RECOMMENDED OIL-CONTROL PRODUCTS

- £ Crabtree and Evelyn Facial Blotting Tissue
- £ Mary Kay Beauty Blotters Oil-Absorbing Tissues
- ££ Ferndale O.C. Eight Oil Control Gel
- ££ Thalgo Intense Regulating Serum
- £££ Cellex-C Betaplex Fresh Complexion Mist
- £££ Dr Brandt Lineless Tone
- £££ Origins Zero Oil

Baumann's Choice: Cellex-C Betaplex Fresh Complexion Mist because it has beta hydroxy acid to smooth skin and remove dark spots.

Treating Dark Spots

If you have dark spots, you can use skin lightening products on them, making sure to use them after cleansing and toning but before other recommended products. Start using the products at the first sign of a dark spot, and continue them until it has completely disappeared. If these nonprescription skin lighteners are not effective enough, consult a dermatologist, who can prescribe a prescription lightener.

In addition, you can use products containing retinol that increase the rate of cell turnover to prevent brown spots from occurring. Use these retinol-containing gels and moisturisers alone when no brown spots are present and with a spot-removing toner or gel containing ingredients that decrease brown spots when spots are present.

RECOMMENDED RETINOL-CONTAINING PRODUCTS

To treat and prevent brown spots:

- £ Roc Retin Ox Anti-Wrinkle Serum max
- ££ Philosophy Help Me

££ Replenix Retinol Smoothing Serum 5x by Topix
££ Sothy's Retinol 15
££ SkinCeuticals Retinol 0.5 or 1.0
£££ Clarins Renew Plus Night Lotion
£££ Estée Lauder Diminish Anti-Wrinkle Retinol Treatment
£££ Jan Marini Factor A Plus Lotion
£££ Lancome Resurface
£££ Prescriptives Skin Renewal Cream

Baumann's Choice: In this case, you have to spend a little more to get a product with active ingredients. I particularly like Philosophy Help Me because it is packaged properly to maintain the stability of the retinol.

Skin Lightening Kits

You're lucky because there are a number of product lines developed especially for you, and some of these prepackaged kits are a good choice.

RECOMMENDED SKIN CARE KITS
FOR DARK SPOTS

££ DDF Holistic Lightening Protocol
££ Dermalogica Skin Brightening System
££ Philosophy Microdelivery Peel
££ MD Forté Normal/Combination Skin Introductory Set
££ Vichy Microabrasion kit
£££ Dr Michelle Copeland Anti-Aging Kit
£££ Obagi System (In US only)
£££ Rodan & Fields Reverse Regimen (In US only)
£££ Skinceuticals Skin Systems III Clarify Kit

Baumann's Choice: Pevonia has a great lightening line, but it's not sold as a kit. Look for their Pevonia Lightening Gel, Fluid and Mask.

Moisturisers

Regular moisturiser use is unnecessary and can make the skin appear more oily. However, in a dry cold, or windy climate, use a moisturiser to protect your skin. If you have dark spots, look for moisturisers that contain soy, niacinamide, mulberry, kojic acid, or licorice extract. In the morning, apply one with SPF or apply a sunscreen over your moisturiser.

For dark circles under your eyes, use eye creams containing retinol and vitamin K.

RECOMMENDED MOISTURISERS

- £ Neutrogena Visibly Refined Moisturiser
- £ Nivea Antiwrinkle Q10 Plus Day Cream
- £ Olay Total Effects 7x Visible Anti-Aging Vitamin Complex
- £ Paula's Choice Skin Balancing Moisture Gel
- ££ Aveda Brightening Moisture treatment
- ££ YonKa Creme PG
- ££ SkinCeuticals Renew Overnight Oily
- ££ SkinMedica Ultra Sheer Moisturiser
- £££ Caudalie Day Fluid SPF 12 with Resveratrol
- £££ Jurlique Day Care Face Lotion

Baumann's Choice: Olay Total Effects 7x Visible Anti-Aging Vitamin Complex because it contains niacinamide.

RECOMMENDED EYE CREAMS AND SERUMS

- £ Avon ANEW Perfect Eye Care Cream SPF 15
- £ Neutrogena Visibly Young Eye Cream
- £ Nivea Antiwrinkle Q10 Plus Day Cream
- £ Olay Regenerist Daily Regenerating Serum
- £ Olay Regenerist Eye Lifting Serum
- ££ Relastin Eye Cream
- ££ Laura Mercier Eyedration
- ££ Clarins Extra-Firming Eye Contour Serum
- ££ Korres Eye Bright Firming Eye Cream
- ££ Quintessence Clarifying Under-Eye Serum
- ££ Thalgo Firming Eye Contour Gel
- £££ Jurlique Eye Gel

Baumann's Choice: Quintessence Clarifying Under-Eye Serum with retinol and vitamin K to diminish dark circles. Since it can be hard to find an effective product in this category, I made sure you can get it at www.Bau-mannstore.co.uk. Until recently, Mary Kay had a great one called Lumi-neyes, but unfortunately, it's no longer being produced.

Masks

Masks, used once or twice a week, can give your skin the strong ingredients it needs. You're better off going to a spa, salon, or dermatologist for a chemical peel or microdermabrasion, and I'll offer specific recommendations in the section called 'Consulting a Dermatologist'. These treatments help improve fine lines and dark spots. But if you don't have the time or the money, try the products listed below. They improve skin oiliness only temporarily, but are helpful for special occasions.

RECOMMENDED MASKS

£ L'Oréal ReNoviste Home Peel Kit
££ Ahava Advanced Mud Masque for Oily Skin
££ DDF Clay Mint Mask
££ Decléor Clay and Herbal Cleansing Mask
££ Gly Derm Gly Masque 3%
££ Jurlique Moor Purifying Mask
££ Laura Mercier Deep Cleansing Clay Mask
££ MD Formulations Vit-A-Plus Clearing Complex Masque
£££ Chanel Précision Masque Pureté Express Instant Purifying Mask
£££ Dr Brandt Poreless Purifying Mask

Baumann's Choice: Gly Derm Gly Masque 3% with glycolic acid

Facial Peels

Although these peels are lower in strength than what you can get at a salon or spa, if used on a daily basis, they do convey some benefits.

RECOMMENDED FACIAL PEELS

£ Avon Anew Clinical 2-Step Facial Peel
£ L'Oréal ReNoviste Home Peel Kit

££ Elizabeth Arden Peel & Reveal Revitalising Treatment
££ MD Skincare Alpha Beta Daily Face Peel
££ Philosophy MicroDelivery Peel
££ Vichy Microabrasion Peel
£££ Lancôme Resurface Peel
£££ Natura Bisse Glyco Peeling 50% Pump

Baumann's Choice: Elizabeth Arden Peel & Reveal Revitalising Treatment combines AHA and grape seed extract.

Exfoliation

You can benefit from gentle exfoliation, but no more than two to three times a week. Overdoing it can cause inflammation and lead to dark spots, especially if you have darker skin – so be careful!

RECOMMENDED EXFOLIATORS

£ Buf-Puf
£ L'Oréal Pure Zone Pore Unclogging Scrub Cleanser
£ Neutrogena Visibly Clear Exfoliating Wash
£ St Ives Swiss Formula Invigorating Apricot Scrub
££ DDF Pumice Acne Scrub
££ Dermalogica Skin Prep Scrub
££ Philosophy The Greatest Love
£££ Dr Brandt Microdermabrasion in a Jar

Baumann's Choice: L'Oréal Pure Zone Pore Unclogging Scrub Cleanser

SHOPPING FOR PRODUCTS

Widen your choice of products by reading labels to select products with beneficial ingredients and avoid ones that tend to cause pigmentation or oiliness. Certain food extracts such as lemon or lime (and essential oils, like oil of bergamot in Earl Grey Tea) may make skin more sensitive to sunlight, resulting in increased tanning and dark spots. People enjoying margaritas while sitting in the sun may notice darkened skin in areas that are splashed by lime juice. Ingredients with 'oestrogenic effects' may worsen hormone-related dark spots such as melasma. If you find products that you like that are not on the list of recommendations, please go to www.DrBaumann.-co.uk and share them with me.

SKIN CARE INGREDIENTS TO USE

For getting rid of dark spots:

- Arbutin
- Bearberry extract
- Cucumber extract
- Kojic acid
- Glycyrrhiza glabra (licorice extract)
- Mulberry extract
- Niacinamide
- Retinol
- Salicylic acid (beta hydroxy acid)
- Vitamin C (ascorbic acid)

To speed up skin renewal:

- Beta hydroxy acid (salicylic acid)
- Retinaldehyde
- Retinol

Alpha hydroxy acids such as:

- Citric acid
- Glycolic acid
- Lactic acid
- Phytic acid

SKIN CARE INGREDIENTS TO AVOID

Due to skin darkening:

- Extracts of celery, lime, parsley, fig and carrot
- Oil of bergamot

Due to oestrogenic effects, increasing pigmentation levels:

- Genistein
- Soy, except when found in Aveeno, RoC, and Neutrogena products (in which oestrogenic fractions have been removed)
- Topical oestrogen (such as estradiol)

Sun Protection for Your Skin

Make sure to use sunscreen to prevent dark spots. Even if you have very dark skin, it's a must! Cream sunscreens can make your skin appear even oilier and will increase makeup streaking. That's why most ORPTs prefer powders and gels. Powder sunscreens are perfect for your type because they absorb oil as well as blocking sunlight. Dark-skinned patients should look for a tinted sunscreen or use a foundation or powder with a sunscreen.

RECOMMENDED SUN PROTECTION PRODUCTS

£ Avon Brighter Days Light Moisture Lotion SPF 15
£ Eucerin Q10 Active Anti-wrinkle Fluid SPF 15
£ Olay Regenerist Rehydrating Lotion SPF 15
£ Olay Touch Sensory Moisturising Fluid SPF 15
££ i.d. bareMinerals Foundation – SPF 15 Sunscreen
££ Mary Kay TimeWise Day Solution with Sunscreen SPF 15
££ Philosophy A Pigment of Your Imagination SPF 18 Sunscreen
££ SkinCeuticals Daily Sun Defence SPF 20
£££ Prada Reviving Bio-Firm Moisture SPF 15
£££ Ultraceuticals Protective Moisturiser SPF30

Baumann's Choice: Philosophy A Pigment of Your Imagination SPF 18 Sunscreen because it contains skin brighteners to get rid of pesky dark spots.

Your Makeup

Makeup can cover dark spots, and give freckled skin a more uniform appearance, but many foundations streak on oily skin. Instead use powders and powder-based foundations. You can also use a foundation and apply a powder on top of it. Look for products that have sunscreen (you can never have too much). Some new facial foundations contain ingredients such as soy that help lighten dark spots.

Foundation is the one product I splurge on. I pick Lancôme Colour ID because of the variety of shades and the texture. Lancôme has several foundations that are appropriate for you. Those with higher O/D scores (30s or above) may prefer Lancôme's Maquicontrôle or Teint Idole.

If oiliness and streaking are your main problems, stay away from liquid foundations; use tinted sunscreens instead and cover them with an oil-control powder. Use these powders dry and apply with a puff to reduce shine.

RECOMMENDED FOUNDATIONS

£ Boots No7 Uplifting Foundation SPF 15

£ Revlon Colourstay Makeup with SPF 6

££ Bloom Compact Foundation with SPF 12

££ Bobbi Brown Oil-Free Even Finish Foundation SPF 15

££ Laura Mercier Oil Free Foundation

£££ Fresh Freshface Foundation with SPF 20

£££ Lancôme Colour ID with SPF 8

Baumann's Choice: Lancôme Colour ID, or Teint Idole

RECOMMENDED FACIAL POWDERS

£ Clean & Clear Shine-Control Invisible Powder

£ CoverGirl Fresh Complexion Pocket Powder

£ Maybelline Shine Free Oil-Control Pressed Powder

££ Bobbi Brown Sheer Finish Loose Powder

££ Laura Mercier Loose Setting Powder

££ MAC Studio Finish Powder/Pressed

£££ Shu Uemura Face Powder Matte

Baumann's Choice: Maybelline Shine Free Oil-Control Pressed Powder is inexpensive and easy to find. In addition, look out for brands that also contain SPF.

CONSULTING A DERMATOLOGIST

If after following my nonprescription protocol for two months, you are still troubled by dark spots, the next step is to see a dermatologist and, with their approval, graduate to retinoids, which help eliminate dark spots and other pigmented areas. You can choose a regimen depending on whether you have active dark spots or wish to prevent them.

With retinoids, you may limit oil production, reduce skin oiliness, and prevent pigmentation that results in dark spots and freckles. You'll be combining them with alpha hydroxy acids (AHAs), such as lactic acid or glycolic acid, and/or beta hydroxy acid (also called BHA or salicylic acid), which enhance cell renewal and prevent clogged pores.

Prescription skin lighteners are ideal for you. Look for ones containing kojic or azelaic acid. Use gel forms to avoid the oiliness of creams.

DAILY SKIN CARE

STAGE TWO: PRESCRIPTION REGIMEN

To get rid of dark spots:

AM	PM
Step 1: Wash with a glycolic acid cleanser	Step 1: Wash with a cleanser
Step 2: Apply lightening gel containing glycolic acid	Step 2: Apply a prescription retinoid
Step 3: Apply sunscreen	

In the morning, wash with a prescription glycolic acid cleanser, then apply a lightening gel. Finally, apply sunscreen. In the evening, wash with cleanser, then apply a prescription retinoid product.

STAGE TWO: MAINTENANCE REGIMEN

To prevent dark spots:

AM	PM
Step 1: Wash with cleanser	Step 1: Wash with same cleanser as in AM
Step 2: Apply glycolic toner or peel product	Step 2: Apply a retinoid product
Step 3: Apply sunscreen	

In this routine, you simply use a retinoid in your basic regimen. In the morning, wash with one of the recommended cleansers, then apply a facial peel. Finally, apply sunscreen.

In the evening, wash with the same cleanser you used in the morning. Next, apply a retinoid.

Retinoid Use for ORPTs

For specific instructions on how to use these products, see 'Further Help for Oily, Resistant Skin'. Unless noted otherwise, all of the prescription products are US brands that may not be available in your country. Please ask your dermatologist for comparable ones.

RECOMMENDED PRESCRIPTION PRODUCTS TO REMOVE DARK SPOTS

- Claripel
- EpiQuin
- Lustra
- Lustra AF
- Solaquin Forte
- Tri-Luma

Baumann's Choice: I prefer Tri-Luma, which, like all these products, contains hydroquinone, an ingredient not used in products in the UK and a number of other countries. Please discuss your available options with your dermatologist.

RECOMMENDED PRESCRIPTION PRODUCTS TO DECREASE OIL AND IMPROVE BROWN SPOTS

- Aknemycin Plus (contains an antibiotic as well)
- Differin gel or cream
- Isotrex
- Isotrexin (contains an antiobiotic as well)
- Retin-A gel, lotion or cream
- Retinova

RECOMMENDED PRESCRIPTION

- Glycolic Acid Cleanser
- Medicis Triaz 3% Cleanser (only in the US)

PROCEDURES FOR YOUR SKIN TYPE

Dark-skinned ORPTs usually find that topical products are effective for eliminating dark spots, which means you can avoid the more costly, unnecessary, and sometimes harmful procedures. But be patient, as topical products will take some time before showing results.

Light Treatments

For those with light skin, light procedures, such as IPL procedures with Metvix, may decrease oil secretion by shrinking the oil-producing glands (for details see the section on light treatments, in 'Further Help for Oily, Resistant Skin Types'). If your skin is medium-dark to dark, I advise against light treatments because they can lead to inflammation and worsen dark spots.

Chemical peels

Chemical peels are an option for those with darker skin tones, or for those who want to stay clear of expensive IPLs. Your dermatologist can perform facial peels with AHAs and BHA in strengths higher than you can find in an over-the-counter product or in spas. These peels contain salicylic acid (BHA) 20 percent or 30 percent, or combinations of glycolic acid and other depigmenting ingredients. I strongly recommend asking your dermatologist about the PCA Peel or Jessner's peel, which are perfect for you. However, if you prefer to go to a spa, ask for peels such as glycolic acid or a modified Jessner's peel.

If you have darker skin, make certain that you go to a dermatologist who is skilled at treating people with similar skin – dark spots can worsen if chemical peels are not done correctly. Peels range from £50 to £100 per peel; a series of five to eight is usually recommended.

Microdermabrasion

Microdermabrasion may help spots disappear faster as well. Dark-skinned people should be extra cautious about getting treatments from anyone other than a dermatologist. Treatments that are too strong can worsen your spots.

Reducing pores

Neither skin care products, facials, microdermabrasion, nor cosmetics can decrease the size of your pores. Any decrease you might observe is caused by ingredients in the products making the skin surrounding the pores swell slightly, so the pores temporarily appear to shrink. Instead, try using products containing AHAs and BHA and vitamin C. You'll find some products I like in the product section. These may help reduce pore size, though only temporarily.

ONGOING CARE FOR YOUR SKIN

By following my oil-decreasing and pigment-prevention regimens, you can get the most out of your easy-care skin. Be thankful you have one of the easier Skin Types, and bask in the glow!

CHAPTER TEN

Oily, Resistant, Non-Pigmented and Wrinkled: ORNW

THE COMPLACENT SKIN TYPE

'What's the big fuss over skin care? Seems like a waste of time. My skin is just like everyone else's. I don't pay that much attention to it, really. Only thing is that I'm noticing some wrinkles lately.'

ABOUT YOUR SKIN

Your skin is so easy, you haven't focused on it. Since the majority of Caucasian Britains have your Skin Type, most skin care products, like over-the-counter toners or face soaps, are geared to you, so they seem to work just fine. Unlike sensitive types, your skin can withstand a wide range of chemicals without experiencing irritation or redness. As a result, you can use any skin care item without worry. When others fuss over skin care, you can't imagine why. You take your skin for granted.

Unlike pigmented types, you don't need to contend with dark spots. Unlike dry types, your need to moisturise is minimal, and until you age, greasy creams hold no appeal. Although you experienced some pimples and oiliness during your teen years, this too seemed perfectly normal. You could handle it with a drugstore pimple treatment product, just like everyone else.

Sunscreen? You probably didn't bother with it. Most sunscreens felt greasy, and a little sun is good for acne, you heard somewhere. If you burned occasionally, so what? So did everyone else. The problem with ORNW skin is that most of your skin problems hit you late in life, and you're not prepared for them. Wrinkles, sags, and other signs of aging seem to appear overnight. You're caught off guard, because you're used to easy skin care. When aging happens to *you*, its effects aren't so pretty. You never thought it could happen, but now when you look in the mirror, you worry – just like everyone else.

ORNW CELEBRITY

Although I'm not privy to her skin care secrets, my guess is that Hollywood actress, television star, and California gal Heather Locklear is an ORNW. Part sex symbol, part all-American beauty, she looks like the girl teens want to grow up to resemble. And like many of her fellow Americans, Locklear is a hybrid of different ethnic groups. Her clean-cut appeal, pale skin, and blue eyes come from Scottish ancestry on her mother's side, while her dad's American-Indian heritage endows Locklear with striking cheekbones, long, lithe legs, and that sparkle in her eyes.

Like her dual ancestry, Locklear's career and persona incorporate some complementary opposites. She came to the fore in the long-running primetime soap *Dynasty* and has made a career of playing sexy, manipulative, determined women in such hit shows as *Melrose Place, Spin City,* and most recently, *LAX.* Yet by all reports, despite her razzle-dazzle looks, this star is unassuming and easygoing and, according to the Biography Channel, she likes Taco Bell, as I do.

In a recent interview, the actress confessed bafflement about the source of her appeal. 'I am clueless,' Locklear is reported as saying. 'I don't know, and I don't want to know, and I don't ask.' Another source quotes her as confessing that, 'When I look in the mirror I see the girl I was when I was growing up, with braces, crooked teeth, a baby face and a skinny body.'

Obviously, television audiences see a lot more! Although photographs early in her career reveal her as an oily type, she seems to avoid the excess acne and dark spots that plague sensitive, pigmented skin, pegging her as a resistant and, most likely, non-pigmented type.

Now in her early forties, Locklear still looks stunning, both on the small screen and the red carpet. I call her a wrinkled type because of her history of excess tanning. A look back through Locklear's publicity and candid photos since her *Dynasty* debut shows photo after photo of an ever-tanned starlet. Also visible are the signs of creases forming around her eyes; but in her case, her beauty and dynamism so entice that she looks cute with wrinkles that might not look so good on the rest of us. In recent years, at last it looks like Locklear has gotten some good dermatological advice and has given up tanning, at least in part. Perhaps she has been persuaded to use a self-tanner or, at the minimum, not to tan that gorgeous face of hers.

Another celebrity whose glowing good looks typify the appeal of oily, resistant, and non-pigmented skin is English actor Jude Law. I can't say for sure whether he is a wrinkled type or not, but my recommendation would be for him to play it safe, and steer clear of the sun. I would give that same advice to beloved actress, Emma Thompson.

CARING FOR YOUR SKIN

Controlling oiliness is your goal before the age of forty, while addressing wrinkles will be your goal thereafter. ORNWs gravitate to facials to clear the pimples, blackheads and whiteheads common to oily skin. Although facials are too drying or irritating for many other Types, Oily, Resistant Skin Types are free to enjoy them. One tip: look for a facial that uses products rich in antioxidant ingredients, which help prevent wrinkles.

Don't permit your facialist to extract your blackheads or whiteheads, which can lead to scarring. Nor should you squeeze them at home. Always resist the urge. Use a cleanser with salicylic acid or adhesive strips such as Bioré to gently clean the pores instead.

In my opinion, skin care products and prescription medications like retinoids do a better job of addressing your type's skin problems than facials. Plus, they are less expensive and less time consuming. Retinoids will also help prevent wrinkles, another problem for your type.

THE DOWNSIDE OF EASY SKIN

Having 'easy' skin has certain disadvantages. To address a variety of skin problems from youth, other types used skin care products, which you never bothered with. These same products may have also conferred antiaging benefits, which you never received.

For example, in your teens, twenties, and thirties, while many of your peers agonised over acne, you had only occasional pimples. As a result, you never used a product like Retin-A, which in addition to lessening acne also has potent antiaging effects. Where many people with oily, sensitive skin covered blemishes with foundation and powder, you never bothered with them, and missed out on the sun protection they provide. Because your skin is oily, you rarely used moisturisers and so you never got the extras they often contain, such as antioxidants, retinoids, sunscreens, or other antiaging ingredients. ORNWs with dark skin never had to consult a dermatologist for help with dark spots, and therefore missed out on antiaging preparations.

Light-skinned ORNWs produce less melanin, a pigment that protects from sun damage. Without either pigmentation or sun protection, your skin is more exposed to harmful rays, and more at risk.

AGING AND ORNW SKIN

Due to all these factors, in your thirties and beyond, many ORNWs are trying to play catch-up. Aging creeps up and catches you unaware. You may notice fine lines beginning to form on your forehead or between your eyebrows. Your jawline or neck begins to sag. Lines etch themselves at the corners of your mouth. While I'll offer skin care and treatment options to address these problems, if you're in your twenties or younger, be fore-warned. Start protecting your skin *now*.

Marion's Story

M arion was a thirty-eight-year-old flight attendant whom I met on a flight to Japan. I worked on this book as the other passengers slept, and when I walked around to stretch my legs, she asked me what I was doing.

'I'm writing a skin care book,' I explained. 'I'm a dermatologist.'

'You are just the person I need to talk to,' Marion replied. Having spent most of her adult life raising her two children while working as a flight attendant, Marion never had the time to worry about her skin. Nor had she cared to, until now.

'Suddenly, I have lines around my eyes and between my eyebrows. Now I finally have time to focus on myself,' she admitted. 'I'd love to have Botox, but it's difficult to afford with two kids who plan to attend college.'

Questioning Marion about her skin care regimen, medical history, and skin concerns, I learned that she never wore sunscreen, moisturisers, powder, or makeup foundation because of her good skin. Nor did she take supple-ments. Serving as a flight attendant for twenty years gave her a higher risk of developing wrinkles, I explained, since before 1994, people were allowed to smoke on aeroplanes, subjecting other passengers, and attendants like Marion, to second-hand smoke, which can activate free radicals that damage and prematurely age the skin. In addition, passing through aeroplane windows, ultraviolet light (UVA) activates destructive enzymes like collage-nase that breaks down skin collagen, leading to wrinkles.

Although her oily skin partially protected her from the drying aeroplane environment, it could not protect her against the ravages of free radicals.

To combat them, I recommended an oral antioxidant supplement, a sunscreen containing z-cote with antioxidants, and the retinoid prescription cream Avage for use at night. Botox could help eliminate the lines around her eyes, but the prevention regimen was just as important.

Her skin care, including oral supplements, Avage prescription (£80), and sunblock would cost about £120 every three months, with an additional £150 per month for the Botox injections to address her crow's-feet and brow furrow lines. With a total bill of about £175 a month, or less than £6 a day, this was the most cost-effective antiaging program for Marion. By saving money on expensive and useless skin creams, she could afford Botox and help prevent future skin aging.

A CLOSE-UP LOOK AT YOUR SKIN

Like Marion, with ORNW skin you may experience any of the following:

- Occasional bouts of facial shininess
- Minimal acne
- History of significant sun exposure in many cases
- No problem with most skin care products
- Difficulty tanning
- Little need to moisturise
- Early signs of wrinkles

HOW WRINKLES FORM

Although wrinkles seem to appear overnight, that's not what really happens. Wrinkle formation occurs in stages. First, typically in your twenties, you will develop temporary 'wrinkles in motion' in areas of facial movement such as around your eyes. These disappear when the corresponding muscle is relaxed. Later, often in your thirties, you will develop 'wrinkles at rest' that remain visible even when the corresponding muscle is relaxed. Don't ignore the warning signs of first-stage wrinkles. The earlier they appear, the greater your tendency for deepening wrinkles over a lifetime. That's why wrinkle prevention is a must for your type.

The good news is that your skin's resilience and oiliness will permit you to tolerate the many treatments I'll recommend. But first and foremost, you must eliminate the ongoing sun exposure that damages skin and accelerates wrinkling.

Now in mid-life, my mum has great skin. It's clear and unlined, and quite youthful for her age. (No worries, Mum, I'm not telling!) Because she's a blonde with light skin that rapidly burns in the sun, she learned when she was young to avoid sun exposure and protect her skin. As a result, she preserved her skin. Her mother, on the other hand, loved the sun and had the wrinkles to show for it. Even though my mother had the genetics to wrinkle, her behaviour protected her skin.

My mother's experience reveals what I will say over and over in this book: genes are only one factor in aging. Equally important is lifestyle. You can turn from a T to a W, depending on lifestyle factors such as smoking and sunning. And vice versa. For example, actresses Renee Zellweger, Cate Blanchett, Naomi Watts and Kim Basinger have the fair skin typical of Non-Pigmented Skin Types. This fair complexion is sensitive to sun damage and can be prone to wrinkling. Genetically Renee, Cate, Naomi and Kim could be wrinkled types. However, strict sun avoidance and good skin care makes them wrinkled types who have beat the odds and maintained their skin in a youthful condition as the years go by. You can do it too!

SELF-TANNERS

All self-tanners, including creams, lotions, gels, sprays, or the types they hose you down with at 'fantasy tan' salons, contain the same active ingredient. It's called dihydroxyacetone (DHA), a sugar that interacts with amino acids in the upper layer of skin. The browning reaction that produces the 'tan' is the same as when sugar-containing foods, like apples, turn brown after they are cut open and left to oxidise. Most self-tanners on the market contain 3–5 percent DHA. Because the upper skin layer is thicker over the elbows, knees, and palms, DHA-containing products cause more browning in these areas, so apply less self-tanner there.

To develop an even tan with these products, always use an exfoliating cream prior to application. Self-tanners provide no appreciable protection from the sun, with an SPF of only 1 or 2, which only lasts for an hour or two following application. Therefore, you should always use sunscreen as well.

Several sunless tanning products also contain antioxidants to ward off sun damage. Studies have shown that when self-tanners contain antioxidants, the end result is a more natural, less orange colour.

INDOOR TANNING

Indoor tanning was originally marketed as the 'safe way to tan'. Does that claim hold up? Not in my opinion. Tanning beds use ultraviolet A (UVA) rays to tan the skin. Since UVA does not cause an immediate skin reddening or sunburn as do UVB rays, people are not aware of the resulting long-term skin damage. UVA rays are more harmful than UVB because they penetrate more deeply into the dermis, the deeper layer of the skin, causing damage to collagen and other important skin proteins. The beautiful tan you see today can lead to premature aging, dark spots and skin cancer tomorrow – or decades from now. If you are visiting a tanning bed, please stop. You are causing irreparable harm to your skin.

SUNLESS TANNING BOOTHS

Sunless tanning booths were first introduced in 1999. These booths employ mobile or stationary misters that move 360 degrees around you to apply uniform amounts of sunless tanning solution to all parts of your body. While this assures a smooth product application that results in an even tan, tanning booth's spray-on self-tanners do have some downsides.

In the US, a recent government advisory cautioned against unwanted exposures to DHA, which may occur in sunless tanning booths. When eyes, lips, and mucous membranes are sprayed with DHA, some of the DHA may be ingested. The FDA advised people to cover and protect sensitive skin areas from receiving the spray, and from inadvertent ingestion or inhalation of DHA-containing products. Who is responsible for making sure you are protected if you go to a sunless tanning booth? Whatever the law may say, *you* are. Obviously, inhalation does not occur when you apply a cream or lotion tanner at home.

In spite of this advisory, research shows that people are not being adequately warned or protected from these dangers by the staff of sunless tanning booths. A recent study published in the *Journal of the American Academy of Dermatology* surveyed facilities that had sunless tanning booths. While most advised clients to close their eyes, that is not sufficient protection. Seventy-seven percent also advised their clients to hold their breath for the duration of misting. Only one business offered clients additional protection, such as protective eyewear, petroleum jelly for the lips, and cotton balls for the nostrils. My advice? If you opt for the spray-on tan, protect your eyes with goggles, your lips with Vaseline, and hold your breath while the spray is being applied. Remember to bring them with you, as they may not be provided at the salon.

WHAT CAN I DO TO PREVENT WRINKLES?

There are other ways to slow down your type's tendency to wrinkle. One key strategy is assuring that you get antioxidants, which combat free radicals and prevent aging. They can be ingested from foods, particularly fruits and vegetables, but I have found that when undertaking diets like the Atkins or South Beach, many people reduce their consumption of fruit. If your diet lacks ample fruits and vegetables, you can obtain them from the foods and supplements I'll recommend later in 'Further Help for Oily, Resistant Skin'. In addition, please check later in this chapter for my lists of anti-oxidant ingredients found in skin care products, as well as my recommendations for products containing these ingredients, well suited to your oily skin. Beyond preventing wrinkles, you need to treat existing wrinkles, and I'll offer a range of suggestions to accomplish that.

YOUR TREATMENT OPTIONS

Facial exercisers that promise to tone the face and prevent wrinkles are sold in various catalogues. Typically, the item is put in your mouth, and then you exercise against its resistance. For certain muscles, increased movement of the face will lead to more wrinkles, as can be seen by the development of lines in areas of movement around your eyes and mouth.

What about facial exercises that you do by yourself at home? Many of my patients have asked me if exercising facial muscles creates more tone, as bodily exercise does, and if that minimises the signs of aging. I cannot recommend that you exercise your facial muscles because there has never been proof that it works. I tend to doubt it, because aging results from loss of fat, collagen, and elastin in the face, which causes the skin to sag. On the other hand, strengthening specific muscles could potentially tone the face somewhat, but it's hard to say whether anyone has been able to isolate the toning muscles without increasing movement in the ones you would want to relax.

Botulinum toxins like Botox inhibit muscle movement where wrinkles form, such as the crow's-feet around the eyes and frown lines, and may prevent the formation of future wrinkles as well. I personally hope it's true since I use them myself.

ORNWs can also use retinoids, prescription medications that help control oiliness and prevent wrinkles. While one particular brand, called Avage (which comes as a cream), is too strong for many types, you can easily tolerate it. In addition, because you don't develop dark spots after trauma and inflammation, you can also tolerate more aggressive wrinkle treatments such as laser resurfacing, dermabrasion, and deep chemical peels that other more pigmented types must rule out. I'll recommend ones you can benefit from in the section on procedures later in this chapter.

Newly advanced wrinkle treatments beyond Botox that are currently in development will also be suitable for ORNWs. These improved treatments may last longer and cost less than Botox. Currently, many dermal fillers, used to fill in wrinkles, are becoming available. Most recently, Captique, made of hyaluronic acid, a natural bodily sugar, was approved as a treatment for facial wrinkles. Often used with collagen-containing fillers such as CosmoPlast, Captique often corrects facial wrinkles. As more fillers and botulinum toxins become available, increasing competition among suppliers will cause prices to come down, making these procedures more affordable.

People with wrinkled skin frequently wonder about a host of newly available and pricey creams advertised as 'better than Botox'. Although it seems appealing to get the same benefit out of a jar, I haven't seen any visible results from these creams beyond hydration, which any skin cream provides. Some of these creams use natural substances called peptides to make the top layer of the skin feel smoother. Their effect is like spackling a wall, which smoothes the surface but does not permanently change it.

My recommendation is that you save money for what you really need: prescription retinoids; botulinum toxins such as Botox; and dermal fillers such as Hylaform, Hylaform Plus, Captique, Restylane, Juvéderm and CosmoPlast.

If you're in your twenties or younger, don't take your skin for granted. Stop age-promoting habits such as smoking and sunbathing now. Take antioxidant supplements and use sunscreen and nonprescription retinol products or prescription retinoids to prevent aging. If you are thirty or older, you probably are beginning to have wrinkles. Using Botox or Reloxin can prevent the wrinkles from worsening by preventing movement of the muscles in wrinkle-prone areas. Wearing sunglasses to prevent squinting will also help minimise the formation of eye wrinkles.

Dr Baumann's Bottom Line: Splurge on the strong wrinkle treatments. Your skin can take it! After you repair the damage, turn your attention to prevention.

Everyday Care for Your Skin

The goal of your skin care routine is to address wrinkles and excess oil with wrinkle- and oil-control products that deliver antioxidants and retinols or retinoids. All the products I'll recommend act to do one or more of the following:

- Prevent and treat wrinkles
- Treat excess oil

In addition, your daily regimen will also help to address your other skin concerns by:

- Preventing skin cancer

ORNWs must address wrinkles and oiliness; a second concern is avoiding skin cancer. To address wrinkles, I'll provide a two-stage regimen consisting of a nonprescription protocol and then a prescription protocol. Many of you will want to see a dermatologist to have one of the many new wrinkle treatments that are available: lasers, dermabrasion, chemical peels, dermal fillers, or other procedures. My two skin care regimens will help prep your skin for these treatments.

These regimens also include products containing retinol and antioxidants that may help decrease your skin cancer risk.

DAILY SKIN CARE

STAGE ONE: NONPRESCRIPTION REGIMEN

AM	PM
Step 1: Wash with antioxidant cleanser	Step 1: Wash with same cleanser as in AM
Step 2: Apply toner, gel, moisturiser, or serum with antioxidants	Step 2: Use a facial scrub

---

Step 3: Apply sunscreen

Step 4: Apply oil-free foundation if you choose to wear it

Step 3: Apply a retinol- or retinaldehyde-containing product

In the morning, wash your face with a cleanser containing antioxidants to help prevent wrinkles. Then apply a toner, gel, moisturiser or serum containing antioxidants such as Prevage by Elizabeth Arden. If your O/D score is very high (over 35), use a toner. If your score is lower (upper 20s or below) pick a serum or gel.

With a high O/D score (over 35), you should next use a mixture of an oil-control product such as Ferndale O.C. Eight and a gel sunscreen.

If your O/D score is between 24 and 34, instead of an oil-control product, apply a lotion sunscreen that contains antioxidants. Finally, apply an oil-free foundation if you would like to wear one.

In the evening, wash your face with the same cleanser you used in the morning, then use a facial scrub. Next, apply a product containing retinol or retinaldehyde, such as Roc Retin Ox Anti-Wrinkle serum. If you choose to use an eye cream, which is not necessary for your type, you can apply after cleansing.

You can remain on this regimen indefinitely. These OTC products are as good for your type as any prescription products – with the exception of the retinol/retinaldehyde product. I suggest instead that you see a dermatologist and get a prescription retinoid such as Retin-A, because the prescription product is stronger.

Cleansers

ORNWs benefit from cleansers containing antioxidants, to help avoid wrinkles.

RECOMMENDED CLEANSERS

£ Clean & Clear Morning Burst Facial Cleanser with Bursting Beads
£ L'Oréal Pure Zone Pore Unclogging Scrub Cleanser Step 1 (with salicylic acid)
£ Neutrogena Clear Pore Wash

£ Olay Daily Facials for Combination or Oily Skin (with salicylic acid)

££ Korres White Tea Facial Fluid Gel Cleanser

££ Laura Mercier Oil-Free Gel Cleanser

££ Mary Kay Time Wise 3-in-1 Cleanser

££ Philosophy Purity Made Simple One-step Facial Cleanser

£££ Chanel Précision Système Éclat – La Gelée

£££ Jurlique Cleansing Lotion

£££ N.V. Perricone M.D. Vitamin C Ester Citrus Facial Wash with DMAE

Baumann's Choice: Korres White Tea Facial Fluid Gel Cleanser. It's from Greece and the packaging is adorable.

Toner Use

Toners are a great oil-free way to give your skin the antioxidants it needs. You can also use a gel or serum with oil-control properties and/or antioxidants.

One very beneficial antioxidant is green tea. Its proven benefits include protection from skin cancer and wrinkle prevention. You'll want to choose a product like Replenix serum, which contains such a high level of green tea that it is brown in colour. But don't let the colour put you off; if it isn't brown it simply doesn't have enough green tea for your purposes.

RECOMMENDED TONERS, GELS AND SERUMS

£ Neutrogena Visibly Refined Facial Toner

££ Avon BeComing Get Supple Hydrating Mist (contains antioxidants)

££ SkinCeuticals Serum 20

££ Topix CRS Cell Rejuvenation Serum

££ Topix Replenix Retinol Smoothing Serum with green tea

£££ Caudalie Face Lifting Serum with Grapevine Resveratrol

£££ Elizabeth Arden Prevage Anti-aging Treatment

£££ N.V. Perricone M.D. Firming Facial Toner

Baumann's Choice: Replenix Retinol Smoothing Serum with green tea by Topix. This contains a higher percentage of green tea than any other product I know.

Oil Control

Toners don't control oil because they don't remain on the skin. Instead use an oil-control powder (recommendations appear later in this chapter) or an oil-control product with oil-absorbing ingredients, like these.

RECOMMENDED OIL-CONTROL PRODUCTS

- £ Simple Oil Control Facial Wipes
- ££ Bobbi Brown Shine Control Face Gel
- ££ Ferndale O.C. Eight Oil Control Gel
- ££ Mary Kay Beauty Blotters Oil-AbsorbingTissues
- ££ Paula's Choice 1% Beta Hydroxy Acid Gel
- ££ Seban pads
- £££ Clarins Mat Express Instant Shine Control Gel
- £££ Korres Lemon Anti-Shine Gel
- £££ Ole Henriksen Grease Relief Face Tonic
- £££ Thalgo Intense Regulating Serum

Baumann's Choice: Ferndale O.C. Eight Oil Control Gel

Moisturisers

You don't need a morning moisturiser. Use one of the recommended serums instead. You may need an evening moisturiser if you have a lower O/D score (below 35).

RECOMMENDED MOISTURISERS

- £ Olay Total Effects Intensive Restoration Treatment
- £ Neutrogena Visibly Young Night Cream
- £ Paula's Choice Completely Non Greasy Moisturising Lotion with Antioxidants
- ££ Aveda Botanical Kinetics Hydrating Lotion
- ££ Clarins Extra Firming Day Lotion SPF 15
- ££ Korres Pomegranate Balancing Moisturiser
- ££ Philosophy Hope in a Jar for all Skin Types
- ££ Replenix CF Cream by Topix
- £££ Alpha H Rejuvenating Cream with 10% Vitamin C and Glycolic Acid

£££ Jurlique Day Care Face Lotion
£££ SkinCeuticals Renew Overnight Oily

Baumann's Choice: Paula's Choice Completely Non Greasy Moisturising Lotion with Antioxidants because it's light enough for oily skin and prevents aging.

Eye Creams

Eye creams are not necessary, but if you choose to use one, select a product with antiaging ingredients.

RECOMMENDED EYE CREAMS

£ Neutrogena Visibly Young Eye Cream
£ Nivea Antiwrinkle Q10 Plus Eye Cream
£ Olay Eye Countour Gel
£ Roc Retin-Ox Correxion Intensive Eye Care
£ Time Dimensions Nourishing Eye Cream
££ Clarins Extra-Firming Eye Contour Cream
££ Cellex-C Eye Contour Gel
££ Laura Mercier Eyedration
££ MD Skincare Firming Eye Lift
££ Origins A Perfect World for eyes
££ Relastin Eye Cream
££ SkinCeuticals Eye Gel
£££ Dr Brandt Lineless Eye Cream
£££ Skinceuticals Eye Gel

Baumann's Choice: Roc Retin-Ox Correxion Intensive Eye Care because it contains retinol.

Wrinkle Prevention

While I'll recommend prescription retinoids later in this chapter, the only effective nonprescription topical products for preventing wrinkles are retinols, but their efficacy depends on the concentration offered in the product. The ones I recommend here are good options.

RECOMMENDED WRINKLE-PREVENTION PRODUCTS

£ Neutrogena Visibly Young Day Cream SPF 30 (with copper peptide)

£ Roc Retin Ox Anti-Wrinkle serum max (with retinol)

££ Philosophy Help Me (with retinol)

££ Prevage by Elizabeth Arden (with idebenone)

££ Rétrinal Cream by Avène

££ Sothy's Retinol 15

££ Topix Replenix Retinol Smoothing Serum 3x

££ Vichy Reti-C Intensive Corrective Care

£££ Clarins Renew Plus Night Lotion

£££ Estée Lauder Diminish Anti-Wrinkle Retinal Treatment

£££ Jan Marini Factor A Plus Lotion

£££ Lancôme Resurface

£££ Prescriptives Skin Renewal Cream

£££ PrevageMD by Allergan (with idebenone)

£££ Skinceuticals Retinol 0.5 or 1%

Baumann's Choice: Prevage by Elizabeth Arden and Roc Retin Ox Anti-Wrinkle serum max. (They each work differently.) You can use the Prevage in the AM and the Roc at night.

Exfoliation

For ORNWs, an at-home exfoliating scrub or microdermabrasion kit will provide the same results as a spa or salon microdermabrasion treatment.

RECOMMENDED EXFOLIATION PRODUCTS

£ Buf-Puf

£ L'Oréal ReFinish Micro-Dermabrasion Kit

£ Olay Daily Facials Intensives Smooth Skin Exfoliating Scrub

££ Laura Mercier Face Polish

££ Philosophy The Greatest Love Microdermabrading Scrub

£££ Dr Brandt Microdermabrasion in a Jar

£££ La Prairie Cellular Microdermabrasion Cream

Baumann's Choice: Buf-Puf. I have always loved this ingenious invention.

SHOPPING FOR PRODUCTS

You can widen your choice of products by reading labels to determine product ingredients; thus, you can select those that contain beneficial ingredients for avoiding wrinkles, while steering clear of ingredients that cause oiliness. If you find favourite products that are not listed in your chapter, please go to www.DrBaumann.co.uk and share your finds with me.

SKIN CARE INGREDIENTS TO USE

To prevent wrinkles:

- Caffeine
- Coenzyme Q_{10} (ubiquinone)
- Copper peptide
- Ginseng Pomegranate
- Grape seed extract
- Green tea
- Humulus lupulus (hops)
- Idebenone
- Lutein
- Lycopene
- Moringa
- Pinus pinaster (pine bark)
- Resveratrol
- Rosemary
- Vitamin C (ascorbic acid)
- Vitamin E

To treat wrinkles:

- Alpha lipoic acid
- Copper peptide
- DMAE
- Glycolic acid (AHA)
- Lactic acid (AHA)
- Phytic acid (AHA)
- Retinol
- Salicylic acid (BHA)
- TGF-Beta
- Vitamin C (ascorbic acid)

SKIN CARE INGREDIENTS TO AVOID

Due to excess oiliness:

- Mineral oil
- Other oils such as safflower oil
- Petrolatum

Sun Protection for Your Skin

Using a sunscreen is especially important for ORNWs. If you have a high O/D score (above 35), you will want to use facial powders with sunscreen. Whether you like to use several different makeup products, such as powder, foundation, and primer, or whether you prefer to simply wear a single product, like sunscreen, make sure you reach the minimum SPF of 15, which I advise for daily use. If your O/D score is between 30 and 34, choose a gel sunscreen. Those with O/D scores lower than 30 may prefer lotion sunscreens.

If you prefer not to use a facial foundation or powder with SPF, use one of the sunscreens listed later in this section.

When and How to Apply Sunscreen

Apply sunscreen every morning, even if you don't expect to go outdoors. Staying indoors will not protect you. UVA easily penetrates windows to send harmful sun rays into buildings, cars and aeroplanes. Keep sunscreen in your car, desk and handbag to reapply if needed.

To use, squeeze out a 10p-size portion of the product and apply it to your entire face, neck, hands, and chest. Make sure the product you choose has a minimum SPF of 15 for daily protection. For prolonged sun exposure outside, at the beach, or in other bright sun conditions, you can use an SPF of 45 to 60 and reapply sunscreen every hour. You can cover the sunscreen with a powder or mix with Clinac O.C. to minimise the oiliness.

Apply sunscreen to your body as well, since clothes provide less protection than most people realise. A normal T-shirt has an SPF of only 5, while tighter-weave fabrics offer more protection.

You can apply sunscreen to the eye area unless you experience itching, burning or irritation. In very hot weather, or if you are involved in active sports, you may find that sunscreen runs into your eyes when you sweat and makes them burn. In that case, don't use it in the eye area. Instead, use a concealer or foundation with sun protective ingredients.

Mexoryl is an ingredient that provides superior UVA protection, but it is not yet approved in the US or the UK, so you have to buy products that contain it in Ireland or France. La Roche-Posay Anthelios Fluid Extreme SPF 60 contains Mexoryl and is right for your type. Be sure to shake it before use.

RECOMMENDED SUN PROTECTION PRODUCTS

£ Neutrogena Visibly Young Day Cream with SPF 20

£ Olay Touch Moisturising Fluid SPF 15

££ Clinique Super City Block Oil-Free Daily Face Protector SPF 25

££ Estée Lauder Multi-Protection Sun Spray (Oil-Free) SPF 15

££ Exuviance Fundamental Multi-Protective Day Fluid SPF 15

££ Exuviance Multi-Defence Day Fluid SPF 15 with AHAs

££ Garnier Ambre Solaire Sheer Protect Shine Free SPF 30

££ Jack Black Oil Free Sun Guard SPF 20

££ La Roche-Posay Anthelios XL SPF 60 Fluide Extreme

££ NeoStrada Oil-Free Lotion SPF 15

£££ Clarins Oil-Free Sun Care Spray SPF 15

Baumann's Choice: Anthelios Fluid Extreme SPF 60 by La Roche-Posay containing Mexoryl and several other sun-blocking ingredients. If you cannot find Anthelios, my second choice is Neutrogena Visibly Young Day Cream with SPF 20.

Your Makeup

Avoid oil-containing foundations and instead use powders that absorb oil. Many foundations are marked 'oil free' on the label, but some that claim to control oiliness actually contain oil. To find out whether yours does, get a piece of 25 percent-cotton bond paper. Place a drop of foundation on it. Oil-containing foundations will leave a ring of oil on the paper. The size of the ring is proportional to the amount of oil in the foundation – the bigger the ring, the more oil the product contains.

RECOMMENDED OIL-FREE FOUNDATIONS

£ Avon Beyond Colour Perfecting Foundation with Natural Match Technology SPF 12

££ Bobbi Brown Oil-Free Even Finish Foundation SPF 15

££ Elizabeth Arden Flawless Finish Skin Balancing Makeup

££ Exuviance CoverBlend Concealing Treatment Makeup SPF 20

££ Laura Mercier Oil-Free Foundation

£££ DiorSkin Compact with SPF 20

£££ Lancôme Maquicontrôle Oil-Free Liquid Makeup

Baumann's Choice: Any with SPF. I like Lancôme Maquicontrôle because it contains antioxidants.

RECOMMENDED OIL-ABSORBING POWDERS

- £ Cover Girl Fresh Look Pressed Powder
- £ Maybelline Shine Free Oil-Control Pressed Powder
- £ Revlon Shine Control Mattifying Powder
- ££ Bobbi Brown Sheer Finish Loose Powder
- ££ Garden Botanika Natural Finish Loose Powder
- ££ Laura Mercier Loose Setting Powder
- £££ Chanel Pureté Mat Shine Control Powder SPF 15

Baumann's Choice: Garden Botanika Natural Finish Loose Powder

CONSULTING A DERMATOLOGIST

PRESCRIPTION SKIN CARE STRATEGIES

My prescription regimen for ORNWs is the same as the nonprescription regimen, but provides stronger ingredients for more aggressive prevention and treatment of wrinkles. That's why you'll use a prescription retinoid in the evening.

DAILY SKIN CARE

STAGE TWO: PRESCRIPTION REGIMEN	
AM	PM
Step 1: Wash with antioxidant cleanser	Step 1: Wash with same cleanser as in AM
Step 2: Apply toner, gel or serum with antioxidants	Step 2: Use same toner as in AM

Step 3: Apply sunscreen either on its own or mixed with an oil-control product

Step 4: Apply oil-free foundation, oil-absorbing powder, or both

Step 3: Layer a moisturiser under the retinoid (optional)

Step 4: Apply a prescription retinoid

In the morning, wash your face with a cleanser containing antioxidants. Then apply an antioxidant-containing toner, gel or serum. Next, if your O/D score is high (over 35), mix together a pea-size dollop of O.C. Eight by Ferndale with a pea-size dollop of a gel sunscreen, and apply.

If your O/D score is between 24 and 34, apply a lotion sunscreen that contains antioxidants. Last, apply an oil-free foundation, an oil-absorbing powder, or both.

In the evening, wash with the same cleanser you used in the morning, then apply a prescription retinoid. I prefer gels for ORNWs, so my choice would be Retin-A gel.

If you wish, you can skip the retinoid every third night, or alternatively you can layer the retinoid over the moisturiser every night. These options will help in case you develop excessive redness or flaking from the retinoid. If you do use a moisturiser, choose one containing antioxidants, like my favourite, Replenix CF Cream.

When following this prescription regimen, you should only use a facial scrub one or two times a week. The retinoid will help exfoliate your skin, so scrubs are less necessary. Use them gently when your skin feels rough or looks dull.

PRESCRIPTION RETINOIDS TO TREAT WRINKLES

- Aknemycin Plus (contains an antibiotic as well)
- Differin gel or cream
- Isotrex
- Isotrexin (contains an antibiotic as well)
- Retin-A gel, lotion or cream
- Retinova

Baumann's choice: Choose the product with highest percentage of active ingredients you can tolerate. Please discuss your options with your dermatologist.

PROCEDURES FOR YOUR SKIN TYPE

Skin care procedures for this type concentrate on treating wrinkles. Follow my skin care recommendations to prevent wrinkles, but to address wrinkles that have already formed, you may want to indulge in the procedures I recommend below to get rid of them.

PROCEDURES TO TREAT WRINKLES

You have a choice of a range of procedures for treating wrinkles. They include injections of botulinum toxin, like Botox, Reloxin, dermal fillers, or dermabrasion. For complete information on these options, please consult 'Further Help for Oily, Resistant Skin'.

Dermabrasion

While the advanced procedures will help with many kinds of wrinkles, stubborn wrinkles around the mouth, called 'smoker's lines', are hard to treat permanently. People with lighter skin (which includes the majority of ORNWs), have an additional option in dermabrasion (which is not to be confused with microdermabrasion).

In the dermabrasion procedure, the physician uses a tiny spinning wheel covered with diamonds to remove the top layer of skin down to the depth of the dermis (the deeper of the two main layers that make up the skin). This level of skin removal is much deeper than occurs in microdermabrasion, which uses tiny crystals that gently abrade the skin, removing only the upper layer of dead skin cells.

Be prepared to take some time off following dermabrasion, since afterwards the treated skin will have an open sore for about four to seven days. Once that heals, you may experience anywhere from a few days to a few weeks of redness. Fortunately, that can be covered by makeup.

The good news is that when the skin heals, it appears much smoother and less lined. However, this procedure does carry some risks, including scarring and lightening of the skin in the treated area. That is why I do not advise this option unless you go to a highly qualified doctor who is experienced in performing the procedure. Admittedly, not many are available. Please consult the Resources section for information on how to find a qualified dermatologist.

Unlike people with pigmented skin, light-skinned ORNWs are good candidates for dermabrasion because they do not develop dark spots in the treated areas. (Someone with tight skin would not require dermabrasion since wrinkles are not an issue.)

Although this procedure may sound scary, I have been amazed by the lack of pain that people report and the results achieved. You may have heard about CO_2 laser resurfacing, which previously was used to get rid of these stubborn lines around the mouth. It has fallen out of favour because many patients reported long-term complications. Dermabrasion has been safely performed for over thirty-five years.

Microdermabrasion

Microdermabrasion, a popular procedure offered in dermatology offices, skin care salons, and spas, removes the upper dead layer of skin to make your skin feel smoother. The practitioner uses a device that sprays micro-crystals to remove the upper surface layer of the skin. As an ORNW, you can freely benefit from microdermabrasion treatments, although frankly, an exfoliating scrub or microdermabrasion home kit will provide the same results, for less cost. (Save the money for what you really need: prescription retinoids and dermal fillers.) Nevertheless, if you want to look radiant for a party, and you have the time and the money – go for it. Or else, try something disposable, like Dove Face Care Essential Nutrients Cleansing Pillows. See the list of exfoliators and microdermabrasion at-home kits for more suggestions.

Thermage

A new technique called thermage can treat droopy lines around the mouth and nose area as well as the under-neck sagging skin, which gives a 'turkey neck' appearance. Please see 'Further Help for Oily, Resistant Skin'.

Spa Procedures

ORNWs are great candidates for spa and cosmetic dermatology services like chemical peels, which help exfoliate skin.

Microcurrent units popular in many facial salons are electrical devices that stimulate the facial muscles to contract or stretch, aiming to relax tight muscles and tone loose ones; but it isn't clear whether this treatment is effective, since the appearance of aging is mostly caused by loss of fat as we age, which causes the skin to lose volume.

As an ORNW considering salon services, be warned: salon services may not be powerful enough for you. Your resistant skin can handle high-strength chemical peels, which are usually not performed in spas, so make sure to ask for a higher concentration than they use on their sensitive-skin clients.

What About Lasers?

Non-ablative lasers and light treatments such as light-emitting diodes and Intense Pulsed Light will probably become important in the future to prevent or treat wrinkles. At this time, the technology is still being improved as far as wrinkles are concerned. I am dismayed by the number of patients I see who have already spent five to six thousand dollars on these treatments and have not seen any difference in their skin.

I believe that some day laser treatments for wrinkles will become effective and worth the expense, but they are not there yet. (Note: these technologies are great for removing blood vessels, redness and dark spots, which are not concerns for ORNWs.)

ONGOING CARE FOR YOUR SKIN

Focus on wrinkle prevention. If it's too late, don't be afraid to bite the bullet and do something that really works! Your RN skin helps protect you from the side effects that other Skin Types develop after more intensive procedures.

CHAPTER ELEVEN

Oily, Resistant, Non-Pigmented and Tight: ORNT

THE GODDESS SKIN TYPE

'I always get compliments on my skin, though honestly, I can't take credit for it. I don't do anything special, so it must be genetic. All the women in my family have beautiful skin. I guess I'm just lucky.'

ABOUT YOUR SKIN

Flawless, even toned, radiant, ageless.

If you're an ORNT, you won the Skin Type lottery – although you probably never knew there was one. You rarely think about your skin. It's easy to care for, plus it always looks great. You don't understand all the fuss about skin care. You wouldn't dream of springing big bucks for procedures or surgery.

Frankly, if you're an ORNT, I'm surprised and flattered that you bought this book. Why? Because you have one of the easiest Skin Types to care for, age in, and live with overall. In you, lucky genes and good skin care habits combine to create age-defying skin. Your oily, tight skin protects you from the visible signs of aging while your skin cells produce colour without any tendency to develop dark spots after trauma or inflammation. If you have a light skin tone, you may have some trouble tanning, but so what? Having youthful skin throughout your life is a good trade-off for the temporary thrill of a tan, especially when you consider that tanning promotes aging. Unlike Sensitive or Dry Skin Types, ORNTs do not get acne, redness, dark spots or dryness.

ORNT CELEBRITY

French film actress and world-class beauty Catherine Deneuve is the quintessential ORNT. Now over sixty, she continues to embody elegance, desirability and feminine seductive power. On-screen in contemporary dramas or classic roles, and off-screen with admirers like Marcello Mastroianni (who fathered her second child), Deneuve exemplifies how ORNT skin flouts the aging process.

As a teenager, Deneuve transformed overnight from a pretty, brunette actress into an enduring icon, whose pale blonde hair, chiseled features, and perfect porcelain skin codified her allure. Deneuve's flawless, non-pigmented, tight skin has helped her embody the cool, remote blondes she so frequently portrays.

Although Deneuve owes her fabulous skin to enviable genes, at least in part, the actress has wisely maintained this treasured heritage. Like many French women, she probably began following a careful skin care regimen early in life and has avoided sun exposure that could have marred her fine complexion.

Having appeared in over ninety films, Deneuve's face has literally been her fortune. Still in demand on-screen, Deneuve's long-lived stardom reveals that resistant, tight skin has staying power. Plus, it helps that this actress works in Europe, where attitudes about aging are more sophisticated, and less youth-oriented, than they are in the United States.

Deneuve is by no means the sole icon to enjoy this type. Many contemporary actresses, performers, and well-known personalities, including Katie Couric, Kelly Ripa and Kate Hudson (as far as I can tell from their public appearances and photos) also have this vibrant Skin Type. You can recognise ORNT skin because it always radiates attractiveness.

Actress Kate Winslet is very likely an ORNT, and it looks like she takes good care of her beautiful skin. With his pale skin, and reddish blonde hair, musician Elton John also looks to be an ORNT, and, he has taken care to safeguard his skin. I've rarely seen photos of him with a tan. His good friend, the late Princess Diana, may very likely have had the same Skin Type. People with her colouring, blonde hair, and rosy complexion, can often be non-pigmented types.

Celebrity couple, David Bowie and his wife, the model Iman, may also both be ORNTs because they both show the smoothness of oily, tight skin, without any spots, freckles or dark spots. Iman, with her breakthrough makeup line for women of colour, is on the leading edge of beauty as were her beauty magnate predecessors. What did Elizabeth Arden, Helena Rubinstein and Estée Lauder, all giants of the cosmetic industry have in common? Like Iman, they too were probably all ORNT types. Although I've never met them, I infer this from photographs, as well as the many reports of their smooth flawless skin. ORNT skin was their best marketing tool in persuading other women to follow their advice. Helena Rubinstein was one of the first to advocate sun avoidance and the use of sunscreen. She observed the sun's detrimental effect well before it was widely recognised or documented by science. Rubinstein never took her good skin for granted. Nor did beauty giants Estée Lauder or Elizabeth Arden whose glowing, unlined skin conferred youth upon them for decades. Although their fabulous skin inspired others to try their products, it didn't mean that their offerings were 100 percent on target for every Skin Type. And that's one reason I want to educate people to the unique needs of their particular skin.

YOUR SKIN HISTORY

In youth, your skin probably tended to be oily, but as you reach your forties, you'll find that your skin begins to normalise and becomes less so. While other forty-year-olds fight dryness, your skin is just right. Some of you are so proud of your skin that you pamper it with various creams and concoctions, avoiding sunning and smoking to preserve your skin's beauty. Others with this type do everything wrong: you smoke, sunbathe, go without adequate sleep, and use whatever soap happens to be lying around, without a thought. In that case, your skin seems to exemplify the power of genetics.

ORNTs with darker skin tones are free of the cycle of acne and dark spots that troubles many people of colour. Though an occasional cut or trauma, like a burn, scrape, or irritation, could lead to a temporary dark spot, this occurs so infrequently that there's little need to prevent it in your Daily Skin Care Regimen. Dark-skinned ORNTs may develop dark spots and temporarily become pigmented types due to the hormonal shifts that occur during pregnancy. However, don't worry, as your skin will return to its native N, or non-pigmented state, soon after your hormones return to post-pregnancy levels. Lighter-skinned ORNTs are not prone to hormonally related pigmentation experienced by people of colour.

Case Story: Heather and Gillian

B est friends and stay-at-home mums, Heather and Gillian met when their daughters were in the same play group. Pretty, blonde, sandy-haired, and blue-eyed Heather was a self-described 'mutt', who laughingly told me that her family heritage was part Scotch-Irish, part Cherokee, and part 'hillbilly'. Petite, coffee-skinned Gillian, on the other hand, was the daughter of an African diplomat. Both in their early thirties, they came to discover what tricks I might have up my sleeve. Neither had any pressing skin problems or questions, which in itself indicated that they were one of the easier Skin Types. Their only concern was whether they should do anything to prevent aging, though neither showed any signs of it.

Sure enough, the questionnaire revealed that they were both ORNTs with no sensitivity to cosmetic products, no skin dryness, and no issues with dark spots. How surprised they were that two friends with totally different colouring could share a Skin Type. But it didn't surprise me. Despite their difference in skin colour, they shared quite a number of ORNT skin qualities.

I explained to them that while the scoring system for the P/N factor in my Skin Type Questionnaire does contain questions that account for ethnicity, it's more concerned with pigmentation problems such as unwanted brown spots. Gillian's skin was darker than Heather's, but, like Heather's, it was uniform in colour, as is typical for ORNTs. I congratulated them both for avoiding the sun; neither of them had any spots, sun damage, or discolouration. When I examined their skin under a special light that reveals underlying damage, they both were wrinkle-free. They were relieved when I told them that their chief skin issues were skin cancer prevention and oil control.

My chief recommendation was to advise Heather to religiously go for a skin exam once a year to make sure she did not have skin cancer. Gillian, because of her darker skin tone, was not at a high risk for skin cancer. Like Heather, ORNTs with a lighter skin tone may be at an increased risk for developing non-melanoma skin cancer, especially if they permit excess, unprotected sun exposure.

A CLOSE-UP LOOK AT YOUR SKIN

Like Heather and Gillian, with ORNT skin you may experience any of the following:

- Smooth, oily skin
- Little need for moisturiser
- Few wrinkles
- Foundation makeup streaks
- Large pores
- Blackheads
- Enlarged oil glands

- Infrequent acne breakouts
- Skin cancers (see below so that you can identify the signs)

Genes determine how much pigment (melanin) your skin produces. Most non-pigmented types produce less than pigmented types, while a light-skinned, non-pigmented type, like Heather, would have even less than a dark-skinned ORNT, like Gillian. Increased melanin lowers your risk of skin cancer. With less skin pigment, there is less protection against the deleterious effects of the sun. As a result, light-skinned ORNTs are more vulnerable to skin cancer than dark-skinned ORNTs. Check yourself, and double-check with a dermatologist regularly.

It's vital to avoid the sun on both sunny days, and overcast ones. Dreary weather can be misleading because many people mistakenly believe that the sun rays cannot penetrate the clouds. But that's not true; sunscreen should be worn at all times. Even a single sunburn can lead to lifelong damage and increased skin cancer risk.

How to Recognise a Non-Melanoma Skin Cancer

A squamous cell carcinoma (SCC) may appear as red, scaling patches that form scabs in sun-exposed areas such as the face, ears, chest, arms, legs, and back. They do not heal. They may be covered by a hard white scale that resembles a wart. Any spot that fits this description and persists for one month or more should be seen by a dermatologist.

A basal cell carcinoma (BCC) may appear as a white, shiny bump, luminous like a pearl. They may have either a central ridge with a little hole or depression, or tiny blood vessels visible in the border. They can also look like a crater or scar that suddenly appears although there has been no prior trauma. Sometimes the border is 'ruffled' or heaped up around the central crater.

Enlarged facial oil glands can be easily confused with BCC, since they both are yellowish bumps. Make sure to check out anything suspicious with a dermatologist. Your skin cancer risk is one of this type's only downsides. Take it seriously, and get regular checkups.

HOW GENES OPERATE IN SKIN AGING

Genes regulate the production of collagen and elastin, the key skin proteins responsible for skin firmness and resilience. Many skin care products contain these ingredients, claiming to deliver them topically. But without studies documenting these claims, I don't find their promises convincing. Cosmetic companies have also tried to capitalise on the emerging science of aging by customising skin care products based on genetic testing. However, we don't yet know how to use that information to create an effective product. Perhaps we will in ten or twenty years, but right now, in my opinion, the promise of individualised genetic-based treatments is just clever marketing and beautiful packaging to sell the same old stuff at higher prices. Until we know how to replicate the genetic factors that make skin great, invest in your future by adopting the positive lifestyle factors that we do know can help.

Most people wonder, 'How gracefully will I age?' While neither I nor this book's questionnaire can predict that absolutely, a few simple certainties and some other subtle tendencies can reveal how well you'll age and what you can and *should* do to maintain youthful skin.

For people with tight, unwrinkled skin, genetics play a key role. Confirming this, you will probably notice that your mother, grandmother, or other relatives aged gracefully and looked younger than their contemporaries even in advanced years.

I commonly hear from my ORNT patients statements like, 'I take after my mother's side of the family. Both my mother and grandmother had great skin,' or, 'My grandmother told people she was sixty when she was really seventy-five and everyone believed her!'

Build on this good foundation with skin-enhancing lifestyle habits like avoiding sun exposure. Don't weaken that foundation with poor ones, like tanning, smoking, or going to tanning beds. Even those with good genes can wind up with more wrinkles if they indulge in the latter habits. I've seen pictures of identical twins, one with sun exposure, one without, and the one without looked much younger.

Some ORNTs do what it takes to preserve skin health. They practise strict sun avoidance and eat plenty of antioxidant-rich fruits and vegetables. In families where beautiful skin is a tradition, a savvy mum will sometimes bring in her daughter to start her out on an antiaging skin care regimen early to preserve and assure her good fortune in having great skin.

Have empathy for the other types since your Skin Type is uncommon. Don't expect your children, guests, or spouses to be able to use skin care products as indiscriminately as you can. One application of that same nicely scented hotel lotion that you use without a second thought, and I, for one, develop red and itching skin for twenty-four hours.

How to take the best care of your skin? Unless you are troubled by oiliness, you don't need to do anything special, other than remembering to apply sunscreen. Overall, my product recommendations will be kinder to your skin than that deodorant soap you happen to use. While maintaining ORNT skin is not hard work, why not treat your skin right with appropriate skin care?

YOUR MOST BASIC SKIN CARE STRATEGIES

If you have excessive oil, use the oil-control products I'll recommend. If you are prone to blackheads, prevent them with prescription retinoids. Use powders instead of makeup foundations when possible. Don't be tricked into wasting money on toners, serums or antiaging night creams, because you don't need them.

Since you have easy, resistant skin, feel free to experiment. You can tolerate fragrant skin creams, all types of ingredients, and preservatives. Getting facials is probably a great treat for you, even when the aesthetician uses products that can irritate many of us. Enjoy, count your blessings, and feel free to add variety to your skin care routine.

Your recommendations include products that are more adventurous than those I suggest to other types. If you develop a problem, recheck your questionnaire responses. You may be an OSNT who in the past has used less adventurous products so that you did not realise that your skin is sensitive. Changing environments, increased stress, or changes in lifestyle habits can also cause your Skin Type to change.

Dr Baumann's Bottom Line: Whatever combination of good genes and good skin care gave you your youthful line-free skin, help out nature and prevent skin cancer through good skin care and avoiding excess sun exposure.

EVERYDAY CARE FOR YOUR SKIN

Your skin care routine focuses on addressing skin oiliness with products that deliver oil-absorbing ingredients or contain ingredients that will to a certain extent decrease oil production. Unfortunately, not many products are able to permanently and totally decrease your skin's production of oil. This makes ongoing control essential.

The products I'll recommend do one or both of the following:

- Prevent and treat oiliness
- Treat oiliness

Your daily regimen will also address your other skin concerns by:

- Preventing pore enlargement
- Treating enlarged pores
- Preventing and treating blackheads
- Preventing occasional acne breakouts

First, look over the regimen and then you can choose the products you'll need from those I recommend in each category later in this chapter.

If after using this regimen for two months, you still have trouble with occasional acne, you may wish to consult a dermatologist who can prescribe retinoids for my Stage Two Regimen.

Since ORNT is the easiest Skin Type to care for, I've built a one-stage regimen geared towards decreasing oil production to help treat and prevent your infrequent acne breakouts as well as minimising enlarged pores. The products you'll use will soak up excess oil and decrease facial shine.

DAILY SKIN CARE

STAGE ONE: NONPRESCRIPTION REGIMEN

AM	PM
Step 1: Wash with cleanser	Step 1: Wash with cleanser
Step 2: Apply oil-control product	Step 2: Use a scrub or exfoliator (optional)
Step 3: Apply oil-free foundation with oil control (optional)	Step 3: Apply a retinol product
Step 4: Apply powder with SPF	

In the morning, wash your face with one of the recommended cleansers. Apply an oil-control product. If you have a higher O/D score (above 35), you may wish to wear oil-free foundation and/or makeup powder with SPF as well. Remember: make sure to wear at least one product that contains SPF 15. Everyone needs sun protection. You may also wish to carry blotting papers with you to absorb oil, whenever needed.

In the evening, wash with cleanser, and then you can use a scrub two to three times per week. Next, use a retinol-containing product to help lessen oil production.

Cleansers

To control your skin's oil production, keep your skin clean. Excess oil clogs pores and stretches them out, resulting in enlarged pores. Products that claim to shrink pores really just irritate the skin, causing the pores to swell so that they look smaller temporarily. Nothing can permanently shrink pores, but products containing beta hydroxy acid (BHA) can penetrate into pores and clear them, thereby minimising pore enlargement. Be sure to use cleanser both morning and evening.

RECOMMENDED CLEANSING PRODUCTS

£ Clean and Clear Daily Pore Cleanser
£ L'Oréal Pure Zone Pore Unclogging Scrub Cleanser
£ Neutrogena Pore Refining Cleanser
£ Olay Daily Facials for Combination or Oily skin
££ Clarins Purifying Cleansing Gel
££ Ella Baché Lotion Adoucissant
££ Kiehls Blue Herbal Gel Cleanser
££ Korres Hamamelis Cleansing Tonic Lotion
££ Lancôme Gel Contrôle Purifying Gel Cleanser
££ Laura Mercier Foaming One-Step Cleanser
££ Origins Mint Wash
££ Philosophy Purity Made Simple One-step Facial Cleanser
£££ Darphin Purifying Foam Gel
£££ Jurlique Cleansing Lotion

Baumann's Choice: Neutrogena Pore Refining Cleanser contains BHA to help keep pores clear.

Toner Use

Some oily types enjoy the refreshing, clean feeling that toners provide. Although they will not control oil as well as the oil-control cleansers, foundations and powder, if you'd like to use a toner, feel free to do so. It will not harm your skin, though in my opinion it's an unnecessary expense. If you do use a toner, you might try any of those I recommend.

RECOMMENDED TONERS

- £ Neutrogena Pore Refining Toner
- £ Nivea Visage Alcohol-Free Moisturising Toner
- ££ Aesop Parsley Seed Anti-Oxidant Facial Toner
- ££ Borghese Acqua Puro Comforting Spray Toner
- ££ Dr Hauschka Clarifying Toner (for oily skin)
- ££ Kiehl's Tea Tree Oil Toner
- ££ Molton Brown Skin Balance Toning Lotion
- ££ Origins Oil Refiner Tonic
- ££ Paula's Choice Final Touch Toner for Normal to Oily/Combination Skin
- £££ Chanel Précision Lotion Tendre Soothing Toner
- £££ Darphin Niaouli Aromatic Care Toner
- £££ Natura Bisse Oily Skin Toner

Baumann's Choice: Dr Hauschka Clarifying Toner

Oil-Control Products

For ongoing oil control, you can use OC Eight Oil Control gel by Ferndale, while to treat pimples when you have them, use Paula's Choice 1% Beta Hydroxy Acid Gel, which contains beta hydroxy acid. Retinol products may also help to decrease oiliness and prevent outbreaks. Applying oil-free makeup foundations, foundation primers, and powders will absorb oil and reduce the appearance of oiliness. Since no ingredients can totally control oil secretion, stay on top of your skin's native oiliness by blotting with the products recommended below. You can address blackheads, when they occur, with Bioré Deep Cleansing Pore Strips.

RECOMMENDED OIL-CONTROL PRODUCTS

- £ Simple Oil Control Facial Wipes
- ££ Mary Kay Beauty Blotters Oil-Absorbing Tissues
- ££ OC Eight by Ferndale
- ££ Paula's Choice 1% Beta Hydroxy Acid Gel
- ££ Clarins Mat Express Instant Shine Control
- £££ Korres Lemon Anti-Shine Gel
- £££ Ole Henriksen Grease Relief Face Tonic
- £££ Thalgo Intense Regulating Serum

Baumann's Choice: Mary Kay Beauty Blotters Oil-Absorbing Tissues are great because they are easy to carry with you.

RETINOL-CONTAINING PRODUCTS

- £ Neutrogena Healthy Skin Cream
- ££ Philosophy Help Me
- ££ Reti-C Intensive Corrective Care by Vichy
- ££ Sothy's Retinol 15
- ££ Topix Replenix Retinol Smoothing Serum 3x
- £££ Clarins Renew Plus Night Lotion
- £££ Estée Lauder Diminish Anti-Wrinkle Retinal Treatment
- £££ Jan Marini Factor A Plus Lotion
- £££ Lancôme Resurface
- £££ Prescriptives Skin Renewal Cream
- £££ SkinCeuticals Retinol 0.5 or 1%

Baumann's Choice: Philosophy's Help Me retinol treatment with a high amount of retinol is packaged properly to ensure stability of retinol.

RECOMMENDED BLOTTERS

- £ Clean & Clear Oil Absorbing Sheets
- £ Crabtree and Evelyn Facial Blotting Tissues
- £ Mary Kay Beauty Blotters Oil-Absorbing Tissues
- £ Paula's Choice Oil Blotting Papers
- £ The Body Shop Facial Blotting Tissues

Baumann's Choice: Any of the above.

Moisturisers

With very oily skin, you generally will not need to moisturise. However, you may find that in drier climates and when the humidity is low, as in winter, your skin feels tight. If so, a light moisturiser can help. If you have a lower O/D score (27 to 35) you may have combination skin and require a moisturiser. If so, choose a light one from among those I suggest and apply it in drier skin areas. Finally, as you age, oiliness will decrease, so that using a light moisturiser becomes an option.

RECOMMENDED MOISTURISERS

£ Neutrogena Ultimate Moisture Day Cream
£ Nivea Antiwrinkle Q10 Plus Day Cream
£ Paula's Choice Skin Balancing Moisture Gel
£ Roc Retin Ox Anti-Wrinkle Serum- Max (with retinol)
££ Clinique Dramatically Different Moisturising Gel
££ La Roche-Posay Effidrate
££ Prescriptives All You Need +
£££ Caudalie Day Fluid SPF12 with Resveratrol
£££ Clarins Skin Beauty Repair Concentrate
£££ Dior Energy Move Skin Illuminating Moisturiser Crème
£££ La Mer Oil Absorbing Lotion

Baumann's Choice: Roc Retin Ox Anti-Wrinkle Serum Max because the retinol may help slow oil production.

Masks

You can apply a mask to temporarily decrease skin oiliness. Use one prior to a party or at any time when you do not want your face to look shiny in photographs.

RECOMMENDED MASKS

£ Ahava Advanced Mud Masque for Oily Skin
£ Botanics Conditioning Clay Mask
£ Olay Daily Facials Intensives Deep Cleansing Clay Mask
£ Queen Helene Natural English Clay Mud Pack Masque
££ Laura Mercier Deep Cleansing Clay Mask
££ Nars Mud Mask
££ Yardley of London Apothecary Firm Deal Face & Body Mask
£££ Dr Brandt Poreless Purifying Mask
£££ Sisley Radiant Glow Express Mask with Red Clays

Baumann's Choice: Olay Daily Facials Intensives Deep Cleansing Clay Mask because of the price, but they are all good.

Exfoliation

ORNTs can benefit from scrubs and microdermabrasion to help keep pores clean and trouble free.

RECOMMENDED FACIAL SCRUBS

- £ Aapri Facial Scrub
- £ L'Oréal ReFinish Micro-Dermabrasion Kit
- £ Nivea Men's Exfoliating Facial Scrub
- ££ Laura Mercier Face Polish
- ££ Philosophy Microdelivery Peel
- ££ The Body Shop Seaweed Foaming Facial Scrub
- £££ Dr Brandt Microdermabrasion in a Jar
- £££ Ella Baché Revitalisant
- £££ Prescriptives Dermapolish System

Baumann's Choice: L'Oréal ReFinish Micro-Dermabrasion Kit. It comes with a moisturiser that those of you with oilier skin may not need. Instead it makes a fantastic hand cream.

SHOPPING FOR PRODUCTS

There are no specific ingredients that you need to look for in skin care products. However, you should choose products labelled oil control and avoid those containing mineral oil and other oils such as sunflower oil and borage seed oil.

SKIN CARE INGREDIENTS TO AVOID

Due to excess oil:

- Borage seed oil
- Mineral oil
- Other oils
- Petrolatum
- Sunflower oil

Sun Protection for Your Skin

For your type, I prefer gels, sprays and SPF-containing powders. Powders are best, because they help absorb oil in addition to providing sun protection. To reach the minimum SPF of 15, which I advise for daily use, use several different kinds of products if needed. I suggest you avoid cream sunscreen, because it tends to make skin feel and appear oilier. However, if you will be receiving prolonged sun exposure, you can use the gel sunscreens I recommend. For complete instructions on sunscreen use, please refer to Chapter Two.

RECOMMENDED SUN PROTECTION PRODUCTS, POWDERS

- £ Boots No7 Uplifting Foundation SPF 15
- £ L'Oréal Air Wear Powder Foundation SPF 17
- £ Revlon Shine Control Mattifying Powder SPF 8
- ££ Colourescience Foundation Powder SPF 20
- ££ Elizabeth Arden Flawless Finish Dual Perfection Makeup SPF 8
- ££ Philosophy Complete Me High Pigment Mineral Powder SPF 15
- ££ Stila Sheer Colour Face Powder SPF 15
- ££ Vichy Capital Soleil
- £££ Bobbi Brown Sheer Finish Loose Powder
- £££ Shu Uemura UV Under Base SPF 8

Baumann's Choice: Colourescience Foundation Powder SPF 20 because I believe you should wear as much SPF as possible.

RECOMMENDED SUN PROTECTION PRODUCTS, LOTIONS, GELS AND SPRAYS

- ££ Aveda Tourmaline Charged Protecting Lotion SPF 15
- ££ Ego Sunsense Clear Mist SPF 30
- ££ Garnier Ambre Solaire Sheer protect SPF 30
- ££ La Roche-Posay Anthelios Fluide Extreme SPF 60 (In Ireland and France)
- £££ Clarins Oil-Free Sun Care Spray SPF 15

Baumann's Choice: Most people with your Skin Type prefer applying a sunscreen powder following the application of one of these gels, lotions or sprays.

Your Makeup

Here you can enjoy and experiment. Unlike some other types, you should not experience reactions to any colours or pigments typically found in makeup products, nor are there any types of makeup you need to avoid.

The powders and foundations I recommend help reduce shine by surrounding the oil, making it less visible on the skin, or else by absorbing the oil. Talc and kaolin in these products help absorb oil. Use oil-control powders to prevent the makeup streaking that often comes with very oily skin. If you have a lower O/D score, you can wear foundations without a problem. If your score is high (above 35), either skip the foundation and use only a powder, or use an oil-absorbing foundation primer.

Foundation primers absorb oil when applied before a foundation and enable the foundation to last longer without streaking. You can also use them on their own, without foundation.

RECOMMENDED FOUNDATION PRIMERS

£ Garden Botanika Skin Perfecting Foundation Primer oily/combo
£ Maybelline Fresh Matte Foundation
£ The Body Shop Matt It Face & Lips
££ Elizabeth Arden Good Morning Skin Serum
££ Laura Mercier Foundation Primer
££ OC Eight Oil Control Gel by Ferndale
£££ Clinique Moisture in Control Oil Free Lotion
£££ Lancôme Hydra Controle Mat Shine control lotion

Baumann's Choice: OC Eight Oil Control Gel by Ferndale

RECOMMENDED FOUNDATIONS

£ Boots No7 Uplifting Foundation SPF 15
£ Bobbi Brown Oil-Free Even Finish Foundation SPF 15
£ L'Oréal Air Wear Powder Foundation SPF 17
£ Maybelline Pure Stay Powder & Foundation SPF 15
££ Colourescience Powder Foundation SPF 20
££ Laura Mercier Oil Free Foundation
££ Philosophy The Supernatural Airbrushed Canvas Powder Foundation
££ Stila Illuminating Powder Foundation

Baumann's Choice: Boots No7 Uplifting Foundation SPF 15

Recommended Oil-Control Powders

£ Maybelline Shine Free Oil-Control Pressed Powder

££ Fashion Fair Oil-Control Loose Face Powder

££ Jurlique Rose Silk Powder

££ Prescriptives Virtual Matte Oil-Control Pressed Powder

£££ Estée Lauder Double Matte Oil-Control Pressed Powder

£££ Shu Uemura Face Powder Matte

Baumann's Choice: Jurlique Rose Silk Powder; it's so elegant.

Consulting a Dermatologist

Earlier in this chapter, I provided a Daily Skin Care Regimen for dealing with oily skin, a common problem for ORNTs. However, if you have acne and tried the nonprescription cleansers and scrubs but feel you need further help, you may want to address the problem with prescription medications. I highly recommend that you do. My Stage Two regimen adds prescription retinoids to your basic daily regimen, along with the nonprescription products I recommend earlier in this chapter.

As I noted before, you should move to this second stage after sticking with stage one for at least two months.

DAILY SKIN CARE

STAGE TWO: PRESCRIPTION REGIMEN

For acne:

AM	PM
Step 1: Wash with cleanser	Step 1: Wash with cleanser
Step 2: Apply a prescription acne product	Step 2: Apply a prescription acne product
Step 3: Apply a sunscreen	Step 3: Apply a moisturiser (optional)
Step 4: Apply facial foundation or powder with SPF	Step 4: Apply a retinoid such as Retin-A gel

In the morning, cleanse and then apply a prescription acne product followed by a sunscreen and facial foundation or powder, if used. In the evening, cleanse, apply the same prescription acne product, and use a moisturiser, if needed. This regimen adds a retinoid in gel form, which is less greasy than a cream. If you have a low O/D score (27–35) you may prefer a retinoid cream instead. Ask your dermatologist for samples of both to see which you like better. Stick with this regimen and you should remain acne free. If redness and rosacea are your problem rather than acne, your dermatologist may give you MetroGel or another rosacea medication rather than the acne prescription products listed below.

PRESCRIPTION ACNE MEDICATIONS

- Benzamycin (contains benzoyl peroxide so it should not be used if you experience redness)
- Duac
- Dalacin T
- Stiemycin
- Topicycline
- Zindaclin
- Zineryt

PRESCRIPTION RETINOIDS

- Aknemycin Plus (contains an antibiotic as well)
- Differin gel or cream
- Isotrexin (contains an antiobiotic as well)
- Retin-A gel, lotion or cream
- Retinova

For advice on retinoid use, please consult 'Further Help for Oily, Resistant Skin'.

PROCEDURES FOR YOUR SKIN TYPE

ORNTs don't need any procedures. Yes, that's right! If you look at the chapters for other Skin Types, you'll see that I don't hesitate to recommend advanced skin options when needed. But you really don't need them. So get yourself a new pair of shoes instead!

That being said, if you want to give yourself some extra pampering, there are a few options you can consider. For instance, you might try microdermabrasion to smooth and soften your skin. Women who have tried it report that their makeup goes on smoother, making pores just a little more refined.

However, I feel that the scrubs suggested above give the same result at a much lower cost and time commitment. Of course, you could always plump your lips with collagen or hyaluronic acid, but – like Alison in the case story below – you probably do not need botulinum toxins, lasers or chemical peels.

Alison was a classic ORNT who also took great care of herself: non-smoker, stayed out of the sun, ate right – had everything going for her. She was in her mid-forties when she came to me. 'I have friends my age who are up to their second or third surgery, they've had Botox and Restylane injections, and they're always talking about what work so-and-so is having – or what work so-and-so *needs* to have. I'm reaching that time in my life where my skin isn't what it used to be. And I feel like I'm behind schedule. So, you're the expert – what do I need?'

What I told Alison was that she didn't need a thing – aside from some advice on a better skin care regimen. I explained how fortunate she was to have the easiest to maintain Skin Type, the type that not only requires little special treatment and can stand up to mild mistreatment, but will usually look even better and require far less maintenance as you age. 'Really?' she asked, looking relieved and a little proud. 'Really,' I said. And I sent her on her way with list of good skin care products, a Differin prescription, and a smile.

ORNTs are very lucky. If you make good lifestyle choices such as sun avoidance, smoking cessation, and consumption of a diet high in antioxidants, you should enjoy many years of good skin. Your skin's oiliness tends to decrease in your forties and fifties, so that, unlike other types, your skin actually gets better with time.

In your late fifties and sixties, you may begin to experience some skin dryness, but using a light moisturiser should be enough to correct this.

Hormone fluctuations can lead to skin oiliness as well. If you are female and this is a troublesome issue for you, you may want to consider an oral contraceptive. Ask your doctor which low-androgen product is right for you.

ONGOING CARE FOR YOUR SKIN

Rejoice! You have the easiest Skin Type. But don't take your good luck for granted. Maintain good skin care habits, and regularly check to assure that new moles or growths are not skin cancers. Plus, keep eating those vegetables.

Further Help for Oily, Resistant Skin

In this section, you'll find follow-up information and instructions on product use and procedures for the Oily, Resistant Skin Types, as well as lifestyle recommendations, diet, and supplements that can help your skin.

HOW RETINOIDS WORK

If retinoid use is recommended in your Skin Type chapter, here's some information about what it does and how to begin using it. A prescription retinoid can address oiliness, brown spots, and wrinkles, making it useful for oily, pigmented, and wrinkled types.

Retinoids speed up the rate at which your skin cells divide, and this improves your skin's appearance in a number of different ways. First of all, enlarged pores are formed by blackheads, which are actually pores clogged with dead skin cells that expand pore size. Retinoids increase cell renewal, reducing the dead skin cell buildup, and thereby decreasing blackhead formation. Goodbye, clogged, enlarged, unsightly pores.

Retinoids may also reduce oil production. Although oral retinoids such as Accutane reduce the size and function of oil glands, doctors can't say for sure if topical use will produce the same effect. However, some patients report that their skin feels less oily following topical retinoid use.

Retinoids also limit dark spot production since the cells that make colour (melanocytes) cannot make the pigment (melanin) fast enough to keep up with rapid cell turnover. Retinoids are vital to prevent wrinkles. They have been proven in multiple studies (on humans, not on cells or animals) to prevent the breakdown of collagen, elastin, and hyaluronic acid that leads to wrinkles.

Finally, retinoids help stimulate skin cells (fibroblasts) to make more collagen and hyaluronic acid. More collagen means more firmness and structure to your skin. More hyaluronic acid means more volume and moisture in your skin. Goodbye, sagging and wrinkles. Although all prescription retinoids will improve wrinkles, in the US, only two retinoids are specifically approved for the treatment of wrinkles (Avage and Renova). However, these products are in a cream form and I prefer a gel form for oily types. Retin-A, Retinova and Isotrex are similar to Renova, so look for those products even though they have not been FDA approved to treat wrinkles. Most people can safely use retinoids. However, pregnant and nursing mothers as well as women who plan to become pregnant should avoid them. Be advised that deep wrinkles and stubborn spots will likely require a medical procedure to improve them.

For pigmented types, I recommend beginning with a prescription skin lightener, which contains a bleaching agent to clear the dark spots faster than a retinoid can do alone. After eight weeks, or when the dark spots disappear, you should switch to other recommended products, such as Retin-A or Isotrex.

HOW TO USE RETINOIDS

Retinoids may irritate even the most resistant skin, so I have several strategies to transition you into retinoid use.

1. In your hand, squeeze out a pea-size portion of retinoid.
2. Apply to face and neck, using upward strokes, and wipe a touch on the backs of your hands. With only a trace of product on your hands, place your fingertips gently on the skin area under the eye (never on top of the eyelid or elsewhere around the eye), being careful not to get too close to the eye.
3. Use once every three days for two weeks or until no redness or flaking is visible.
4. At the end of two weeks, begin applying the mixture every other night. Continue this use for another two weeks.
5. Once your skin has adjusted to retinoid use, you can apply nightly and indefinitely. The longer you use it the better it works.

During the process of introducing retinoids, on the nights when you don't use it, apply instead one of the products (such as serums, moisturisers, or retinol-containing creams) recommended in your Skin Type chapter. After two applications of retinoids (over the course of six days), check to see how your skin feels. If you are not experiencing irritation, dryness or redness, you can begin using it every other night, while continuing to use the non-retinoid product on alternate nights. If your skin flakes initially (which is quite common), you can exfoliate with one of the scrubs recommended for your Skin Type in the Exfoliation section of your chapter. Once you no longer experience skin irritation, you may begin to use the retinoid every night.

If you choose to have light treatments and chemical peels (see 'Procedures' below), this regimen will make those procedures work better. Retinoids speed healing time by making your skin cells divide faster.

PROCEDURES

LIGHT TREATMENTS

Light-skinned, Oily, Resistant Skin Types can benefit from light procedures to remove dark spots, eradicate blood vessels, and help improve tiny wrinkles; however, darker-skinned people should avoid them and rely upon topical products and other treatments.

If your skin tone is light to medium-light (ranging from someone with a light skin tone like Nicole Kidman to someone with a medium-range skin tone like Jennifer Lopez) you'll benefit from light therapy in the form of Intense Pulsed Light treatments (IPL). When combined with a light sensitising agent (I prefer Metvix), this therapy is called photodynamic therapy, or PDT. First, the Metvix is placed on the skin for thirty to sixty minutes to make both the skin and the sebaceous glands light sensitive. A special light (usually a blue light or Intense Pulsed Light) is then directed onto the skin. Depending on the light source used, the effects of this treatment may vary. Because there are many light machines available, and they are not all created equal, make certain to have these treatments performed by a doctor. Unless supervised by a physician, salons and spas are not allowed to use the stronger machines. I personally prefer the IPL (or Quantum) machine made by a company called Lumenis or the blue light by a company called Dusa. The light shrinks the sebaceous glands, resulting in decreased sebum oil secretion, which in turn will help prevent acne breakouts. For maximum results, your dermatologist can combine IPL with chemical peels. Please see 'Further Help for Oily, Sensitive Skin' for a complete description of what you will experience if you opt for this treatment.

Ranging in cost from approximately £100 to £400 (depending on the light source used), four to ten treatments are usually required. The number will depend on the severity of your skin's condition and how closely you follow your prescribed skin care regimens. Use of retinoids, such as Isotrex or Differin gel, will improve the treatment's results and shorten the recovery time. While most people experience no downtime after the procedure, some do find their skin turning red and flaky for three to seven days afterwards.

IPL and pigmented lesion lasers effectively remove dark spots, but in order to prevent the spots from returning, you must use sunscreen, even indoors (UVA can penetrate windows). IPL and vascular lasers are effective at removing visible red and blue blood vessels.

BOTOX/RELOXIN

Resistant, wrinkled types with mild, moderate, or deep wrinkles may choose a medical procedure such as Botox, Reloxin or dermal fillers. These can be done by your dermatologist. To find out how to locate a doctor in your area, please consult the 'Resources' section. For more information about these treatments and what to expect, please consult 'Further Help for Oily, Sensitive Skin'. Don't waste money on 'pore minimising' treatments. These really don't work. They only cause the skin to swell, which makes the pores look temporarily smaller.

WHAT THE FUTURE HOLDS

Newly advanced wrinkle treatments beyond Botox will also be suitable for wrinkled types when they become available following adequate research and testing. It's anticipated that new treatments, which may last longer and cost less than Botox, may soon become available. Current trends include treatments that add volume to skin by injecting fat or other naturally occurring substances like hyaluronic acid and collagen. If you opt for fat injections, there is another benefit that I have not mentioned. The fat has to be taken from somewhere. The fat is first removed from another bodily area (usually the hips) via liposuction, and then injected into the face to plump out drooping or thinning areas.

In the past, most treatments were aimed at wrinkles, but upcoming treatments will be directed at restoring facial volume and shape. For example, comparing a grape to a raisin, the raisin not only has wrinkles but also volume loss. To make it look like a grape again we need to plump up the volume, not just treat the wrinkles. That's why the trend is towards combining treatments. Doctors are now combining skin care, light treatments, Thermage, Botox, or Reloxin injections, fillers, and New-Fill to re-create the youthful look.

LIFESTYLE RECOMMENDATIONS

Since you are less prone to breakouts or acne than many other types, you can try different spa services that other types must avoid. Aromatherapy facials, chemical peels, masks geared towards wrinkles and pigmentation, as well as masks containing antioxidants are all typical services that you can enjoy without worry. Decreasing stress may help oil secretion, so avail yourself of relaxing treatments that feature products that your resilient skin can handle, while more sensitive types must avoid them. Pamper yourself with baths or body lotions using essential oils, like lavender, sandalwood, rose or chamomile. Facials can cause breakouts in some types, but should not be a problem for you. You can use some of the money you saved on skin care and skin procedures and splurge on a facial.

Avoiding sun exposure, using self-tanners, and avoiding tanning beds are key for you. And if self-tanners are not for you, hey, a little blusher and lipstick go a long way. Find creative ways to give your complexion vibrancy without harming your skin.

DIET

What you eat can also have an impact on your skin, which is why I recommend foods that help minimise wrinkling and pigmentation. These nutritional suggestions can also help reduce oil production, especially during your oilier, younger years.

Vitamin A has been shown to be associated with decreased oil secretion. That's why you may want to increase your dietary intake of foods rich in vitamin A such as liver, shellfish, cod liver oil (taken as liquid or capsules), butter, and other full-fat dairy products. In addition, although vegetables do not contain vitamin A, many are an excellent source of beta-carotene, which helps the body make, utilise, and store vitamin A. It can be found in sweet potatoes, mangoes, spinach, cantaloupe, kale, dried apricots, egg yolks and red peppers. Some foods, including milk, instant oats, breakfast cereals and meal replacement bars, are also vitamin A fortified. In addition, other plant phytonutrients have also been shown to offer some protection against skin cancer, with spinach, kale and broccoli containing lutein, while tomatoes contain cancer-fighting lycopene.

To fight wrinkles, antioxidants are helpful in combating free radicals, renegade oxygen molecules that cause cellular aging within the body. While an Australian study showed that blueberries are the number one source, they are also found in such foods as cranberries and pomegranates. Out of season, you can obtain the benefits of these fruits via unsweetened juice concentrates. A tablespoon or two can be mixed with water and sipped to deliver both hydration and antioxidant benefits. Artichokes also have antioxidant activity, helpful in preventing wrinkles, while both ginseng and cucumber are thought to prevent pigment formation and help prevent wrinkles.

Other sources of antioxidants are ginger, which can be added to stir-fries or enjoyed as a tea, tomatoes and basil, which can be enjoyed in salad and pasta. Antioxidants are also amply present in vegetables such as spinach, kale, collard greens, turnips, romaine lettuce, broccoli, leeks, corn, red peppers, peas and mustard greens, while egg yolks and oranges contain the antioxidant lutein.

Grapes and grape seed extract also rate high in antioxidants. Grape seed extract can be obtained via supplements. While red wine and tea have high antioxidant capacity, I have good news for chocolate lovers. One study showed that cocoa had a higher antioxidant capacity than black tea, green tea, or red wine. However, because of the sugar content in cocoa, you may prefer to drink tea more regularly.

Apple peels have higher antioxidant levels than the flesh of the apples eaten alone. You can enjoy apples raw, or make them into apple-sauce and baked apples.

It's better to get antioxidants through natural food sources, rather than supplements; however, when this is not feasible, supplements are likely to be of value. If nothing else, they will not cause any harm and may help prevent wrinkles and brown spots.

SUPPLEMENTS

Look for supplements containing vitamin C and L-selenomethionine (selenium) as well as antioxidants. Murad's APS Pure Skin Clarifying Supplements with L-selenomethionine; vitamins A, C, E, B5; alpha lipoic acid; and grape seed extract. The instructions are to take two tablets in the morning and two in the evening. However, I recommend taking only one tablet each morning and evening. I advise that you discontinue use for ten days prior to surgery or collagen, hyaluronic acid, or Botulinum toxin injections.

Ultraceuticals Ultra Active C Cell Protect contains vitamin C to help build collagen, and other helpful supplements are Olay's Ester-C Alpha Lipoic Collagen Support, which contains vitamin C and alpha lipoic acid (vitamin C 500mg); Olay's Total Effects Beautiful Skin & Wellness Vitamin Pack, with Coenzyme Q_{10} lutein, Vitamins C and E, and zinc. Stiefel's DermaVite Dietary Supplement contains Vitamins A, C and E, as well as zinc, selenium, copper and lycopene. Avon's VitAdvance Acné Clarifying Complex contains Vitamins A, C, and E, as well as zinc, selenium and alpha lipoic acid.

Vitamin A supplements are also an option to decrease oil production. Although there have been some concerns about vitamin A toxicity at high doses, one study showed that getting your vitamin A from a food source, like cod liver oil, with its naturally occurring vitamin D (and its oil-based delivery), makes it safe at normal dosage levels. Nordic Naturals Arctic Cod Liver Oil is available in gel caps or liquid. Ultraceuticals Ultra Active Clear Skin has vitamin A as well as Evening Primrose Oil.

Heliocare, an oral supplement found behind the pharmacist's counter and available without prescription, contains PL extract from ferns, shown to be a powerful antioxidant. If you have trouble locating this or any supplement, please check at www.baumannstore.com where I'll offer some choices, while also referring you to other places where they are readily obtainable.

PART FOUR

Skin Care for Dry, Sensitive Skin

CHAPTER TWELVE

Dry, Sensitive, Pigmented and Wrinkled: DSPW

THE DESPERATE SKIN TYPE

'I have to be so careful what I use on my face. My skin reacts to everything. Finding skin care products is like searching for the Holy Grail. How do I get rid of these spots and wrinkles?'

ABOUT YOUR SKIN

A DSPW Skin Type gives you no slack. Your skin is dry, flaky, parched and crying out for moisturisers. Yet you react with pimples or stinging, burning and itching to so many ingredients that few products can help. Synthetic ingredients in skin care (such as fragrances, detergents and preservatives) can trigger a reaction. Natural ingredients in skin care (such as essential oils, coconut oil or cocoa butter) can also trigger a reaction.

When using a product to treat your dark spots, it may sting and turn your pigmented skin red. Even though you avoid the sun, people frequently ask if you've been to the beach, because your red flushed face makes you look sunburned even in the dead of winter. Antiaging creams make you look like a burn victim, leaving inflamed red patches that turn brown over time and take months to heal.

Though improving your skin will be a careful step-by-step process, it can be done, so do not give up. The good news is that of all the types, DSPWs will gain the most from this book. Fortunately, there has been a great deal of research into your type that I'll translate into clear recommendations to help you improve your skin and with it your quality of life.

DSPW CELEBRITY

Katharine Hepburn, who died in 2003, was both a screen legend and one of the first 'modern women'. She had a successful career, several romances, and a great love. Her beauty, talent, energy and wit were allied to a freedom to be herself and a devotion to those she loved. She will never cease to inspire. The classic films in which she starred, like *Philadelphia Story*, *The African Queen* and *On Golden Pond*, tell great stories with great casts of actors, like Cary Grant, Humphrey Bogart and Henry Fonda. But most important, they bring us Kate herself. Recently immortalised by Cate Blanchett's performance as her in *The Aviator*, Hepburn lives on, a classic Hollywood icon.

It's quite likely that Hepburn was a DSPW. Her skin was clearly dry, highly pigmented and wrinkled. At the recent auction of her possessions, private photos revealed that she was freckled from head to toe. In fact, the noted skin care expert Erno Laszlo is said to have refused her request to remove them, saying they were part of her beauty. But in the days before laser treatments, I'm not sure how he could have done so anyway. In her early films and photos, the Hollywood makeup experts covered them with foundation to give her a clear complexion. But later films reveal a tanned Hepburn, and, later still, the wrinkles to show for it. Warren Beatty recounts that he persuaded Hepburn (then in her eighties) to see a dermatologist to help her sensitive skin.

But we still love her, freckles and all.

Another favourite actor, whose freckles have only served to endear him to his legions of fans is talented actor-director, Kenneth Branagh. His freckled, wrinkled skin points to his most likely being a dry, pigmented and wrinkled type. I am guessing that his skin is sensitive as it can be for many redheads with his appealing colouring.

THE DSPW DOUBLE BIND

Your skin's hyperreactivity is not your imagination. With one of the most distressing Skin Types, you find it difficult to care for properly. Though friends with easier types don't understand, I can validate your experience. Unless you're a millionaire who can afford to buy dozens of products, then use and discard them when they don't work, it's nearly impossible to find your way through the labyrinth of skin care products to the select few that work for your skin.

DSPWs often have eczema, also called atopic dermatitis, a skin condition in which dry skin becomes irritated, reddened and inflamed before developing patches that itch and take a while to heal. If allowed to persist, the condition is both physically uncomfortable and psychologically embarrassing, since it's visible to others. In fact, many people may mistakenly believe that this condition is contagious, which it's not. A recent international survey revealed that eczema seriously impacts quality of life, with many sufferers reporting that they had been bullied, teased and even suffered job discrimination due to this unsightly condition. Social life was also impacted, as the condition disturbed the ability to make friends and even attract romantic partners, 20 percent of those surveyed said. Seventy-five percent of the survey participants maintained that achieving effective treatment for their eczema would be 'the single most important improvement to their quality of life'.

Most other types have no idea what DSPWs go through. But I know very well, and what's more, I know what to do about it. However, I won't promise you that your skin will ever be trouble free. You'll always have to put a lot more effort into skin care than most other types. But with the right care, you can manage your skin problems and enhance your skin's appearance as well.

Julie, a beauty editor with dry, resistant skin, attended many beauty conferences, heading home with a suitcase of sample face and body products, which she loved to use. After she married Will, a witty fellow magazine editor, Julie discovered that her DSPW husband was unwilling to sample these products. Will would nervously read the label, sniff the product, try a little dab on his arm, and then reject it firmly.

Julie began to buy special moisturisers that promised to address various skin problems, but Will wouldn't use them. Once the weather turned cold and the heat came on, Will's dry skin worsened, becoming itchy, red and irritated, as well as reacting to many ingredients, fabrics and even foods. His skin reacted to the easy-care chemicals used in their pretty flowered sheets, so Julie replaced them with all organic cotton undyed sheets. When Julie bought them matching sweatshirts, Will wouldn't wear his because it was made of polyester. Moisturisers turned him bright red. Eating acidic foods (like tomatoes, oranges or grapefruits) seemed to worsen his condition. Anything spicy was a no-no. When the couple went out to a restaurant, people would see his bright red head, neck, and forearms and jokingly tell Julie, 'Don't let him get too much sun.'

Julie slowly realised that Will had a major skin problem. Then, during an interview with me, she asked for my help. After we had determined that Will was a DSPW, it was evident that he had eczema and rosacea, with frequent flare-ups. He had a damaged skin barrier and rebuilding it was key. He also needed to get his rosacea under control. With my guidelines, he was able to find products that worked for him, and began to include omega-3 fats in his diet. He also decided to follow my recommendations and use a prescription medication for his rosacea. 'This is a miracle,' he told me a few months later. 'My skin was a mystery before, but now I have the confidence to read a product ingredient list and know what I am looking for.' Will still refuses to wear polyester and insists on organic cotton sheets, but he no longer looks like he's sunburned in November, and Julie knows what kinds of moisturisers to get him at Christmas.

A DISTURBED SKIN BARRIER

Dry, sensitive types have a disturbed skin barrier. The cells that maintain the integrity of the skin have broken down as a result of different causes – including allergies, sensitising products and ingredients, and environmental conditions, like dryness and cold. As a result, the barrier doesn't keep water in, so skin lacks the hydration it needs. On the other hand, it also doesn't keep allergenic ingredients out. When these ingredients invade, they trigger inflammation.

DSPWs have no protection. You are literally thin-skinned. The resulting dryness, irritation, redness and itchiness give you the urge to scratch, but scratching further attacks your skin barrier. Next, pigmentation causes skin darkening at irritated areas, such as the back of the knees and inside of the elbows. Scratches, cuts and scrapes are more than uncomfortable: they can result in dark spots at the site of injury because your skin's high pigment levels react to any inflammation. It's a vicious cycle.

Dark spots can result from many causes, including cuts, scratches, oral contraceptive use, pregnancy and sun exposure. The dark spots appear darker in the summer if the skin is tanned. Dark patches resulting from injury more commonly occur in dark-skinned people. Dermatologists call them post-inflammatory pigmentation alteration (PIPA). Both dark- and light-skin-toned DSPWs can suffer from melasma (also called 'the mask of pregnancy'), which results from sun exposure and higher oestrogen levels.

Eczema can occur anywhere on your body. To find out if you suffer from this problem, please go to 'Do I Have Eczema?' in Chapter Thirteen. Skin dryness, redness and irritation can appear on your face and neck, while scaling dry patches frequently crop up behind the ears. As if all this were not stressful enough, eczema *worsens* with stress. In more severe cases, sufferers may experience sleep problems due to discomfort. Given the frequency of flare-ups, sleep loss is more than occasional. One study revealed that those with a moderate form of eczema suffer flare-ups for three months a year, while severe patients may experience flare-ups for five months a year. Irritable, uncomfortable, embarrassed and sleep deprived, you may also suffer from depression. Yet the steroids and cortisone topical creams often recommended provide only temporary relief, while worsening the problem long-term, since the skin is progressively thinned by them.

Not knowing what leads to a flare-up keeps sufferers on edge. Any provocation, physical or emotional, can throw you off and result in itching and irritation.

The bottom line is that eczema-prone DSPWs need to avoid irritating ingredients *and* irritating life situations. Cultivate calm, meditate, and have a cup of anti-inflammatory green tea. One brand calls their green tea 'Zen'. No one needs it more than you.

Dorothy dressed for church in her Sunday finest, putting on her favourite pink lipstick and her favourite perfume, 'Eternal Gardenia'. Unfortunately, her perfume was *too* eternal, causing a rash on her neck. The lace of her blouse further irritated her skin, and this unsightly condition persisted for a month. When Dorothy came in to see me, I determined that she was a DSPW. Since fragrances are frequently sensitising, instead of spraying her neck or wrists, I recommended that she spray the air in front of her and then walk into the perfume mist, lessening the possibility of reactions. Another option would be to forego the perfume altogether. Once triggered, eczema can become progressive, so why not avoid the problem before it becomes serious?

A COMPLEX SKIN TYPE

DSPW is one of the most challenging and complex of the Baumann Skin Types because you have (or have the potential for) every kind of skin problem.

Your skin is dry, putting you at risk for eczema and related dry skin conditions. Your skin is sensitive, causing redness, irritation, stinging and rashes in reaction to many skin care ingredients and other provocations. Your skin is pigmented, producing freckles, brown spots and sunspots. And your skin is wrinkled; so that later in life, you are likely to get wrinkles and show the signs of aging more than certain other types.

The way these factors interact is highly individual, and what manifests for you will depend on how you score in each of the four categories. Dryness combined with skin sensitivity can result in acne, rosacea and eczema. For more information on how your scores interact to create your particular skin problems, you may wish to reread Chapter Two.

Fortunately, the right regimen can help. But given all of these possible skin issues, there is no single prescription, so I have created a number of different and individualised skin care regimens which you can find in a later section of this chapter.

Wrinkling may result from genetics, lifestyle factors (like sunning and smoking), diet, or any combination of these factors. In some people, eczema may result from an autoimmune condition. Therefore, some eczema sufferers find that sun exposure helps their skin, because it can downshift the hyperreactivity of the autoimmune response. But sunbathing to control eczema can increase skin's wrinkling and dryness, further contributing to eczema. Sun exposure and hot climates will also worsen rosacea.

Is there anything good about your skin? Well, your risk for non-melanoma skin cancer may be lower than many other types. However, please consult 'How to Recognise a Non-Melanoma Skin Cancer' in Chapter Seven to learn to distinguish potentially harmful signs – and make sure to go to a dermatologist for annual checkups in any case.

Ava's Story

Ava's friends pitched in and bought her a gift of expensive antiaging skin care products after her recent divorce. 'I feel insecure about dating again,' Ava told me. 'After all, I'm forty, with wrinkles and stretch marks from pregnancies with my two kids.' Although the products were from a well-known, high-end line sold at Neiman Marcus, they were not right for Ava's skin. 'The first night I luxuriated in the sweet-smelling, heavenly feeling cream and massaged a thick layer into my skin,' Ava reported. But Ava's delight was short-lived. Ava awoke to find that her skin felt sore and sunburned. 'When I looked in the mirror,' she told me with horror, 'I looked red and swollen.' Ava's skin didn't get over it quickly. It took three days to recover from the redness, and then the reddened areas turned brown, which lasted for four weeks.

A CLOSE-UP LOOK AT YOUR SKIN

Like Ava, with DSPW skin you may experience any of the following:

• Dryness and flaking
• Itching skin

- Pink scaled patches
- Dark patches and spots in response to injury or trauma
- Facial redness and flushing
- Broken blood vessels in the face
- Acne
- Dark circles under the eyes
- Increased susceptibility to skin allergies
- Dry lips
- Skin darkening at irritated areas, such as the back of the knees and inside of the elbows

Both light- and dark-skinned people can be DSPWs. Lighter skin-toned DSPWs may suffer from dark spots, melasma, or freckles from previous sun exposure. Please refer to the section on pigmentation in Chapter Two to learn more about melasma and see if you might have it.

Melasma can be treated with bleaching creams, but it's most effective to stop taking any form of hormones (like birth control pills or HRT), as they tend to increase pigmentation. Avoid sun exposure since that will worsen it. Choose the right sunscreen because some products fail to block UVA rays, which contribute to melasma. Wear a UVA-blocking sunscreen indoors, and even in a car or on an aeroplane, because UVA rays penetrate glass. The good news about melasma is that it tends to improve after menopause.

Although darker-toned DSPWs do not freckle, they have complex issues for other reasons. Darker-skinned people often get dark patches after inflammation. Once the redness and itching has gone, it's replaced by a dark patch, which can last, increasing irritation and dryness.

On darker skin, flaking dry skin may look like grey scales. Many people call this 'ashy skin' and several skin care products are marketed to address it – though it's simply dryness and can be treated with any good moisturiser. Choose the right body product or face cream, depending on where the dryness occurs.

ADJUSTING YOUR SKIN CARE

Your ideal climate is humid. In the winter, the drop in humidity may increase dryness and skin sensitivity, leading to skin scaling and itching. Drying environments, such as aeroplanes or desert locales, can further dehydrate your thirsty skin. DSPWs may also develop dryness, itching and increased sensitivity to heavy winter clothes made from fabrics like wool, because they rub against and irritate the skin.

You need to alter your skin care regimen with the seasons. Don't just blindly stick to one regimen. Pay attention to your skin's condition, and adjust as needed. In dry climates, moisturise more frequently, using a heavier cream product. In more humid locales, you can get away with a lighter product. When dark spots develop, treat them, and when they leave, return to a maintenance programme. Later in this chapter, I'll offer you several options.

For DSPWs, skin problems will often increase with age. After forty, skin dryness can worsen, especially in women going through menopause, requiring frequent moisturising and richer moisturisers. Skin sensitivity increases with age, because as you are exposed to more topical skin care ingredients, more allergies can develop – until you reach your eighties and nineties, when allergies lessen due to diminished immune function. There-fore, find a few products that work for you and stick with them. Freckles, sunspots, visible blood vessels (sometimes seen with rosacea) and wrinkles also worsen with age, while acne and melasma tend to lessen. With your range of skin problems, I can't promise a permanent solution, but I can promise improvement if you stick with the strategies I'll offer in the next section of this chapter.

Dr Baumann's Bottom Line: Your skin options must be right on the money. You have no room for error, so follow my advice to a T. If you think that you suffer from eczema, see your dermatologist. In many cases of eczema, moisturisers and routine skin care are not enough. Luckily, new prescription medications such as Elidel are very effective at treating this condition.

EVERYDAY CARE FOR YOUR SKIN

The goal of your skin care routine is to address skin dryness, skin sensitivity and dark spots with products that deliver ingredients that hydrate your skin, decrease its sensitivity and reduce dark spots. All the products I'll recom-mend will do one or more of the following:

- Prevent and treat dryness
- Prevent and treat sensitivity
- Prevent and treat dark spots

In addition, your daily regimen will also help to address your other skin concerns by:

- Rebuilding skin barrier
- Lessening inflammation
- Preventing and treating wrinkles
- Preventing and treating acne

Because DSPW skin can potentially suffer from so many different kinds of problems, adjust your regimen to your skin's current condition. Here you'll find regimens to use if you are experiencing dark spots, redness and stinging, or acne. You'll find three nonprescription regimens to get you started and seven prescription regimens to cover every combination of these conditions – as well as regimens for maintenance when dark spots, redness, stinging and acne have cleared.

If you suffer from acne, it is best to see a dermatologist. Ingredients in acne products such as benzoyl peroxide and salicylic acid will only further dry and irritate your skin. Your dermatologist can prescribe sulphur-containing and antibiotic topical medications or even oral medications that can treat your acne without irritating your skin. Light treatments (*not* sun exposure, which can worsen acne) can be useful as well.

If your skin problems are troublesome, I suggest you only try your nonprescription regimen for two weeks, or until you can get into a dermatologist's office. Make your appointment today.

DAILY SKIN CARE

STAGE ONE: NONPRESCRIPTION REGIMEN

For treating dark spots:

AM	PM
Step 1: Wash with a cleanser	Step 1: Wash with a cleanser
Step 2: Rinse with facial water	Step 2: Rinse with facial water
Step 3: Apply a lightening gel	Step 3: Apply a lightening gel
Step 4: Apply a moisturiser with sunscreen	Step 4: Apply an antioxidant-containing night cream
Step 5: Apply a foundation with sunscreen (optional)	

In the morning, wash your face with a cold cream or oil cleanser, which is less drying than other cleansers. Rinse your face with facial water. (See page 294 for more information on facial water.) Then quickly apply a lightening gel to your dark spots, and next apply a moisturiser containing SPF. Try to apply the moisturiser while your face is still moist to trap water into your skin. Finally, use a foundation with SPF, if you wish.

In the evening, wash with a cold cream or oil cleanser, then rinse with facial water. Apply a lightening gel to dark spots, then quickly apply a night cream containing antioxidants.

If you have acne, you can also follow this regimen, plus add a sulphur-containing mask once or twice a week. Apply the mask after cleansing, leave it on as per the instructions, and wash it off. Then continue with the rest of the regimen.

For maintenance once dark spots have cleared

AM	PM
Step 1: Wash with cleanser	Step 1: Wash with cleanser
Step 2: Apply antioxidant serum	Step 2: Spray facial water
Step 3: Spray facial water	Step 3: Apply antioxidant-containing cream
Step 4: Apply an SPF-containing moisturiser and/or sunscreen	
Step 5: Apply a foundation with sunscreen (optional)	

In the morning, wash your face with cleanser. You can use a cold cream, facial oil, or soothing cleanser or lotion. Next, apply an antioxidant serum. Spray facial water, then quickly apply a moisturiser-containing SPF. Finally, apply a foundation with SPF.

In the evening, wash with the same cleanser and spray facial water. While your skin is still moist, apply an antioxidant-containing night cream.

*For use after spots have cleared but when you
have redness and stinging:*

AM	PM
Step 1: Wash with cleanser	Step 1: Wash with cleanser
Step 2: Rinse with facial water	Step 2: Rinse with facial water
Step 3: Apply anti-inflammatory product	Step 3: Apply anti-inflammatory product
Step 4: Apply an SPF-containing moisturiser and/or sunscreen	Step 4: Apply antioxidant-containing cream
Step 5: Apply a foundation with sunscreen (optional)	Step 5: Once or twice a week use a sulphur-containing mask

In the morning, wash with your choice of cleanser and rinse with facial water. Apply an anti-inflammatory product (see the following list). Next, apply moisturiser with SPF, and follow with a foundation containing SPF if you wish.

In the evening, wash with cleanser and rinse with facial water. Apply the same anti-inflammatory product, then a night cream containing antioxidants.

Once or twice a week, use a mask containing sulphur. Apply the mask after cleansing, leave it on as per the instructions, and wash it off. Then continue with the rest of the regimen.

Cleansers

DSPWs should avoid any cleansers that foam. Best for you are oil-based cleansers or cold creams.

RECOMMENDED CLEANSERS

£ Eucerin Gentle Cleansing Milk
£ Lutsine Gentle Cleansing Cream
£ Nivea Gentle Cleansing Cream Wash
£ Quintessence Skin Science Purifying Cleanser

££ Aesop Purifying Facial Cream Cleanser
££ Avène Extremely gentle Cleanser
££ Clarins Extra-Comfort Cleansing Cream
££ Elizabeth Arden Millennium Hydrating Cleanser
££ Kiehl's Oil-Based Cleanser and Make-Up Remover
££ La Roche-Posay Toleriane Demo-Cleanser
££ L'Occitane Olive Harvest Daily Face Cleanser
££ L'Occitane Shea Butter Extra Moisturising Cold Cream Soap
££ Oilatum-AD Cleansing Lotion
££ Vichy Detoxifying Cleansing Milk–Dry
£££ Darphin Intral Cleansing Milk
£££ Leaf and Rusher Green Tea Wash
£££ Pevonia Dry Skin Cleanser

Baumann's Choice: Nivea Gentle Cleansing Cream Wash. If you come to the US, look for the Dove Essential Nutrients products that are perfect for your skin type.

RECOMMENDED COLD CREAMS AND OIL CLEANSERS FOR VERY DRY SKIN

£ Dove Essential Nutrients Deep Cleansing Cream (not in UK)
£ Noxzema Cleansing Cream, Sensitive
££ Aesop Camellia Nut Facial Hydrating Cream
££ Kiehl's Ultra Moisturising Cleansing Cream
££ Shu Uemura Skin Purifier Cleansing Oil
££ SK II Facial Treatment Cleansing Oil
£££ Decléor Cleansing Oil
£££ Ella Baché Floral Oil
£££ Jurlique Face Wash Cream

Baumann's Choice: SK II Facial Treatment Cleansing Oil (I prefer the Dove but you cannot get it in the UK.)

Anti-Inflammatory Products

Anti-inflammatory products are often serums and gels. While the most effective ones are prescription products, a few over-the-counter options are available.

RECOMMENDED ANTI- INFLAMMATORY PRODUCTS

£ Olay Total Effects 7x Visible Anti-Aging Vitamin Complex (Fragrance Free)

£ Paula's Choice Skin Relief Treatment

££ Avène Skin Recovery Cream

££ Cutanix Dramatic Relief for Sensitive Facial Skin

££ La Roche-Posay Rosaliac Hydrante Perfecteur

££ Mary Kay Calming Influence

££ Prescriptives Redness Relief Gel

£££ B. Kamins Booster Blue Rosacea Treatment

£££ Pevonia Rose RS2 Concentrate

Baumann's Choice: Paula's Choice Skin Relief Treatment has willow herb.

Antioxidant Serums

Use these antioxidant serums as called for in some of the regimens unless you experience frequent redness and stinging in response to skin care products. If so, they're too irritating for you.

RECOMMENDED ANTIOXIDANT SERUMS

££ Elizabeth Arden Ceramide Advanced Time Complex Capsules

££ Korres Royal Jelly and Grape Seed Capsules

££ La Roche-Posay Active C

££ SkinCeuticals C + E

££ Vichy Reti-C

£££ Pevonia Vitaminic Concentrate

£££ Chanel Precision Age Delay Regeneration Serum

Baumann's Choice: Korres Royal Jelly and Grape Seed Capsules because they are best for very sensitive skin. Serums are a time to splurge. I could not find any £ products that I liked.

Facial Water

A DSPW should never use toners, which usually have drying ingredients designed to remove lipids from the skin. Your skin needs all the lipids it can get. Toners also contain ingredients that will further irritate your sensitive skin.

If your skin is super sensitive, it may benefit from special waters. In a recent study, skin that was irritated by detergent cleared faster when rinsed with CO_2-enriched tap water for one minute once daily, as compared to rinsing with regular tap water. This result suggests that washing your face with Pellegrino or another carbonated water may be beneficial. You may find this impractical, but it is an interesting idea.

Spray facial water on your face just before applying eye cream and moisturiser. The moisturiser and eye cream will help trap the water on the skin, giving the skin a reservoir to pull water from. This is particularly beneficial in low-humidity environments such as the dry winter air or an aeroplane.

Facial waters come from thermal springs. They do not contain chemicals such as chlorine that are added to our tap water to keep it free from algae and other organisms. The constituents of the water vary according to the source. Vichy water contains sulphur, while the La Roche-Posay water contains selenium and has been shown to be effective in treating eczema. Both selenium and sulphur can be anti-inflammatory.

RECOMMENDED FACIAL WATERS

- £ Evian Mineral Water Spray
- ££ Aesop Immediate Moisture Facial Hydrosol
- ££ Avène Thermal Water Spray
- ££ Chantecaille Pure Rosewater
- ££ Fresh Rose Marigold Tonic Water
- ££ Korres Hamamelis Hydrating Face Water
- ££ La Roche-Posay Thermal Spring Water
- ££ Molton Brown Skinboost 24-hour Moisture Mist
- ££ Shu Uemura Depsea Therapy
- ££ Vichy Eau Thermal
- £££ Jurlique Rosewater
- £££ Susan Ciminelli Seawater

Baumann's Choice: Eau Thermale by La Roche-Posay contains selenium, which soothes the skin.

Treatments for Dark Spots

I really prefer prescription products for lightening dark spots, but here are some suggestions if you want to try over-the-counter products. Products in the US contain hydroquinone, which is not found in products in the UK. Visit www.Baumannstore.co.uk to find more options to treat dark spots.

RECOMMENDED LIGHTENING PRODUCTS

- ££ B. Kamins Skin Lightening Treatment
- ££ L'Occitane Immortelle Brightening Serum
- ££ Laura Mercier Multi Vitamin Serum
- ££ Obagi 'Clear'
- ££ Philosophy A Pigment of Your Imagination
- £££ DDF Intensive Holistic Corrector Swabs
- £££ Dr Brandt Lightening Gel
- £££ Dr Michelle Copeland Skin Care Pigment Blocker 5
- £££ Pevonia Lightening Gel
- £££ SkinCeuticals Phyto + Botanical Gel for Hyperpigmentation
- £££ Thalgo Unizones
- £££ TYK White Glow Retinol, Kojic, Mag-C Absolute Skin Brightener

Baumann's Choice: DDF Intensive Holistic Corrector Swabs. There are cheaper, better options in the US.

Moisturisers

Apply moisturiser frequently throughout the day – in the morning after gently cleansing your face, again in the later afternoon or early evening, and finally at bedtime. With a very low O/D score, or during times of low humidity, use creams rather than lotions. Your skin needs the extra moisture. If you have a medium O/D score of 17–26, or during times of high humidity when you prefer a lighter product, use lotions. Avoid heavily fragranced moisturisers and those containing essential oils.

RECOMMENDED DAYTIME
MOISTURISERS (WITH SPF)

- £ Neutrogena Ultimate Moisture Day Cream
- £ Olay Regenerist Replenishing Cream

£ Olay Total Effects with VitaNiacin

££ Elizabeth Arden Ceramide Plump Perfect Moisture Cream SPF 30

££ Jurlique Day Care Face Cream

££ Laura Mercier Mega Moisturiser with SPF 15

££ L'Occitane Face and Body Balm (SPF 30)

££ Vichy Nutrilogie 1 – Intensive Care for Dry Skin

£££ Pevonia Rejuvenating Dry Skin Cream

Baumann's Choice: Neutrogena Ultimate Moisture Day Cream. Although it does not contain a sunscreen, it contains a form of soy that helps prevent dark spots. Be sure to apply a sunscreen on top of your skin after application of the moisturiser if your selection does not contain sunscreen.

RECOMMENDED NIGHTTIME MOISTURISERS

£ Burt's Bees Healthy Treatment Marshmallow Vanishing Crème

£ Eucerin Lipo Balance Cream with Ceramide

£ Neutrogena Ultimate Moisture Night Cream

££ AtoPalm MLE Face Cream

££ Cutanix Dramatic Relief for Dry to Normal Skin

££ Elizabeth Arden Ceramide Moisture Network Night Cream

££ Kiehl's Creme d'Elegance Repairateur

££ La Roche-Posay Toleriane Soothing Protective Facial

££ Laura Mercier Night Nutrition Renewal Crème

£££ Freeze 24/7 IceCream Anti-Aging Moisturiser

£££ La Prairie Cellular Face Moisturiser

Baumann's Choice: Cutanix Dramatic Relief for Dry to Normal Skin. If redness is your problem, this is the product for you. Find out where to buy it at www.DrBaumann.co.uk. If dark spots are more of a problem, choose Neutrogena Ultimate Moisture Night Cream with soy.

Eye Creams

You have enough skin problems already, so why not make life easy and skip the eye cream? Instead you can apply your regular moisturiser around the eyes. If you really want to try one, select one of these products and apply it prior to moisturiser.

RECOMMENDED EYE CREAMS

£ Neutrogena Visibly Young Eye Cream
£ Nivea AntiWrinkle Q10 Plus Eye Cream
£ Olay Regenerist Eye Lifting Serum
££ Aveda Pure Vital Moisture Eye Cream
££ Dermalogica Intense Eye Repair
££ Elizabeth Arden Ceramide Plump Perfect Eye Moisture Cream SPF 15
££ L'Occitane Immortelle Eye Balm
££ Nivea Visage Anti Shadow Eye Cream
££ Relastin Eye Cream
£££ Dr Brandt Lineless Eye cream
£££ SkinCeuticals Eye Balm

Baumann's Choice: Olay Regenerist Eye Lifting Serum because it contains niacinamide, a soothing ingredient that help prevent aging and dark spots.

Masks

Here are recommended masks containing sulphur, as called for in two of the nonprescription regimens.

RECOMMENDED SULPHUR-CONTAINING MASKS

££ DDF Sulphur Therapeutic Mask
££ Peter Thomas Roth Therapeutic Sulphur Masque Acne Treatment

Exfoliation

DSPWs should never exfoliate since it can make your skin more sensitive and hurt your skin barrier. Concentrate instead on moisturizing.

SHOPPING FOR PRODUCTS

Reading product labels is particularly important for DSPWs, whose sensitive skin can be irritated by so many types of ingredients. Other ingredients are beneficial, so you should choose products containing them. Below, I've listed ingredients that are helpful for preventing and treating dark spots, hydrating the skin, improving wrinkles, and preventing inflammation – as well as ingredients to avoid. If you find skin care products that are not on my lists, please share them with me at www.DrBaumann.co.uk.

SKIN CARE INGREDIENTS TO USE

To improve dark spots:

- Arbutin
- Cucumber extract
- Kojic acid
- Glycyrrhiza glabra (licorice extract)
- Magnesium ascorbyl phosphate
- Mulberry extract
- Tyrostat

To prevent dark spots:

- Cocos nucifera (coconut extract), unless you have acne
- Cucumber
- Niacinamide
- Pycnogenol (a pine bark extract)
- Saxifraga sarmentosa extract (strawberry begonia)

To moisturise and hydrate:

- Ajuga turkestanica
- Aloe vera
- Apricot kernel oil
- Borage seed oil
- Canola oil
- Ceramide
- Cholesterol
- Cocoa butter (not if you have acne)
- Colloidal oatmeal
- Dexpanthenol (provitamin B_5)
- Dimethicone
- Evening primrose oil
- Glycerin
- Jojoba oil
- Macadamia nut oil
- Olive oil
- Safflower oil
- Shea butter

To prevent wrinkles:

- Basil
- Caffeine
- Camilla sinensis (green tea, white tea)
- Carrot extract
- Ginseng
- Grape seed extract
- Idebenone
- Lutein
- Lycopene

- Coenzyme Q_{10} (ubiquinone)
- Copper peptide
- Curcumin (tetrahydracurcumin or turmeric)
- Ferulic acid
- Feverfew
- Ginger
- Punica granatum (pomegranate)
- Pycnogenol (a pine bark extract)
- Rosemary
- Silymarin
- Yucca

To improve wrinkles:

- Copper peptide
- Ginkgo biloba
- Vitamin C (asorbic acid), may be too irritating for you

Anti-inflammatory:

- Aloe vera
- Chamomile
- Colloidal oatmeal
- Cucumber
- Dexpanthenol (provitamin B_5)
- Evening primrose oil
- Feverfew
- Green tea
- Licochalone
- Mirabilis
- Perilla leaf extract
- Pycnogenol (a pine bark extract)
- Red algae
- Trifolium pretense (red clover)
- Thyme
- Epibolium angustifolium (willow herb)
- Zinc

SKIN CARE PRODUCTS TO AVOID

For all DSPWs:

- Cleansing products that foam
- Scrubs
- Toners

If you have acne:

- Cinnamon oil
- Cocoa butter
- Decyl oleate
- Octyl stearate

- Cocos nucifera (coconut oil)
- Isopropyl isostearate
- Isopropyl myristate
- Isopropyl palmitate
- Butyl stearate
- Isostearyl neopentanoate
- Myristyl myristate

- Octyl palmitate or isocetyl stearate
- Propylene glycol-2 (PPG-2)
- Myristyl propionate
- Lanolin
- Peppermint oil

If you have skin redness:

- Alpha hydroxy acids (lactic acid, glycolic acid
- Alpha lipoic acid
- Benzoyl peroxide
- Gluconolactone
- Phytic acid

- Polyhydroxy acids
- Retinaldehyde
- Retinol
- Retinyl palmitate
- Vitamin C (ascorbic acid)

SUN PROTECTION FOR YOUR SKIN

Use creams. If you have dark spots, there are a few sunscreens with depigmenting agents, such as Philosophy A Pigment of Your Imagination. When possible, look for sunscreens that also contain antioxidants.

RECOMMENDED SUN PROTECTION PRODUCTS

£ Eucerin Q 10 Active Antiwrinkle Fluid SPF 15
£ Olay Regenerist Rehydrating Lotion with UV Protection
££ La Roche-Posay Fluide Extreme SPF 60 (available in Ireland)
££ Philosophy A Pigment of Your Imagination
££ SkinCeuticals Ultimate UV Defence SPF 30
£££ Darphin Ultra Sun Protection Cream SPF 30
£££ Decléor Écran Très Haute Protection SPF 40
£££ La Prairie Age Management Stimulus Complex SPF 25
£££ Orlane B21 Soleil Vitamines SPF 15 Anti-Wrinkle Cream for the Face Vitamins
£££ Sisley Broad Spectrum Sunscreen, SPF 40

Baumann's Choice: A Pigment of Your Imagination, as it also contains depigmenting agents, a must if you have dark spots. If you don't have dark spots, choose Eucerin Q 10 Active Antiwrinkle Fluid SPF 15.

CONSULTING A DERMATOLOGIST

PRESCRIPTION SKIN CARE STRATEGIES

If you think you have eczema, see a dermatologist for prescription medications that can treat this condition. These medications can be used temporarily to relieve redness and itching, giving your daily skin care regimen time to rebuild the skin barrier.

Below you will find seven different prescription regimens. Choose them depending on what combination of dark spots, acne, and facial redness and stinging you are experiencing. One of these protocols is a maintenance regimen to use when acne, dark spots, and facial redness and stinging have cleared. In addition, I've also tried to direct you to products I consider most helpful for each condition.

DAILY SKIN CARE

STAGE TWO: PRESCRIPTION REGIMEN

For spots but no acne or facial redness:

AM	PM
Step 1: Wash with a cleanser	Step 1: Wash with a cleanser
Step 2: Apply a prescription lightening gel to dark spots only	Step 2: Apply a prescription lightening gel to dark spots only
Step 3: Apply a moisturiser with SPF and/or sunscreen	Step 3: Apply a night cream
Step 4: Apply a foundation with sunscreen (optional)	Step 4: Apply a prescription retinoid

In the morning, wash with a cleanser, then apply a prescription lightening gel just to your dark spots. Apply a moisturiser with SPF, then if you wish, a foundation-containing SPF.

In the evening, wash with a cleanser and apply a prescription lightening gel to dark spots only. Next, apply a night cream, and finish with a prescription retinoid.

This regimen does not include antioxidants, so please include an antioxidant oral supplement.

How to Use Retinoids

Please go to 'Further Help for Dry, Sensitive Skin' for instructions on retinoid use.

STAGE TWO: PRESCRIPTION REGIMEN

For dark spots and acne but no facial redness or stinging:

AM	PM
Step 1: Wash with cleanser	Step 1: Wash with cleanser
Step 2: Apply a prescription lightening gel to dark spots only	Step 2: Use a prescription mask once or twice a week
Step 3: Apply prescription topical prescription to entire face	Step 3: Apply a prescription lightening gel to dark spots only
Step 4: Spray facial water	Step 4: Apply prescription topical antibiotic to entire face
Step 5: Apply a moisturiser with SPF and/or sunscreen	Step 5: Apply a prescription retinoid cream as directed below
Step 6: Apply a foundation with sunscreen (optional)	

In the morning, wash with cleanser and apply a prescription lightening gel just to your dark spots. Then apply a prescription topical antibiotic to your entire face. Next, spray facial water, followed by a moisturiser containing SPF. Finish with a foundation containing sunscreen, if you wish to wear one.

In the evening, wash with a cleanser. Once or twice a week, use a prescription mask, which contains sulphacetamide and sulphur. Following the product directions, apply after cleansing. After rinsing it off, proceed with the skin lightening gel to the dark spots only. Apply a prescription topical antibiotic to your entire face, then a prescription retinoid cream.

This regimen does not include antioxidants, so please include an antioxidant oral supplement.

STAGE TWO: PRESCRIPTION REGIMEN

For dark spots, acne, and facial redness or stinging:

AM

Step 1: Wash with a prescription
sulphacetamide cleanser

Step 2: Rinse with facial water

Step 3: Apply a prescription
lightener to spots only

Step 4: Apply a prescription
topical antibiotic

Step 5: Apply a moisturiser with
SPF and/or sunscreen

Step 6: Apply a foundation with
sunscreen (optional)

PM

Step 1: Wash with a prescription
sulphacetamide cleanser

Step 2: Rinse with facial water

Step 3: Apply a prescription
lightener to spots only

Step 4: Apply a prescription
topical antibiotic

Step 5: Apply a night cream with
antioxidants

In the morning, wash your face with a prescription sulphacetamide cleanser, then rinse with facial water (*not* tap water). Apply a prescription lightener just to your dark spots, then apply a prescription topical antibiotic. Next, apply a moisturiser containing SPF, and finally, a foundation with SPF if you wish.

In the evening, wash with a prescription sulphacetamide cleanser and rinse with facial water. Apply a prescription lightener to your dark spots, then apply a prescription topical antibiotic Finish with a night cream containing antioxidants.

This subset of DSPW is quite difficult to treat. It is likely that your dermatologist will put you on an oral antibiotic like minocycline or tetracycline to help improve the acne and facial redness.

STAGE TWO: PRESCRIPTION REGIMEN

For dark spots and facial redness and stinging, but not acne:

AM

Step 1: Wash with a prescription
sulphacetamide cleanser

PM

Step 1: Wash with a cold cream or
oil cleanser

Step 2: Rinse with facial water

Step 3: Apply a prescription
lightening gel to dark spots only

Step 4: Apply a prescription
topical anti-inflammatory

Step 5: Apply a moisturiser with
SPF and/or sunscreen

Step 6: Apply a foundation with
sunscreen (optional)

Step 2: Rinse with facial water

Step 3: Apply a prescription
lightening gel to dark spots only

Step 4: Apply a prescription
topical anti-inflammatory

Step 5: Cover with a night cream

In the morning, wash your face with a prescription sulphacetamide cleanser, then rinse with facial water (*not* tap water). Apply a prescription lightening gel just to your dark spots, then apply a prescription topical anti-inflammatory medication. Next, apply a moisturiser containing SPF. Last, if you wish, apply a foundation with SPF.

In the evening, wash with a cold cream or oil cleanser and rinse with facial water. Apply a prescription lightening gel to dark spots only, then apply a prescription topical anti-inflammatory. Last, apply a night cream.

This regimen does not include antioxidants, so please include an antioxidant oral supplement.

STAGE TWO: PRESCRIPTION REGIMEN

*For maintenance after dark spots, acne,
and redness have cleared:*

AM

Step 1: Wash with a prescription
sulphacetamide cleanser

Step 2: Apply an antioxidant serum

Step 3: Apply a moisturiser with
SPF and/or sunscreen

Step 4: Apply a foundation with
sunscreen (optional)

PM

Step 1: Wash with a cold cream or
oil cleanser

Step 2: Apply a night cream

Step 3: Apply a prescription
retinoid as directed below

In the morning, wash your face with a prescription sulphacetamide cleanser, then apply an antioxidant serum. Next, apply a moisturiser with SPF, and finally, if you choose, apply foundation with SPF.

In the evening, wash with a cold cream or oil cleanser. Apply a night cream, and then apply a retinoid over the night cream.

Look for moisturisers with niacinamide or active soy that will help prevent dark spots from returning such as Neutrogena Ultimate Moisture with active soy, Olay Total Effects, or Olay Regenerist with niacinamide

For this regimen, I suggest the retinoid Differin, which can be applied every third night for two weeks. If you do not develop redness or stinging, apply it every other night for two weeks. If there is still no redness, apply the retinoid every night.

STAGE TWO: PRESCRIPTION REGIMEN

When dark spots have cleared but there is still acne and minimal facial redness and stinging:

AM	PM
Step 1: Wash with a cleanser	Step 1: Wash with a cleanser
Step 2: Apply prescription antibiotic medication	Step 2: Apply prescription antibiotic medication
Step 3: Apply a moisturiser with SPF and/or sunscreen	Step 3: Apply night cream
Step 4: Apply a foundation with sunscreen (optional)	Step 4: Apply a prescription retinoid cream as directed below

In the morning, wash your face with cleanser. Apply a prescription antibiotic medication, then a moisturiser containing SPF. Last, apply a foundation with SPF if you wish.

In the evening, wash with cleanser and apply prescription antibiotic medication. Apply night cream, then apply a prescription retinoid over the night cream. Ask your doctor about Isotrexin which contains a retinoid and an antibiotic, thus allowing you to omit step 4. For instructions on gradually introducing retinoid use, please refer to 'Using Retinoids' in 'Further Help for Dry, Sensitive Skin'.

STAGE TWO: PRESCRIPTION REGIMEN

*When dark spots have cleared but there is
still facial redness or stinging:*

AM

Step 1: Wash with a prescription
sulphacetamide cleanser

Step 2: Rinse with facial water

Step 3: Apply an antibiotic cream

Step 4: Apply a moisturiser with
SPF and/or sunscreen

Step 5: Apply a foundation with
sunscreen (optional)

PM

Step 1: Wash with a cold cream or
oil cleanser

Step 2: Rinse with facial water

Step 3: Apply an antibiotic cream

Step 4: Apply a night cream

In the morning, wash with a prescription sulphacetamide cleanser. Rinse your face with facial water (*not* tap water). Next, apply a prescription antibiotic cream, then a moisturiser with SPF. Last, apply a foundation with sunscreen if you wish.

In the evening, wash with a cold cream or oil cleanser and rinse with facial water. Apply an antibiotic cream, then a night cream.

Look for moisturisers with niacinamide or soy that will help prevent dark spots from returning. Good choices include Neutrogena Ultimate Moisture with soy, and Olay Regenerist with niacinamide.

Prescription Products for Your Skin

Listed below are examples of prescription products called for in the prescription regimens. For some of the categories below there are many products available, so my lists are not inclusive. In any case, you should discuss prescription choices with your dermatologist.

RECOMMENDED PRESCRIPTION LIGHTENING PRODUCTS

- Claripel
- EpiQuin Micro

- Generic prescription hydroquinone
- Lustra or Lustra AF
- Solaquin Forte
- Tri-Luma

The above-mentioned products are US name brands that may not be available in your country. Please ask your dermatologist for a substitution.

RECOMMENDED PRESCRIPTION TOPICAL ANTIBIOTICS

- Benzamycin (contains benzoyl peroxide which you should not use if you have redness)
- Duac
- Dalacin T
- Stiemycin
- Topicycline
- Zindaclin
- Zineryt

RECOMMENDED PRESCRIPTION RETINOID CREAMS

- Aknemycin Plus (contains an antibiotic as well)
- Differin gel or cream
- Isotrex
- Isotrexin (contains an antiobiotic as well)
- Retin-A gel, lotion or cream
- Retinova

Fortunately, these retinoids are available in the UK.

RECOMMENDED PRESCRIPTION MASK

- Plexion

This mask available in the US is one that I like very much. I was not able to locate any comparable masks in the UK, but check with your dermatologist.

RECOMMENDED PRESCRIPTION SULPHACETAMIDE CLEANSERS

- Rosac
- Rosanil
- Rosula

These prescription cleansers are available in the US, but you may be able to find something comparable.

RECOMMENDED PRESCRIPTION TOPICAL ANTI-INFLAMMATORIES

- Elidel
- MetroCream
- Protopic

Ask your dermatologist for topical anti-inflammatories comparable to these US brands.

RECOMMENDED ORAL MEDICATIONS

- Erythromycin
- Minocycline
- Tetracycline
- Azithromycin

PROCEDURES FOR YOUR SKIN TYPE

There are no procedures that can improve the dryness and sensitivity of your skin. These problems are best treated with skin care products, lifestyle changes, and dietary recommendations. Please see 'Further Help for Dry, Sensitive Skin'. However, your dark spots can be treated and there are more options to get rid of wrinkles than ever before.

Lasers and Light Treatments

For DSPWs with light skin, a number of types of lasers and light treatments are specifically designed to remove brown spots such as freckles. Please see 'Further Help for Dry, Sensitive Skin' for your options.

Lasers and light treatments work by targeting a particular colour. For example, pigmented lesion lasers such as the Ruby laser, the Alexandrite laser, or the Nd:Yag emit a specific wavelength of light that can only be absorbed by the colour brown. The Intense Pulsed Light treatments emit different wavelengths of light that target several skin features, such as dark spots and blood vessels.

When the laser or light is focused on a brown spot, the brown pigment (melanin) absorbs the energy of the light until the pigment becomes so hot that the cells containing melanin burst. The surrounding non-melanin-containing cells are unharmed. Patients with darker skin cannot use this technology because their normal skin cells contain higher amounts of melanin and would also be affected.

For more details on how light treatments work, see the procedures section of 'Further Help for Oily, Sensitive Skin'.

Chemical Peels

DSPWs with darker skin can use light chemical peels on their dark spots. Glycolic acid- and lactic acid-containing peels are best for your type because they hydrate the skin as well as exfoliating it. In addition, these peels have been shown to improve fine wrinkles. Although you can get these alpha hydroxy acid peels at a salon, a dermatologist will be able to use a higher concentration of AHA, giving you better results.

Botox/Reloxin

Your type may also benefit from Botox or reloxin treatments for wrinkles. Please see 'Further Help for Oily, Sensitive Skin' for details on Botox treatments and on the methods for treating different kinds of wrinkles.

Dermal Fillers

There are many good dermal fillers available to treat wrinkles. I prefer those containing collagen or hyaluronic acid. These fillers are ideal for DSPWs (and DSNWs) because collagen and hyaluronic acid are naturally occurring substances that look and feel natural and give instantaneous results. Please see the dermal fillers section of 'Further Help for Oily, Sensitive Skin'.

Mesotherapy

Mesotherapy is a new technique that is not yet perfected, so I am not recommending it at this time. In the future, I believe that it may well prove interesting because it has the potential to improve the skin's appearance by tightening it, without addressing wrinkles specifically. In this procedure, various vitamins, collagen, elastin or HA are injected superficially, or into the top part of the skin, all over the face, not just where there are wrinkles.

Right now each physician defines this treatment individually, with one injecting vitamin C mixed with collagen, while another uses HA. I plan to do studies of the various recipes to determine exactly which ones are helpful, which are harmful, and which do nothing, in order to try to define and standardise effective treatment.

ONGOING CARE FOR YOUR SKIN

Your skin may seem high maintenance now, but with a clear plan and these easy-to-follow regimens, you can finally manage your skin. Avoid cleansers that foam. Instead use an oil-based cleanser or a cold cream. Moisturise at least twice a day. Apply sunscreen daily, and use more often (reapplying hourly) if you are out in the sun.

CHAPTER THIRTEEN

Dry, Sensitive, Pigmented and Tight: DSPT

THE CHALLENGED SKIN TYPE

'Flaking, redness and under-eye dark circles – when my skin itches, it drives me crazy because scratching makes it worse.'

ABOUT YOUR SKIN

If your questionnaire results reveal you as a DSPT, you probably face a variety of skin issues. Your skin can be prone to eczema, dryness, acne, flaking, redness, itching and rosacea. The problems that plague DSPTs are more than visually disturbing. Having itchy skin, redness, rosacea or acne is just plain uncomfortable. You can't forget about it. It's a constant irritation and distraction. DSPTs feel helpless in managing their skin's dryness and sensitivity. Remember the old expression 'Walk a mile in my shoes?' Well, most other Skin Types wouldn't want to spend a day in your skin. And few people can imagine the ongoing distress that DSPTs experience every minute of their lives.

Even though your reddened, dry, and flaky skin cries out for moisturisers, your skin's sensitivity produces reactions to so many ingredients that you don't feel confident trying out products. Fragrance in skin care products, detergents in soaps, rough fabrics, and blustery weather can cause disturbances. Heavy moisturisers may cause acne. What can you feel happy about? Well, your risk for non-melanoma skin cancer may be slightly lower than for other types, but it is always best to get regular checkups.

All four Dry, Sensitive Skin Types have a disturbed skin barrier. To learn how dryness, sensitivity and pigmentation interact to create the skin issues you experience, please read 'A Disturbed Skin Barrier' in Chapter Twelve.

Many people of medium-tone skin have the DSPT type, which includes people of Latin American, Spanish, Mediterranean, or Middle Eastern ancestry. This type is also quite common among African-Americans and Asians.

DSPT CELEBRITY

For country singer Shania Twain, platinum albums and music industry awards are the public response to an unmatched musical outpouring that moves people to dance and to feel deeply. But even as Twain reigns as a music supernova, she never forgets her roots in poverty or the hard times she survived to become who she is today. Having endured hunger and her parents' early deaths, in her rise to fame, Shania has always remembered those who are less fortunate, championing charities like 'Second Harvest', which feeds hungry children, and participating in Purina's campaign to 'Adopt a Homeless Pet'.

Her love for animals and her simple country roots are also apparent in her choice of moisturiser. To help her dry skin, according to Internet gossip, Shania favours Bag Balm, a moisturising product used for udder soreness in cows and chapped hands in farmers. Known for its ability to address eczema, psoriasis, and other dry skin conditions, the product (packaged in the same green tin since its inception in 1899) contains petrolatum, lanolin and an antiseptic. Growing up with the cold and hard Canadian winters, Shania likely has dry, sensitive skin, and if so, heavy moisturising is definitely right for her. Her skin also appears to be pigmented and tight. In the past, Shania has certainly had her share of stress, which can contribute to dry skin conditions like dermatitis and eczema. However, today, she has *good* stress: the stress of meeting creative challenges and living in partnership with her husband, record producer Robert John 'Mutt' Lange. Her husband could very possibly be a DS*N*W to Twain's DS*PT*. Sharing dry, sensitive skin could help them understand each other, while being on opposite sides of the other skin factors could spell enduring attraction – and clearly has for them.

DEALING WITH DRYNESS

Dark-skin-toned DSPTs may have dry, sensitive skin for genetic reasons, but their skin's dryness can also result from environmental conditions and chemical exposures. Many of the products and chemical treatments used on black hair can undermine the skin barrier and contribute to allergies.

An allergy occurs when the immune system makes antibodies that react to a substance. For example, some people have antibodies to poison ivy and they develop a rash when exposed to it, while others do not have this antibody and don't react to it. Ingredients can penetrate a compromised skin barrier to reach the bloodstream, where they can produce an allergic reaction. Irritant rashes are different, though often confused with allergies. An irritating substance causes a skin rash but, unlike an allergy, is not caused by antibodies. An impaired skin barrier makes you more susceptible.

Rashes, redness and itching are all responses to inflammation, which further undermines the skin barrier. Once your skin is inflamed, you need to calm it by avoiding irritants and accessing skin soothers. Continued damage can lead to eczema, to which DSPTs are prone.

DSPTS AND ECZEMA

Over twelve million people have eczema, also known as atopic dermatitis (AD), a severe form of dry skin that tends to recur in the same place, such as behind the knees, on the wrists, knuckles and ankles, and in the bend of the arm. It begins as an itching patch that becomes red and inflamed. Scratching of the area can cause the skin to tear and become infected. In DSPT and DSPW Types, the affected areas become dark and can take months to fade to your natural skin colour. Eczema results from a combination of dryness and sensitivity, and sometimes allergies play a part. These may include both topical allergies to substances that touch the skin and internal reactions to foods, inhalants, and other substances that produce an allergic reaction via the skin. For more information about how skin barrier damage can lead to problems like eczema, please refer to Chapter Two, 'Allergic Subtype'.

Do I Have Eczema?

If you have any of the following symptoms, you may have eczema:

- Itching skin anywhere on the face or body
- Irritation and need to frequently scratch behind the knees, elbows, wrists or ankles
- Areas of itching turn into darkened or reddened patches that remain after itching has calmed
- Cracking of the skin over areas of redness and dryness, especially over joints

- Itching and redness that tend to recur in the same areas of the body
- Itching, redness and scaling behind the ears
- History of allergies or asthma in you or your family

One key rule is that it's important not to scratch when you feel the itch because the friction of scratching further degrades the skin barrier. Instead I'll provide you with both over-the-counter and prescription medications to calm eczema flares.

Predisposed to Eczema?

Eczema can often be an inherited condition, striking people with a family history or medical history of asthma and allergies. The onset of eczema usually occurs within the first year of life and most people who are going to get it develop it by age five. Luckily, many 'grow out of it'. plagued in the future by just routine dry skin. Adults with atopic dermatitis usually have excessively sensitive skin.

A recent study reveals that breast-fed infants have a lower incidence of atopic dermatitis, most likely because breast-fed infants are not exposed to common allergens like dairy products and soy before their young immune systems have developed. Interestingly, another study showed that babies who were breast-fed by mothers who eliminated common allergic foods (such as eggs, dairy, fish, peanuts and soybeans) from their diets had a lower incidence of eczema than breast-fed babies whose mothers were not on restricted diets.

Avoiding Irritants

The three key interventions for addressing both dryness and eczema are:

- Calming inflammation
- Rebuilding the barrier
- Hydrating the skin

Although there is no cure for eczema, it can be controlled. It's important to avoid sun exposure and use skin care products designed to strengthen the skin's barrier. My selections will include ingredients that hydrate the skin and repair the skin's barrier, allowing the skin to better hold on to water.

DSPT ENVIRONMENTAL IMPACT REPORT

The problems DSPTs suffer also change with the seasons, as weather conditions can assault your dry, sensitive skin. It's hard to say which season is best for your Dry, Pigmented Skin Type. In the summer, sun exposure may darken dark spots. As a result, sun protection and skin lightening are often needed. When the temperature drops, so do humidity levels, with wintry cold and low humidity increasing dryness and skin sensitivity. Heavy winter clothes, made with rough fabrics like wool, may cause skin friction that worsens dryness and sensitivity. For DSPTs, the ideal climate is a cool, humid environment. Moving to Arizona is not recommended.

Jessica's Story

Forty-eight-year-old Jessica was a Hawaiian employed by a national banking group who came to the clinic to enrol in a melasma study to test the effectiveness of a new topical cream for facial dark spots. For several years, Jessica had had a band of darkened skin that looked a bit like a mud pack covering her forehead. Planning her wedding in three months, Jessica was desperate to deal with this skin problem. 'I was planning to wear white gardenias in my hair,' she confided. 'But at this rate, I'll be wearing a heavy veil that covers my whole face.'

For Christmas, Jessica's best friend gave her a series of six facial chemical peels at a local spa. The peels, which contained glycolic acid and resorcinol, worsened her darkened forehead. I began to wonder if pigmentation was the source of her problem.

In conducting her physical examination, I noticed that behind her knees and in the bend of her arms (on the opposite side of her elbow), the skin was dry, thickened and darkened. Enquiring further into her medical history, I learned that she'd had asthma as a child. In fact, asthma and dry skin ran in her family. Now the cause of her problem was clear. Jessica did not have melasma after all: she had eczema.

In eczema, itchy dry skin can result in darkened skin areas in Pigmented Types like Jessica. The area on her forehead was a dry area with eczema, which had been exacerbated both by the hair-colouring product she used to hide her grey and by the depigmenting treatments she'd tried that were too harsh for her damaged skin barrier.

To help address the dryness and rebuild the skin barrier, I put Jessica on a diet rich in essential fatty acids and gave her a skin care regimen geared to improve her skin barrier. I prescribed a steroid-free medication called Elidel that reduces inflammation. I advised her to have her hair colourist apply Vaseline petroleum jelly to her affected area prior to colouring her hair to prevent the hair colour from irritating her facial skin.

One month later, she returned for a follow-up visit. With the wedding just two months away, she was thrilled with her skin's smoothness and clarity. With the darkened eczema area on her forehead nearly healed, she was able to stop using the Elidel while maintaining her recommended diet and skin care regimen. A few months later, I got a bridal photo of Jessica and her new husband on their wedding day. She looked stunning, with perfect skin and gardenias in her hair.

A CLOSE-UP LOOK AT YOUR SKIN

Like Jessica, with DSPT skin you may experience any of the following:

- Eczema (atopic dermatitis)
- Scaling skin
- Thick rough patches of skin
- Itching
- Dryness that worsens in winter or low-humidity climates
- Sensitivity to fragrances that can cause skin rashes
- Dryness from detergents, creating 'dish pan hands'
- Dark patches in areas of inflammation or trauma such as after a cut
- Dark patches in areas of sun exposure
- Dark eyelids
- Dark circles under the eyes

With tight skin, you won't experience that much wrinkling as you age, while other problems *will* worsen with aging. Your dry skin gets drier as the years go by. Winter is harder on skin than in youth, resulting in redness, flaking, and cracking. Going without a moisturiser is usually not an option over the age of fifty. Heavier night creams will feel good to older DSPTs; however, don't be fooled into buying expensive ones with antiaging ingredients you don't need. I'll offer the right moisturisers later in this chapter. For women, melasma and dark spots will improve with declining oestrogen levels in perimenopause and menopause. However, lower oestrogen levels also contribute to dry skin. In the eighties and nineties, as the immune system weakens, any condition arising from allergies or autoimmune conditions (such as certain cases of eczema) may improve.

ETHNICITY AND DSPT SKIN

Like Jessica, many DSPT Asians have a higher incidence of eczema and melasma, but a lower incidence of wrinkles and skin cancer than do Caucasians. As a result, Asian product lines focus more closely on treating dryness and pigmentation. Due to biochemical differences, Asian skin also reacts differently to products than Caucasian and black skin.

For example, several studies have demonstrated that Japanese skin is more reactive to detergents. This may be why many Asians prefer oil-based cleansers. While detergents (contained in most cleansers, shampoos, face and body soaps, laundry and dish-cleaning products) are drying and should be avoided by all Dry, Sensitive Types, those of Asian ancestry in particular should steer clear of soaps, shampoos, and cleaning products that vigorously foam. Pick milder products, rinse thoroughly after cleansing, and re-moisturise after use. Also wear rubber gloves when using household cleaning products. Although in the US, I recommend skin care products that contain hydroquinone, an ingredient used in skin care to lighten dark spots, it's not widely used elsewhere in the world; what's more some Asians with dry, sensitive skin and a history of ochronosis (a hereditary enzyme deficiency) should avoid it, as they may develop the blackish patches characteristic of this condition. Instead, Asian DSPTs can receive hydroquinone-free peels, light treatments, or microdermabrasion from a dermatologist or spa professional. I recommend you request a 'light' rather than strong treatment, proceeding gradually to assure that your skin does not become irritated.

PRODUCT CHOICES FOR DSPT SKIN

DSPTs benefit from constant moisturiser use, and you also need products and treatments that lighten dark patches and melasma. However, DSPTs react negatively to a wide range of products and ingredients. Fragrances are the most common allergens, instigating rashes more than anything else, including parabens and other chemical preservatives used in skin care. Obviously, you should avoid dousing yourself in perfume, although you may be able to find a single essential oil that does not cause a reaction. Still, the search to find one can create so much havoc, it may not be worth it. As mentioned earlier, most skin care products, even those marketed as fragrance free, contain some perfume to mask the unpleasant smell of the ingredients. The perfume used for this purpose is often a mix containing as many as forty or more different ingredients, so identifying the culprit can be next to impossible. One patient of mine developed a rash from the perfume samples stapled inside magazines. Now before she reads a magazine, she asks her boyfriend to remove the offending samples.

Not knowing which ingredients cause reactions makes skin care shopping a danger-fraught experience. You may find that when you use your new skin purchases, your skin flares up, with rashes and redness that can persist for days, weeks, and months. Don't think that you can use the cream you bought on a less critical area, like your hands, feet or legs. When you're at risk for eczema, you have to be ultra careful. Many DSPT patients report that it's an achievement to find even a single product that they can safely use.

Anita Lopez was a slender fifty-four-year-old who worked in a newspaper's high-stress newsroom. With brown hair and lively, light brown eyes, Anita had a medium-fair skin tone, but suffered from dark spots. In her youth, her skin was more combination; with age, it became drier. Although her dry, pigmented skin got dark spots and increased dryness from sun exposure, Anita couldn't find a sunscreen that did not irritate her skin. Whenever she used products containing benzophenone, she'd react with redness, especially around the eyes and cheeks.

Anita also had trouble finding the right night cream. Fruit acids, for example, made her itch. Antiaging creams made her skin turn red and burn. She had to completely avoid perfume. Having tried many products, she had come to distrust salespeople. 'They don't know what they are selling,' she told me. One recent skin care book recommended an expensive serum to lighten her dark spots; but when she purchased the author's products, she developed red scaled spots everywhere she applied it. When one of her friends told her that I supply specific skin care regimens based on each individual's Skin Type, she decided right away to come and see me.

First of all, I recommended that Anita try a cream sunscreen product containing titanium dioxide, which is less irritating to sensitive skin than benzophenone. 'I love this product,' Anita enthused. 'At last, I can wear sunscreen.' In addition, since both acupuncture and massage can help sensitive skin by calming stress, I recommended that Anita consult a doctor of traditional Chinese medicine and a massage therapist. Finally, I prescribed a cleanser and a moisturiser that she could use to soothe and hydrate.

KNOWING YOUR SKIN

Beauty companies design skin care products that are effective for the largest segments of the public, but what works for many people won't work for you because even a tiny amount of one harsh ingredient can cause your skin to hyperreact. That's why I've spent weeks sifting through product offerings to find the select few that meet your exacting needs. Then I've spent years ensuring that they work for my DSPT patients.

THE MOISTURE CURE

DSPTs, if I have one message to you, it's this: hydrate, hydrate, hydrate.

Moisturisers with an SPF factor blended into simple beneficial ingredients, like shea butter, cocoa butter, olive and jojoba oils, are best for you. When I was in my dermatology residency, one of my colleagues used to cover her skin with lard nightly. Although the trans fats it contains make it unhealthy to eat, as they can displace needed skin-building fats like the omega-3 fatty acids, it certainly moisturised her dry skin. Why? Because hydrogenated or trans fats are occlusive, which means that they hold water in, much like cling film.

Your skin care products should either contain or cause the skin to produce ceramides, fatty acids and cholesterol. These three different forms of fat are needed to create a healthy skin barrier. In addition, you must apply a moisturiser at least twice a day. Notice that I said *at least*. In your case, more is better. I also advise you use both a sunscreen and a moisturiser, because sunscreens alone will not provide enough hydration. Heavy night creams are good but should not contain fragrances that will further irritate and dry your skin. Beware of the expensive creams that do contain fragrances. Sunscreens must be worn daily, for two reasons. First, the sun disrupts the skin's barrier; and second, the sun causes dark spots.

Unfortunately, there are no in-office dermatological procedures that I know of that will improve the skin's barrier. In many cases, dark spots in lighter-skinned individuals can be treated with laser and light therapies. Both dark- and light-skinned individuals may be treated with chemical peels or microdermabrasion to hasten the resolution of dark spots and to temporarily improve the roughness of the skin. Prescription medications can be used to treat eczema flare-ups and to lighten dark spots. But above all, you must take control and be vigilant about moisturising your skin and avoiding irritants.

Dr Baumann's Bottom Line: For you, moisturising as often as four times a day isn't too much. Apply moisturisers immediately after bathing, dish-washing, or facing the elements. Do it whenever you change clothes. You cannot over-moisturise your skin.

EVERYDAY CARE FOR YOUR SKIN

The goal of your skin care routine is to heal your skin's barrier to make it stronger, helping it hold on to moisture (so that your skin becomes less dry) and keep out allergens and irritants (so that your skin becomes less sensitive). To accomplish these goals, you'll use products that deliver barrier repair ingredients. This will also help prevent inflammation that leads to dark spots.

All the products I'll recommend act to do one or both of the following:

• Prevent and treat skin dryness
• Prevent and treat skin redness and itching

In addition, your daily regimen will also help to address your other skin concerns by:

• Preventing and treating dark spots
• Preventing and treating acne

While not everyone with this type will get acne, having dry skin does not protect you from outbreaks. I'll provide optional treatments for pimples.

Products designed for 'sensitive skin' are for dry, sensitive types. How-ever, if you have a high P/N score (over 40), there are few sensitive skin products that contain depigmenting agents. I will point you towards products that will give your skin an even tone in addition to hydrating it, building its barrier, and decreasing its sensitivity.

I'll provide both a Stage One nonprescription regimen and a Stage Two prescription regimen in this chapter. Try the nonprescription one first for eight weeks. If it doesn't help your skin, move to the prescription regimen.

DAILY SKIN CARE

STAGE ONE: NONPRESCRIPTION REGIMEN

AM	PM
Step 1: Wash with cleanser	Step 1: Wash with cleanser
Step 2: Spray facial water	Step 2: Spray facial water
Step 3: Apply eye cream (optional)	Step 3: Apply eye cream (optional)
Step 4: Apply skin lightener to spots (optional)	Step 4: Apply skin lightener to spots (optional)
Step 4: Apply moisturiser	Step 4: Apply moisturiser
Step 6: Apply sunscreen	
Step 7: Apply foundation (optional)	

In the morning, wash your face with a cleanser, then spray on facial water. Eye cream use is optional, you can use one if you want. In that case, be prepared to apply your eye cream, skin lightener, and moisturiser in rapid sequence while your face is still damp from the facial water. Have all your products out and ready for use to assure you apply them all before your face dries. If the water evaporates prior to moisturiser application, this will dry your skin, which is totally counterproductive. Skin lightener should be applied to dark spots only. Then apply moisturiser, sunscreen, and finally, foundation if you wish.

In the evening, wash with a cleanser, spray facial water, and apply an eye cream and a skin lightener if needed. Last, apply moisturiser.

Although you may never before have heard of spraying your face with specially packaged facial waters prior to moisturising, it's a great secret for hydrating dry skin. You'll find more information about it in this chapter in my section on facial water.

After eight weeks on this regimen, if your dryness and skin sensitivity fail to resolve, try *different* products from my list of recommendations. If your skin still does not improve in another four weeks, see a dermatologist who can prescribe medication for severe dryness, itching and eczema that can be used along with this Stage One regimen.

Cleansers

Cleansing and moisturising are the two most important aspects of your skin regimen. Using the wrong cleanser can aggravate your condition even if you are doing everything else right. Cleansers that contain detergents (which produce a lot of foam and suds) strip your skin of necessary lipids, causing dryness and increased sensitivity. DSPTs should never use soap, shampoo, moisturiser, or hair conditioner that you haven't selected yourself to assure they do not contain irritating ingredients.

Did you know that you can wash your face with oil? It's very popular in Asia, since so many people there have dry skin. If you have acne, this may not work for you; but if you're like me (very dry and scaling), it's a great way to moisturise. I *love* cleansing oils for DSPTs. Try Shu Uemura Skin Purifier Cleansing Oil, being sure to follow the directions that tell you to apply it to a dry face and then add water with your fingertips.

RECOMMENDED CLEANSERS

- £ Eucerin Gentle Cleansing Milk
- £ Lutsine Gentle Cleansing Cream
- £ Nivea Visage Gentle Cleansing Cream Wash
- ££ Bobbie Brown Rich Cream Cleanser
- ££ Dermalogica Ultra-Calming Cleanser
- ££ Eleusian Facial Hydrating Cleanser (do not use if acne is your complaint)
- ££ Ella Baché Gommage Délicat
- ££ Gly Derm Gentle Cleanser 2% (do not use if skin stinging is your complaint)
- ££ La Roche-Posay Toleriane Dermo-Cleanser
- ££ L'Occitane Shea Butter Extra Moisturising Cold Cream Soap
- ££ Organic Pharmacy Rose & Chamomile Cleansing Milk
- ££ Stiefel Oilatum-AD Cleansing Lotion
- £££ Darphin Intral Cleansing Milk
- £££ Dermalogica Ultra Calming Cleanser

Baumann's Choice: Eucerin Gentle Cleansing Milk

RECOMMENDED CLEANSING OILS

- £ Jojoba Cleansing Oil
- ££ Shu Uemura Skin Purifier Cleansing Oil

££ SK II Facial Treatment Cleansing Oil
£££ Decléor Cleansing Oil
£££ Seikisho Cleansing Oil

Baumann's Choice: Seikisho Cleansing Oil has safflower oil to improve skin hydration and licorice extract, which may help reduce pigment. Go to www.DrBaumann.co.uk to learn where to find these products.

Facial Water

DSPTs should *never* use toners, which usually have drying ingredients that remove lipids from the skin. Your skin needs all the lipids it can get. Instead of a toner, use a facial water. Spray it on your face immediately prior to applying an eye cream and moisturiser. The moisturiser and eye cream will help trap the water on the skin, giving the skin a reservoir to pull water from. This is especially important in low-humidity environments such as in the winter air, on aeroplanes, in air-conditioning, or in windy locales.

Facial waters come from thermal springs. They do not contain chemicals such as chlorine that are added to our tap water to keep it free from algae and other organisms. The constituents of the water vary according to the source. Vichy water contains sulphur, while the La Roche-Posay water contains selenium, which has been shown to be effective in treating eczema. Both selenium and sulphur can be anti-inflammatory.

RECOMMENDED FACIAL WATERS

£ Evian Mineral Water Spray
££ Avène Thermal Water Spray
££ Chantecaille Pure Rosewater
££ Fresh Rose Marigold Tonic Water (with chamomile)
££ Korres Hamamelis Hydrating Face Water
££ La Roche-Posay Thermal Spring Water
££ Organic Pharmacy Rose Facial Spritz
££ Shu Uemura Depsea Therapy
££ Vichy Thermal Spa Water
£££ Jurlique Rosewater Freshener

Baumann's Choice: Eau Thermale by La Roche-Posay because it contains selenium.

Acne Treatment

DSPTs who have acne are a minority, but I haven't forgotten about you. Learning to properly hydrate your skin will actually improve your acne. It is a myth that the skin must be dried out to improve acne. Based on recent studies, dermatologists now believe that acne clears better with a hydrating cleanser than with a drying one. If your acne does not improve, you may add an over-the-counter retinol cream such as Philosophy Help Me, followed by a moisturiser in your nighttime regimen. In most cases, this will be enough to clear your skin. If not, please see your dermatologist.

Treatments for Dark Spots

Any allergenic product can cause inflammation, which in turn can lead to dark spots. For instance, some accessories or cosmetics worn by Indian women are known to cause skin reactions. The *bindi,* a circular plastic disc attached to the forehead, contains an adhesive that can cause inflammation and skin darkness. *Sindoor,* a red powder sprinkled on the scalp along the parting to denote (female) marital status, and *surma,* a fine black powder usually applied to the eyelid margins, have also caused skin irritations.

When dark spots are present, use a skin lightening gel. Several over-the-counter products are suggested below, but I highly recommend getting a stronger prescription product from your dermatologist.

RECOMMENDED SKIN LIGHTENERS

££ B. Kamins Skin Lightening Treatment
££ L'Occitane Immortelle Brightening Serum
££ PCA Skin pHaze 23 A&C Synergy Serum
££ Peter Thomas Roth Potent Skin Lightening Lotion Complex
££ Philosophy A Pigment of Your Imagination
£££ DDF Intensive Holistic Corrector Swabs
£££ DDF Intensive Holistic Lightener
£££ Dr Brandt Lightening Gel
£££ Pevonia Lightening Gel
£££ Rodan and Fields Reverse Prepare Skin Lightening Toner
£££ SkinCeuticals Phyto + Botanical Gel for Hyperpigmentation
£££ Thalgo Unizones
£££ TYK White Glow Retinol, Kojic, Mag-C Absolute Skin Brightener

Baumann's Choice: In the US, there are many more options in skin lighteners. See www.Baumannstore.co.uk for other choices. My favourite in the UK is SkinCeuticals Phyto + Botanical Gel.

Moisturisers

You need to moisturise frequently, at least three times daily. The ideal would be in the morning after gently cleansing your face, again in the later afternoon or early evening, and at bedtime. If you have a very low O/D score of 11 to 16, use creams. If you have a medium O/D score of 17 to 26, use lotions. Avoid gels, which are better for oily types.

Assure that every day you are covered with a minimum SPF of 15. You can obtain this degree of protection via a single product, such as moisturiser, or via several used in combination, such as moisturiser and foundation.

RECOMMENDED EYE CREAMS

- £ Olay Regenerist Eye Lifting Serum
- £ Neutrogena Visibly Young Eye Cream
- £ Nivea Antiwrinkle Q 10 Plus Eye Cream
- ££ DDF Nutrient K Plus
- ££ MD Skincare Lift & Lighten Eye Cream
- ££ Peter Thomas Roth AHA/Kojic Under Eye Brightener
- ££ Relastin Eye Cream
- £££ La Prairie Cellular Eye Moisturiser
- £££ Sisley Eye and Lip Contour Cream

Baumann's Choice: Olay Regenerist Eye Lifting Serum because it contains niacinamide which may help dark circles.

RECOMMENDED DAYTIME MOISTURISERS

- £ Boots No7 Uplifting Day Cream
- £ Olay Regenerist Rehydrating Lotion with UV Protection
- £ Neutrogena Ultimate Moisture Day Cream
- £ Neutrogena Visibly Young Day Cream with SPF 15
- ££ Elizabeth Arden Prevage
- ££ Laura Mercier Mega Moisturiser with SPF 15
- ££ L'Occitane Face and Body Balm with SPF 15

£££ Dermalogica Barrier Repair
£££ Pevonia Evolutive Eye Cream
£££ Sisley Broad Spectrum Sunscreen, SPF 40

Baumann's Choice: Neutrogena Ultimate Moisture Day Cream

RECOMMENDED EVENING MOISTURISERS

£ Boots No7 Uplifting Night Cream
£ Neutrogena Ultimate Moisture Night Cream
£ Neutrogena Visibly Young Day Cream
£ Olay Total Effects 7x Visible Anti-Aging Vitamin Complex
££ Atopalm MLE Cream
££ D R Harris Almond Oil Skin Food
££ Elizabeth Arden Perpetual Moisture 24 Cream
££ Ferndale Nouriva Repair Moisturising Cream
££ L'Occitane Shea Butter 24 Hours Ultra Rich Face Cream
££ Osmotics Tri Ceram
££ Sekkisei Cream Excellent
££ SkinCeuticals Renew Overnight Dry
££ Vichy Nutrilogie 2
£££ Dior Energy-Move Skin Illuminating Moisturising Crème
£££ La Prairie Skin Caviar Luxe Body Cream
£££ RéVive Moisturising Renewal Cream
£££ Sisley Botanical Moisturiser with Cucumber
£££ Z. Bigatti Re-Storation Enlighten Skin Tone Provider

Baumann's Choice: Neutrogena Ultimate Moisture Night Cream because it contains active soy to help diminish dark spots.

Exfoliation

As a rule, people with DSPT skin shouldn't exfoliate, unless your dermatologist recommends it. I have seen many DSPT patients who over-exfoliated, leading to skin redness, tiny red bumps, and inflammation-induced pigmentation. Concentrate instead on moisturising. Many at-home microdermabrasion kits are available, but I feel you are much better off doing these treatments under the supervision of a dermatologist.

SHOPPING FOR PRODUCTS

With your sensitive skin, you need to read labels carefully in order to avoid ingredients that may aggravate dryness and pigmentation. Look for ingredients that prevent and improve dark spots, hydrate the skin, and prevent inflammation. If you find favourite products that are not on my recommended lists, please go to www.DrBaumann.co.uk and share your discoveries with me and others of your Skin Type.

RECOMMENDED SKIN CARE INGREDIENTS

To prevent dark spots:

- Cocos nucifera (coconut extract), unless you have acne
- Niacinamide
- Pycnogenol (a pine bark extract)
- Soy, with oestrogenic components taken out

To improve dark spots:

- Arbutin
- Bearberry extract
- Cucumber extract
- Glycyrrhiza glabra (licorice extract)
- Mulberry extract

To prevent inflammation:

- Aloe vera
- Chamomile
- Colloidal oatmeal
- Cucumber
- Dexpanthenol (provitamin B$_5$)
- Epilobium angustifolium (willow herb)
- Evening primrose oil
- Feverfew
- Licochalone
- Perilla leaf extract
- Pycnogenol (a pine bark extract)
- Red algae
- Thyme
- Trifolium pretense (red clover)

To help skin hold on to water:

- Borage seed oil
- Castor oil
- Ceramide
- Cholesterol
- Cocoa butter (avoid if you have acne)
- Dimethicone
- Evening primrose oil
- Glycerin
- Jojoba oil
- Olive oil
- Pumpkin seed oil

- Colloidal oatmeal
- Dexpanthenol (provitamin B$_5$)
- Safflower oil
- Shea butter
- Sunflower oil

SKIN CARE INGREDIENTS TO AVOID

Due to irritating detergents:

- Dimethyl dodecyl amido betaine
- Lauryl sulphates
- Sodium dodecyl sulfate
- Sodium laurel sulfate

Due to increasing acne or skin redness:

- Cinnamon oil
- Cocos nucifera (coconut oil)
- Cocoa butter
- Isopropyl isostearate
- Isopropyl myristate
- Peppermint oil

Due to problematic preservatives:

- Benzalkonium chloride
- Bronopol
- Chloroacetamide
- Chlorocreso
- Chlorhexidine
- Chloroquinaldol
- Diazolidinyl urea
- Dibromodicyanobutane (phenoxyethanol)
- Dichlorophen
- DMDM hydantoin
- Formaldehyde
- Glutaraldehyde
- Imidazolidinyl urea
- Kathon CG
- Parabens
- Phenylmercuric acetate
- Quaternium-15
- Sorbic acid
- Thimerosal
- Triclosan

Due to stimulating skin pigmentation:

- Achillea millefolium (yarrow)
- Cananga odorata (ylang ylang)
- Dandelion
- Geranium
- Jasmine
- Lavender
- Lemongrass
- Lemon oil
- Neroli
- Peppermint
- Rose oil (Bulgarian)
- Rosemary
- Sandalwood
- Tea tree oil

Sun Protection for Your Skin

To prevent dark spots and dryness, wear sunscreen regularly. Since sunscreen products can cause redness and irritation and each person reacts to different ingredients, you may have to try several of my recommended products (chosen to minimise skin reaction) before you find one that works for you. Make sure that your combined use of moisturiser, sunscreen, and foundation provides you with a minimum SPF of 15 for daily use.

RECOMMENDED SUN PROTECTION PRODUCTS

£ Eucerin Q 10 Active Antiwrinkle Fluid SPF 15
£ Olay Regenerist Rehydrating Lotion SPF 15
££ Garnier Ambre Solaire Ultra Protect Face Cream SPF 50
££ Glycolix Elite Sunscreen SPF 30 by Topix
££ La Roche-Posay Anthelios Fluide Extreme SPF 60 (found in Ireland)
££ L'Occitane Shea Butter Ultra Moisturising Care SPF 15
££ Molton Brown Active Defence City Day Hydrator
££ Origins Out Smart Sunscreen SPF 20
££ Philosophy A Pigment of Your Imagination SPF 18 Sunscreen
£££ SkinCeuticals Ultimate UV Defence SPF 30

Baumann's Choice: L'Occitane Shea Butter Ultra Moisturising Care SPF 15 is excellent for dry skin because it contains shea butter. However, for prolonged sun exposure use a higher SPF such as Garnier Ambre Solaire Ultra Protect Face Cream SPF 50.

Your Makeup

DSPTs often become irritated by ingredients in makeup, but may not recognise that their cosmetics are the source of the problem. DSPTs with an Asian background are especially prone to develop darkness of the skin resulting from a reaction to cosmetic products. Experts believe that this problem, called pigmented contact dermatitis, is induced by very small amounts of allergens that come into almost daily contact with the patient's skin. Eyeshadows and blushers are frequent culprits.

If you tend to have darkness on the eyelids, under the eyes, or on the cheeks, consider eliminating cosmetic products that contain ingredients listed previously under 'Skin Care Ingredients to Avoid'.

You may also find that eye makeup remover can irritate your eyelids, leading to redness and then dark pigmentation. If you suspect that this is your problem, use an eye makeup remover for sensitive skin such as Toleriane Eye Makeup Remover by La Roche-Posay to remove eye makeup.

Choose foundations containing oil and avoid those labelled oil free. With your dry skin, you should not be using face powders. And if your skin is very dry, use cream eyeshadows and blushers.

RECOMMENDED FOUNDATIONS

£ Boots No7 Radiant Glow Foundation with SPF 15
£ Botanics Fresh Face Tinted Moisturiser
£ CoverGirl CG Smoothers All Day Hydrating Make-Up for Normal to Dry Skin
££ Bloom Foundation
££ Bobbi Brown Moisture Rich Foundation SPF 15
££ Chantecaille Real Skin Foundation
££ Laura Mercier Moisturising Foundation
££ Origins Original Skin More Coverage (To hide dark spots)
£££ Chanel Vitalumière Satin Smoothing Crème Makeup with SPF 15
£££ DiorSkin Liquid SPF 12

Baumann's Choice: Boots No7 Radiant Glow Foundation with SPF 15. If you have many dark spots, choose a heavier product such as Origins Original Skin More Coverage.

CONSULTING A DERMATOLOGIST

PRESCRIPTION SKIN CARE STRATEGIES

My prescription regimen for DSPTs focuses on preventing and treating dark spots. If you suffer from eczema or atopic dermatitis, properly moisturising your skin by following the tips in this chapter will help prevent the condition from worsening. If eczema is problematic and you have exhausted the resources available through your GP, I suggest that you consult a dermatologist, who can prescribe drugs such as Elidel and Protopic that can help treat your skin's redness and itching.

DAILY SKIN CARE

STAGE TWO: PRESCRIPTION REGIMEN

For dark spots:

AM	PM
Step 1: Wash with cleanser	Step 1: Wash with cleanser
Step 2: Spray facial water	Step 2: Spray facial water
Step 3: Apply prescription skin lightener to spots (optional)	Step 3: Apply prescription skin lightener to spots (optional)
Step 4: Apply moisturiser	Step 4: Apply moisturiser
	Step 5: Apply sunscreen
	Step 6: Apply foundation (optional)

In the morning, wash your face with a cleanser and spray facial water. Although it's not necessary, you can apply eye cream after your facial water. Then, if dark spots are present, apply a prescription skin lightener. If the facial water has dried, you can add another spritz at this time. Next, apply moisturiser, then sunscreen. Foundation should be the last product you apply before going out, if you wear it.

In the evening, wash with cleanser, spray facial water, apply prescription skin lightener to dark spots if needed, and finish with moisturiser.

I recommend combining daily use of prescription skin lighteners with micro-dermabrasion treatments in your dermatologist's office once every week or two, or as the dermatologist prescribes. (See the section on microdermabrasion below.)

It usually takes eight weeks on this regimen before you'll notice results. But stick with it because it will improve your complexion.

If acne is a significant problem for you, you could help alleviate that condition by following the Stage Two regimen for improving acne or rosacea in the DSNT chapter.

PROCEDURES

Although your dermatologist can help treat acne, facial flushing, and dark spots, no skin care procedures currently available can improve your skin's dryness and sensitivity. Avoid facials, since they will most likely expose your skin to irritating agents. You may, however, benefit from chemical peels or microdermabrasion to improve dark spots.

Chemical Peels

Your prescription regimen will show results faster if you combine it with dermatologically administered chemical peels, since the retinoids used in the regimen will enhance the penetration of the peel and will help you heal faster afterwards by speeding up cell division. I always advise DSPTs to go to a dermatologist for the peels rather than having them at a spa or salon because your pigmented skin is at risk for developing dark spots with any potentially irritating treatment.

There are many different chemical peel preparations on the market and it is important that you be given the proper one to prevent skin irritation and resulting pigmentation. If you have dark skin or are of Asian ancestry, make sure you see a dermatologist who specialises in skin of colour.

Microdermabrasion

If your S/R score is low (below 40) and you suffer from dark spots on your face, you may benefit from combining microdermabrasion with your depigmenting agent. In microdermabrasion, the practitioner uses a device that sprays microcrystals to remove the upper surface layer of the skin, making it easier for the depigmenting ingredients to penetrate.

If the microdermabrasion is too strong, however, your skin will become inflamed, producing more pigment and worsening your condition. So it's important that you see a dermatologist for these procedures.

ONGOING CARE FOR YOUR TYPE

Fighting dry, sensitive skin will be a lifelong challenge. But putting the proper dietary and skin care routines in place will help. So remember to decrease sun exposure, get enough sleep, avoid irritating products and ingredients, increase humidity in your environment, and use skin care with barrier repair ingredients. Hydrate, hydrate, hydrate.

CHAPTER FOURTEEN

Dry, Sensitive, Non-Pigmented and Wrinkled: DSNW

THE REACTIVE SKIN TYPE

'My skin is so changeable, I never know how I'll look from day to day. Some seasons, it looks fine, while at other times, it reacts to just about everything. Is there any logic to managing reactive skin?'

ABOUT YOUR SKIN

Relax, DSNW, you *can* manage your reactive skin although, admittedly, yours is not an easy Skin Type.

There's no predicting your skin condition. One day you're fine, and the next, inexplicably, you're having a bad skin day – just when you have that big meeting or date. It's hard to plan and feel confident when you have changeable skin. Dry, flaking, dull, itching and reddened, often your skin feels uncomfortable and looks irritated. You're puzzled because your desert-dry skin craves moisture, but many products you try cause itching, stinging and burning. Skin dryness makes wrinkles look worse. If you're in your thirties or older, you may imagine you can see your skin aging day by day. Although moisturisers can help by plumping out fine lines, your sensitive skin won't tolerate most products, even ones designed for sensitive skin.

Antiaging creams are often irritating. When you try a retinoid, your skin may not tolerate the redness and flaking that develop. You're in a double bind: you wrinkle if you don't moisturise, and react if you do. I can identify because I'm a DSNT and it's a close cousin to your Skin Type; so never fear, I know what will work for you.

The good news is that the proper skin care regimen with the right products and ingredients can make a huge difference. In fact, daily skin care is key to addressing your problems. With the right regimen, your skin condition will stabilise, and I'll provide several options to assure that you can care for your skin whatever your particular problem.

DSNW CELEBRITY

By playing outcasts, cowboys, blue-collar guys and outsiders, Clint Eastwood became not only an international movie star, but the most enduring screen actor and director of his generation – not to mention the mayor of Carmel. This man of few words is a prolific filmmaker whose credits include *Unforgiven*, *The Bridges of Madison County*, and *Mystic River*.

Eastwood is a man's man whom women consider a total hottie. According to *CBS 60 Minutes*, he has 'seven children with five women'. That tells you something.

All of this, in spite of the condition of his skin. Eastwood's trademark scowl, sunburnt tan, and lined face contrast with his innate good looks. Decades of sun exposure have turned his non-pigmented skin into a weathered leather, with deeply etched lines and dryness. A woman of his age and skin condition would most likely not be considered a sex symbol. Despite all that sunning, Eastwood's skin has a reddish cast, with no freckles or sunspots, pegging him as a Non-Pigmented Type. The wrinkles are obvious, and I'm guessing that his skin may be sensitive, whether due to genes or all that sun exposure degrading the skin barrier. In recent years, I do note some improvement, signalling that perhaps at last Clint has learned to apply sunblock when he heads out to golf, one of his current passions. Still, without some interventions, those wrinkles are here to stay.

Chris Martin, the lead singer of Coldplay, looks as though he might have the sensitive, non-pigmented skin of a DSNW. It's also possible that the husband of actress Gwyneth Paltrow could have oily skin and be an OSNW. Actress Maggie Smith could also have this Skin Type, as her skin appears delicate, wrinkled, but unblemished in her photographs. However they must all take the Baumann Skin Type Questionnaire for the most accurate assessment of their Skin Type.

SKIN SENSITIVITY AND THE DSNW

Sensitivity contributes to such skin issues as product and ingredient allergies, rosacea, acne, as well as burning and stinging in response to various substances. Learning to manage your skin's reactivity is a challenge, but understanding why it's occurring can help.

Your key problems result from a damaged skin barrier. The barrier, the outer layer of your skin, is your body's boundary between you and the world. When that boundary is overly permeable, you cannot keep *inside the barrier* important things that you need (such as moisture), and you cannot keep *outside the barrier* problematic things (such as irritants, allergens and bacteria). Once the skin barrier is damaged, a cycle begins. Lack of protection leads to invasion of substances that cause inflammation; inflammation leads to itching and further breakdown of the protective barrier. As a result, the skin cannot hold on to water, and dehydration results. Dehydration then triggers further inflammation, itching and dryness.

A whole host of insults can initiate or worsen the barrier breakdown. Preservatives, perfumes, detergents, and other chemicals in skin care products can cause inflammation and damage cells. Ingredients in shampoos, conditioners, hair dyes, shaving products, toners and soaps can be a problem. Dry-cleaning fluids, chemicals in building materials, carpets, furniture finishes, and industrial and auto pollutants can potentially cause problems in individuals who are allergic.

An allergy patch test performed by a dermatologist or allergist can identify your specific triggers, but the first step is addressing the symptoms by avoiding sensitising ingredients and using helpful ones. Once the reactive cycle begins, all substances you use must soothe and desensitise. Otherwise, they may further damage your skin barrier and increase your overall skin sensitivity. Later, in the product recommendation section of this chapter, I'll enumerate what to look out for and avoid. If avoiding the most common sensitisers does not produce results, it's advisable to keep a food and product diary, which will help narrow the field if you eventually decide to test for allergies.

Alex's Story

A lex, the eight-year-old-son of friends of mine, was a good kid with a bad case of eczema. Although it's easier for adult eczema sufferers to control the urge to scratch, little kids will often scratch even in their sleep, and it's nearly impossible to get them to stop. As a result, Alex got a bacterial infection and was at risk for a form of skin discolouration that may result. His parents (who were in the cosmetics business) followed my advice and gave him the topical medication Elidel, which nearly always works, but it didn't help Alex.

I was baffled. One day my family and I were visiting their home, and I decided to investigate. I excused myself and went upstairs, where I looked through the family's medicine cabinet (after obtaining permission, of course). There was an assortment of products that Alex's mum readily obtained from the company where she worked. These were fine products, quite a few that I recommend, and that many people find helpful – but they were totally wrong for anyone with dry, sensitive skin, like Alex.

When I questioned his parents, I learned that they used a foaming cleanser, a bubble bath, and a shampoo on Alex – what a disaster. Products that bubble and foam contain drying detergents, which Dry, Sensitive Types must take care to avoid, especially if they are prone to eczema. These products stripped valuable fats from his skin, drying it and exposing its deeper layers to allergens and irritating agents. To make matters worse, this was a family that valued 'squeaky clean', so poor Alex was shampooed and given a bubble bath daily. Since his skin was dry, after his bath, they coated him with a moisturiser, which though labelled as fragrance free did in fact contain a perfume mix, a leading allergic trigger for many people.

I urged his parents to avoid all perfumed products, detergents, and chemicals, and to limit his baths to ten minutes, shampooing Alex's hair at the end of the bath so he would not sit in shampoo-filled water. Afterwards, they applied a rich moisturiser while his skin was still damp. A few weeks after his parents made these changes, Alex's skin problem resolved.

A CLOSE-UP LOOK AT YOUR SKIN

With DSNW skin, you may experience any of the following:

- Dryness
- Scaling and flaking
- Redness
- Burning or stinging
- Wrinkles
- Makeup cakes in wrinkles
- Eye shadows look flaky
- Dry lips with flaking skin
- Rough skin on face

- Lack of skin radiance
- Irritated skin when coming into contact with wool and other rough fabrics
- Mild acne
- Broken blood vessels on face

Most DSNWs are Caucasians from a northern European background. The majority have light skin, which shows every blood vessel, making facial flushing and redness much more obvious. Though annoying, redness is a secondary problems, while dryness, crepiness and wrinkles are primary skin issues.

DSNW: A COMPLEX SKIN TYPE

Because DSNW is one of the two most complex Skin Types (the other is DSPW), DSNWs may manifest a variety of different skin problems. Some DSNWs may have few issues – or none. Some may be troubled by one major problem. And some may have the entire range of possible skin problems. It all depends on how you score in each of the four factors measured on the questionnaire. For example, skin sensitivity can result in acne, rosacea and eczema. If you score high on the sensitivity scale, with a score over 34, you are more likely to have one, two – or all of these three conditions. On the other hand, if your skin is only slightly sensitive, with a score of 24 or less, you may have none of these conditions.

Your O/D score interacts with your S/R score to produce the problems your skin expresses. You may have very dry skin (with a score between 11 and 15), slightly dry skin (with a score between 15 and 18), or combination skin (with a score between 18 and 26). If your skin is combination, your skin sensitivity is more likely to express as acne than as eczema. If your skin is very dry, you are far less likely to get acne, but are more prone to eczema. And once again, if your skin is very sensitive, you could potentially have eczema, acne and rosacea.

Treating the acne that some (but not all) DSNWs experience can be problematic. Many acne ingredients, such as salicylic acid, benzoyl peroxide, retinol, retinoid and glycolic acid are drying. Your over-the-counter treatment options are very limited. Fortunately, a few things I'll recommend later in this chapter can help. Because of your type's complexity, I'll offer a greater range of skin care regimens than I have for most other types. Choose the one right for you, depending upon your skin care needs.

ROSACEA

Rosacea can be a problem for sensitive, non-pigmented types. To find out if you have any of its symptoms, please consult 'The R-Word, Rosacea' in Chapter Six. If you experience any of the rosacea symptoms detailed in Chapter Six, seek help from a dermatologist sooner rather than later because receiving treatment can prevent rosacea from developing to its later stages.

In treating rosacea, several over-the-counter products marketed as 'redness relief' contain hydrocortisone or other steroids. Steroids are temporarily effective in shrinking the blood vessels to control redness and calm irritation, but they create a boomerang effect, as blood vessels rebound and enlarge further, worsening the problem. I don't recommend steroid use for that reason. Recently, a friend of my mother's used an 'anti-redness' moisturiser; in a week, she developed a beet-red face and dermatitis. After a complete review of her skin care regimen, I recognised that the problem was caused by the steroid-containing cream. The tipoff? When she stopped using it, the redness would get worse; when she resumed its use, the redness would stop. This is the 'rebound' reaction that occurs with steroid use, creating a dependency on the product. I weaned her from this vicious cycle by introducing a moisturiser with soothing ingredients, like aloe and licorice extract.

Sean, an architect in his late thirties, was the DSNW brother of a good friend of mine. When he heard I was a dermatologist, he shared with me his saga in finding the right skin care. Around the time of his thirtieth birthday, Sean had vacationed in Puerto Rico, where he partied on the beach with his friends without adequate sun protection. Everyone else tanned, so why couldn't he? Like many non-pigmented types, Sean didn't know that his was a Skin Type that can't, won't, and shouldn't tan.

On his vacation, Sean burned in the harsh Caribbean sun, and though he never achieved the golden tan he'd hoped for, he did succeed in damaging his skin barrier, which is most vulnerable in dry, sensitive types.

To make matters worse, after his vacation, Sean returned home to Montreal, where a cold, dry winter further battered his skin. Once the final remnants of his sunburn had flaked off, Sean was left with reddened, itchy skin in the area below his eyes at the top of his cheeks. This area of skin damage was now sensitised to ingredients, and products that Sean previously used without a problem now stung and burned his skin. At first, Sean tried to resolve his skin care issue himself, but once the problem had persisted for several months, he consulted a dermatologist, who diagnosed him with a mild form of eczema and prescribed a cortisone cream and moisturiser. Although his skin cleared up temporarily, once he ceased using the cortisone, the reddened irritation on his cheeks returned and worsened.

This pattern persisted for several years, as Sean consulted different dermatologists whenever he had a flare-up. Some would recommend their own product formulations, which often contained small amounts of cortisone. Sean came to realise that the cortisone was not resolving the problem, nor did he wish to use steroids long-term. (He also learned that using steroids long-term on the face could actually thin the skin and cause wrinkling.) On his own, he gradually decreased his use of them, while searching for skin care products that would calm rather than irritate his skin. In his profession, Sean had learned to be meticulous and thorough. Now he proceeded like a scientist, trying product samples to narrow down to a skin care line that worked for him. Eventually, he found a moisturiser that soothed his skin, and gradually incorporated more offerings from the same company, including a facial wash and shaving cream. Once he confirmed that these products worked for him, he stuck with them – no more experimentation.

This was fortunate, since he was therefore limiting his exposure to a wider range of other ingredients that might possibly have triggered further sensitivity.

In looking through the ingredients in his product choices, I was able to validate what Sean had discovered through personal experience. However, since not everyone possesses the same kind of persistence, my product selections for DSNWs will supply a shortcut to the same result.

Like Sean, you need to rebuild the skin barrier and use anti-inflammatory ingredients to help lessen skin reactivity. To find out if you too could be suffering from eczema, please consult 'Do I Have Eczema?' in Chapter Thirteen for more information about this condition.

DRY SKIN, DRY ENVIRONMENTS

Dry, sensitive skin can be reactive to ingredients, environmental conditions, fabrics, and stress. Summer can be a challenge because sun exposure worsens redness, dryness, and aging. Your skin doesn't love autumn or winter either: blustery winds; parched climates; cold weather; overheated homes, offices and cars all worsen dry skin. I come from Lubbock, Texas, and its ultradry climate was the bane of my dry, sensitive skin. Who knows? That may be why I learned all about skin care ingredients: to treat *my* skin.

After an aeroplane flight, during the winter, or in low-humidity environments, your skin will often appear even more dry and wrinkled. When fun-loving friends want to head out onto the slopes for a ski trip, you'd rather stay home or in the nearby ski lodge. Scaling icy peaks is not for you. You'd have to carry your body weight in moisturisers – and even that wouldn't help. Your lips chap, your heels crack. Your face turns red and peels after exposure to icy winds. You try heavy-duty moisturisers, and either they aren't powerful enough or they cause a reaction.

In my Florida practise, we call our many patients from colder climates 'snow birds' because they fly down to Miami to escape the cold. Often these patients show up with red, flaking cheeks. One year I read in the newspapers that it had been a particularly harsh winter up north, with many days of severe cold, wind and snow, especially hard on people with dry skin.

Hal, an eighty-six-year-old retired magnate, came into my office complaining of stinging, due (he thought) to an allergy to moisturiser or sunscreen. He was the fifth person with the same complaint, and I realised that all of these patients had three things in common: First, they had dry, sensitive skin. Second, they'd flown in the last three days. Third, they'd been in a harsh, cold weather climate prior to that flight. DS types react more strongly to cold weather, low humidity, and wind, which can strip moisture out of their already parched skin because they lack the protective skin barrier. Flying worsens the problem due to low humidity in the aeroplane cabin. These three factors had resulted in the redness, flaking and discomfort reported.

Once sensitive skin has sustained these insults, it's important to avoid exacerbating the problem. I warned Hal off of foaming soaps, shampoos, and conditioners, as products that foam contain drying detergents. I recommended a cold cream for cleansing.

After cleansing, I recommended a moisturiser for sensitive skin containing ingredients to help the skin retain moisture. Plus, I advised him that if at any future time he were exposed to harsh weather conditions, he should take action to protect his face from the cold.

'I can take the cold!' this retired executive told me.

I had to use all of my powers of persuasion to get this feisty gentleman to use a hat and scarf and apply a heavy night cream, or Vaseline petroleum jelly, when he next flew north to see his new great-grandson. But at his follow-up visit, he reported no further skin dryness or flaking.

As a dry, sensitive type myself, I always moisturise before, during and after air travel, making sure to apply ample sunscreen as well. I may not look that elegant, but I am protecting my skin. In addition, I try to persuade my seatmate to allow me to pull down the shade on the aeroplane window. Although most people don't realise it, harmful sun rays penetrate the glass at high altitudes. Always wear sun protection on a plane.

DSNWS AND AGING PREVENTION

I counsel strict sun avoidance for everyone, even those who tan well, because harmful sun rays accelerate aging and worsen skin conditions like pigmentation and rosacea. However, if I had to single out a type for whom sun exposure produces the most aging effects, it would probably be you. Your non-pigmented skin may have less melanin to handle sun exposure and that's why you burn in the sun. Plus, sun exposure increases rosacea and makes dry skin even drier. Worst of all, your sensitive skin reacts to many sunscreens, causing you to bypass sunscreen – and the end result is premature aging and wrinkling. It's entirely likely that a few bad episodes of burning, along with other genetic and lifestyle factors, have resulted in your scoring as a Wrinkled Type on the questionnaire. So you know what to do: use sunscreen at all times, indoors and out, and use higher SPFs (45 or above) when you receive direct sun exposure. The products I'll recommend should not cause irritation.

Some DSNWs suffer from acne and/or eczema, and sun exposure is often recommended for these conditions. Although acne was long thought to be 'dried out' by the sun, many studies show that acne actually worsens in hot weather. So don't sun to treat your acne.

In some people, eczema arises from an underlying autoimmune condition in which the protective immune system overreacts and attacks itself. Sun exposure temporarily suppresses the immune response, which can lead to a lessening of symptoms for some, but not all, eczema sufferers. Still, since sun exposure contributes to skin aging, why mess around?

Many DSNWs go to tanning beds, which deploy harmful UVA rays that penetrate deeper into the skin layers, causing aging. When I see someone like Paris Hilton, who could possibly be a DSNW, I worry about her perpetual tan. I hope for her sake it comes from a bottle, because if it does not, she'll be paying for it later. DSNWs don't tan well, so my advice is: give it up. Use strong sun protection, and use it consistently; it's your key step to prevent aging. If you want to tan, use a self-tanner. For more on self-tanners and how to apply them, please refer to 'Self-Tanners' in Chapter Ten.

If you needed yet another reason to quit smoking, researchers found that cigarette smoke stimulated an *increased breakdown* of collagen, while lowering collagen production by as much as 40 percent. The more concentrated the smoke, the worse the impact on the skin's collagen. Quit now and your skin will thank you.

HOW YOUR SKIN TYPE AGES

DSNW skin does not age well, overall. People who experience acne in youth find relief in mid-life. But facial flushing, redness, visible veins, sensitivity to skin care products, dryness and wrinkling are all conditions that worsen with age. People who've failed to follow preventative skin care before their forties feel it now.

Luckily new advances in skin care such as dermal fillers and Botox can address your wrinkles. Advanced skin care products will help treat your skin dryness. Whatever your skin's current condition, it's never too late to take care of your skin.

For postmenopausal women, as oestrogen levels go down, you may notice that your skin becomes thinner, drier and more wrinkled if you do not take hormone replacement therapy. If you wish to consider HRT, first discuss its use with your physician, especially if you or someone in your family has a history of breast cancer or endometrial cancer. Luckily there are some naturally occurring phytooestrogens that can help. Adding phytooestrogen supplements or foods to your diet can be beneficial.

MOISTURISING

Moisturise at least twice daily, and don't hesitate to apply creams more often, especially in winter or in low-humidity environments. Because of your skin's tendency to wrinkle, you may be tempted by certain face creams claiming to produce the same results as Botox. These claims are based on the action of skin peptides that in the lab relax muscle cells (or are believed to relax skin cells). Although some research indicates that muscle cells can 'relax' in lab settings, it's hard to re-create that same effect outside of the lab. A substance would need to penetrate the epidermis, the dermis, and the fat layer to get to the muscle layer. I've not seen convincing evidence that that can happen. If it could, diabetics could apply their insulin topically rather than injecting it because insulin is a protein, which is composed of peptides. Nor am I convinced that skin cells can 'relax', or that it would be beneficial.

Why pay a steep price for a jar of cream? Many who do may be DSNWs or DRNWs, with dry, wrinkled skin that any moisturiser can improve – temporarily. However, I've yet to see a cream that will deliver the same benefits as Botox. So if you think you need Botox, get Botox. Here in the US, it costs about £300 to £600 per treatment and although its effects are also temporary, it lasts four to six months.

Dr Baumann's Bottom Line: Rebuild your skin barrier and moisturise, avoid harsh ingredients, and protect against drying environments.

EVERYDAY CARE FOR YOUR SKIN

The goal of your skin care routine is to address skin dryness, wrinkles and sensitivity (resulting in stinging and redness) with products that deliver hydrating, moisturising ingredients that do not irritate your skin. All the products I'll recommend act to do one or more of the following:

- Prevent and treat dryness
- Prevent and treat wrinkles
- Prevent and treat stinging and redness

In addition, your daily regimen will also help to address your other skin concerns by:

- Preventing and treating acne

To address your type's different issues, I've provided two nonprescription regimens and two prescription regimens. My first nonprescription protocol is a hydrating maintenance regimen that may also help acne. Studies show that in many cases, moisturising the skin will improve acne, even without acne medications, so this regimen concentrates on moisturising.

The second nonprescription regimen is designed for those of you who frequently experience redness and stinging in response to skin care products. It uses products with anti-inflammatory and antioxidant ingredients to help rebuild the skin barrier and prevent wrinkles. Select the regimen right for your needs at this time, and you'll find product recommendations for each category of product later in this chapter.

If hydrating your skin does not resolve acne, I've provided a prescription regimen that includes prescription antibiotics to treat acne. Finally, I've created a second prescription regimen that uses an anti-inflammatory medication to treat redness and stinging resulting from reactions to ingredients in skin care products and from exposure to cold, dry weather.

DAILY SKIN CARE

STAGE ONE: NONPRESCRIPTION REGIMEN

Hydrating regimen for maintenance (and for acne):

AM	PM
Step 1: Wash with a cold cream or oil cleanser	Step 1: Wash with a cold cream or oil cleanser
Step 2: Apply a moisturiser with SPF and/or sunscreen	Step 2: Apply antioxidant-containing night cream
Step 3: Apply a foundation with sunscreen (optional)	Step 3: Once or twice a week use a sulphur-containing mask

In the morning, wash your face with a cold cream or oil cleanser. Apply a moisturiser containing SPF; then, if you wish, apply a foundation with sunscreen. If your skin feels a little oily after using these products, that's all right. You need the protection. Although I don't consider it essential, you can elect to use an eye cream as well, applying it before your moisturiser. In general, I try to avoid exposing your skin to products that are not of real benefit, but if your skin isn't irritated, you can opt to use one.

In the evening, wash with a cold cream or oil cleanser, then apply a night cream that contains antioxidants. Once or twice a week, finish with a mask containing sulphur.

If hydrating your skin with this regimen does not improve your acne, you need to see a dermatologist. Unfortunately, the over-the-counter ingredients available to treat acne will dry your skin out. DSNWs do well with a prescription topical antibiotic or light treatments (see 'Procedures', later in chapter) to treat acne.

STAGE ONE: NONPRESCRIPTION REGIMEN

For facial redness or frequent stinging:

AM	PM
Step 1: Wash with a cold cream or oil cleanser	Step 1: Wash with a cold cream or oil cleanser

Step 2: Rinse with facial water

Step 3: Apply anti-inflammatory serum or lotion

Step 4: Apply a moisturiser with SPF and/or sunscreen

Step 5: Apply a foundation with sunscreen (optional)

Step 2: Rinse with facial water

Step 3: Apply an antioxidant and/or anti-inflammatory night cream

Step 4: Once or twice a week, use a hydrating mask with antioxidant and/or anti-inflammatory ingredients

In the morning, wash your face with a cold cream or oil cleanser, then rinse with facial water, not tap water. Next, apply a moisturiser containing SPF, and finish with a foundation-containing sunscreen. I do not recommend eye cream when your skin is reddened and reactive.

In the evening, wash with a cold cream or oil cleanser, and rinse your face using facial water. Apply a night cream that contains antioxidant and/or anti-inflammatory ingredients (see the lists below for product and ingredient recommendations).

Once or twice a week, use a hydrating mask that also contains antioxidant and/or anti-inflammatory ingredients.

Cleansers

As a DSNW, you need gentle, hydrating cleansers. To use, apply a small amount to your face with a soft, clean washcloth, using gentle circular motions over your entire face. To rinse, spray facial water over your face and tissue off whatever cleanser remains. If your skin is only slightly sensitive, you can rinse with regular tap water.

RECOMMENDED CLEANSING PRODUCTS

- £ Cetaphil Gentle Facial Cleanser
- £ Eucerin Gentle Cleansing Milk
- £ Lutsine Gentle Cleansing Cream
- £ Nivea Gentle Cleansing Cream Wash
- £ Noxzema Cleansing Cream, Sensitive
- ££ La Roche-Posay Toleriane Derma-Cleanser
- ££ L'Occitane Shea Butter Extra Moisturising Cold Cream Soap
- ££ Oilatum-AD Cleansing Lotion

££ Organic Pharmacy Rose & Chamomile Cleansing Milk

££ Shu Uemura Skin Purifier Cleansing Oil

££ SK II Facial Treatment Cleansing Oil

£££ Darphin Intral Cleansing Milk

£££ Decléor Cleansing Oil

£££ Ella Baché Crème Douce Démaquillant

Baumann's Choice: For frequent redness and stinging, I prefer Toleriane Dermo-Cleanser by La Roche-Posay.

Facial Waters

DSNWs should never use toners, which are drying. Instead, use these special facial waters either to remove cleansers or to spray on the face after cleansing, before applying moisturiser. Water, especially hot hard water, has been shown to irritate the skin. For skin that is not raw and sensitive, you can use tap water but make sure it's lukewarm.

RECOMMENDED FACIAL WATERS

£ Evian Mineral Water Spray

££ Avène Thermal Water Spray

££ Chantecaille Pure Rosewater

££ Fresh Rose Marigold Tonic Water

££ Korres Hamamelis Hydrating Face Water

££ La Roche-Posay Thermal Spring Water

££ Molton Brown Skin Boost 24 Hour Moisture Mist

££ Organic Pharmacy Rose Facial Spritz

££ Shu Uemura Depsea Therapy

££ Vichy Thermal Spa Water

£££ Jurlique Chamomile Floral Water

Baumann's Choice: La Roche-Posay Thermal Spring Water

Serums

Anti-inflammatory serums and lotions contain powerful ingredients to help calm sensitivity. Use them before you apply a daytime moisturiser with SPF.

RECOMMENDED ANTI-INFLAMMATORY
SERUMS AND LOTIONS

£ Mary Kay Calming Influence
£ Olay Regenerist Daily Regenerating Serum
£ Paula's Choice Skin Relief Treatment
£ Paula's Choice Super Antioxidant Concentrate
££ La Roche-Posay Rosaliac Perfecting Anti-Redness Moisturiser
££ L'Occitane Immortelle Precious Fluid
££ Prescriptives Redness Relief Gel
£££ Babor Calming Sensitive Couperose Serum
£££ Joey New York Calm and Correct Serum
£££ Neocutis Bio-restorative Skin Cream
£££ Pevonia Rose RS2 Concentrate

Baumann's Choice   La Roche-Posay Rosaliac Perfecting Anti-Redness
Moisturiser

Moisturisers

Dry, sensitive skin needs to be moisturised at least twice a day. When your
skin is especially dry, moisturise more often. For daytime use, I've included
products with antioxidant and anti-inflammatory ingredients. Use a product with SPF.

RECOMMENDED DAYTIME MOISTURISERS

£ Neutrogena Visibly Young Day Cream
£ Nivea Anti-Wrinkle Q10 Plus Day Cream
£ Olay Regenerist Replenishing Cream
££ Bloom Hydrating Day Cream with SPF 8
££ Clinique Weather Everything Environmental Cream SPF 15
££ Emollience by SkinCeuticals (no SPF, so use with a sunscreen)
££ Estée Lauder DayWear Plus Multi Protection Anti-Oxidant Crème
   SPF 15 for Dry Skin
££ Laura Mercier Moisturising Cream with SPF 15
££ L'Occitane Shea Butter Ultra Moisturising Care SPF 15
££ Vichy Nutrilogie 1 SPF 15 Sunscreen Lotion
£££ Bobbi Brown EXTRA SPF 25 Moisturising Balm

Baumann's Choice: L'Occitane Shea Butter Ultra Moisturising Care SPF 15, which I found while researching this book. It's soothing to dry, sensitive skin, and I now use it myself.

RECOMMENDED EVENING MOISTURISERS

- £ Boots No7 Advanced Hydration Night Cream
- £ Eucerin LipoBalance cream with Ceramide
- £ Neutrogena Visibly Young Night Cream
- £ Nivea Anti-Wrinkle Q10 Plus Night Cream
- £ Olay Regenerist Replenishing Cream
- ££ Alchimie Forever Kantic + Ultra Nourishing Cream
- ££ Atopalm MLE Cream
- ££ Cutanix Dramatic Relief for Sensitive Facial Skin
- ££ Clinique Moisture On-Line
- ££ La Roche-Posay Toleriane Soothing Protective Facial Cream
- ££ Laura Mercier Night Nutrition Renewal Crème
- £££ Dior Energy-Move Skin Illuminating Moisture Crème
- £££ Freeze 24/7 IceCream Anti-Aging Moisturiser
- £££ Jurlique Wrinkle Softener Beauty Cream
- £££ Guerlain Issima Successlaser Night Care
- £££ Susan Ciminelli Super Hydrating Cream

Baumann's Choice: Cutanix Dramatic Relief for Sensitive Facial Skin is available online at www.Baumannstore.co.uk.

Masks

Masks can be very helpful for DSNWs; a sulphur mask will help reduce inflammation and acne, while hydrating masks help repair the skin barrier.

My favourite mask for improving acne is actually a prescription product: Plexion SCT mask by Medicis, which contains sulphacetamide to help reduce inflammation. These sulphur-containing masks are not found in the UK so look for them on the internet.

RECOMMENDED MASKS FOR ACNE SUFFERERS

- ££ DDF Sulphur Therapeutic Mask
- ££ Peter Thomas Roth Therapeutic Sulphur Masque Acne Treatment

Baumann's Choice: DDF Sulphur Therapeutic Mask

RECOMMENDED MASKS TO HYDRATE SKIN

£ Botanics Quenching Mask
££ Aveda Intense Hydrating Mask
££ Boscia Moisture Replenishing Mask
££ Caudalie Revitalizing Moisture Grape-seed Cream Mask
££ Elizabeth Arden Hydrating Mask
££ Laura Mercier Intensive Moisture Mask
££ L'Occitane Immortelle Cream Mask
££ MD Formulations Moisture Defence Treatment Masque
£££ Dr Hauschka Firming Mask

Baumann's Choice: MD Formulations Moisture Defence Treatment Masque has barrier repair ingredients and antioxidants.

SHOPPING FOR PRODUCTS

Look for products containing ingredients that will effectively hydrate and protect your skin. Avoid products that will irritate your sensitive skin. I can't list all detergents to avoid because much depends on their concentrations and formulations, so the easiest guideline is to avoid any products – be they cleansers, shampoos or bubble baths – that foam. If you feel you must use a foaming cleanser, make sure it has minimal rather than thick foam. You should also avoid fragrances, which can lead to skin allergy.

Below, I've listed other ingredients to avoid. If you have a favourite skin care product that is not on my recommended list, please go to www.DrBaumann.-co.uk and tell me what it is. I am always looking for the next new thing!

RECOMMENDED SKIN CARE INGREDIENTS

For wrinkle prevention:

- Basil
- Caffeine
- Camilla sinensis (green tea, white tea)
- Grape seed extract
- Idebenone
- Lutein
- Lycopene

- Carrot extract
- Coenzyme Q_{10} (ubiquinone)
- Copper peptide
- Curcumin (tetrahydracurcumin or turmeric)
- Ferulic acid
- Feverfew
- Genistein (soy)
- Ginger
- Punica granatum (pomegranate)
- Pycnogenol (a pine bark extract)
- Rosemary
- Silymarin
- Ginseng
- Yucca

To improve wrinkles:

- Copper peptide
- Ginkgo biloba

Anti-inflammatory:

- Aloe vera
- Chamomile
- Colloidal oatmeal
- Cucumber
- Dexpanthenol (provitamin B_5)
- Epilobium angustifolium (willow herb)
- Evening primrose oil
- Feverfew
- Green tea
- Licochalone
- Perilla leaf extract
- Pycnogenol (a pine bark extract)
- Red algae
- Thyme
- Trifolium pretense (red clover)
- Zinc

For moisturising:

- Ajuga turkestanica
- Aloe vera
- Apricot kernel oil
- Borage seed oil
- Canola oil
- Ceramide
- Cholesterol
- Cocoa butter (not if you have acne)
- Colloidal oatmeal
- Dexpanthenol (provitamin B_5)
- Dimethicone
- Evening primrose oil
- Glycerin
- Jojoba oil
- Macadamia nut oil
- Olive oil
- Safflower oil
- Shea butter

SKIN CARE INGREDIENTS TO AVOID

If you have acne:

- Butyl stearate
- Cinnamon oil
- Cocoa butter
- Coconut oil
- Decyl oleate
- Isocetyl stearate
- Isopropyl isostearate
- Isopropyl myristate
- Isopropyl palmitate
- Isostearyl neopentanoate
- Lanolin
- Myristyl myristate
- Myristyl propionate
- Octyl palmitate
- Octyl stearate
- Peppermint oil
- Propylene glycol-2 (PPG-2)

If you have skin redness:

- Alpha hydroxy acids (lactic acid, glycolic acid)
- Alpha lipoic acid
- Benzoyl peroxide
- Gluconolactone
- Phytic acid
- Polyhydroxy acids
- Retinaldehyde
- Retinol
- Retinyl palmitate
- Salicylic acid (beta hydroxy acid)
- Vitamin C (L-ascorbic acid)

Due to allergy or irritation:

- Bismuth oxychloride (found in eye shadow)
- Castor oil and eosin (both found in long-lasting lipsticks)
- Chromium hydroxide and chromium oxide compounds (give makeup the green colour but can cause allergy)
- Cobalt
- Lead
- Nickel
- Propyl gallate
- Ricinoleic acid

Sun Protection for Your Skin

Use cream sunscreens to give your skin extra moisture. If you react to chemical sunscreen ingredients like avobenzone and benzophenone with redness and sensitivity, look for sunscreens containing dimethicone and cyclomethicone, which may prevent irritation from other sunscreen ingredients in those with easily irritated skin.

RECOMMENDED SUN PROTECTION PRODUCTS

£ Eucerin Q 10 Active Antiwrinkle Fluid SPF 15
£ Olay Regenerist Rehydrating Lotion SPF 15
£ Segreti Mediterranei SPF 10 Moisturising Facial Lotion
££ Dermalogica Ultra Sensitive Face Block SPF 25
££ L'Occitane Shea Ultra Moisturising Care SPF 15
££ Mario Badescu Aloe Vera Moisturiser SPF 15
££ Origins Sunshine State SPF 20
££ Philosophy When Hope Is Not Enough SPF 20
££ SkinCeuticals Physical UV Defence SPF 30
£££ Darphin Sun Block SPF 30
£££ Decléor Écran Très Haute Protection SPF 40
£££ Sisley Broad Spectrum Sunscreen, SPF 40

Baumann's Choice: Eucerin Q 10 Active Antiwrinkle Fluid SPF 15 because it contains Coenzyme Q10, a strong antioxidant to help prevent wrinkles.

SUNSCREEN INGREDIENTS TO SUSPECT IF REDNESS OR STINGING OCCURS

• Avobenzone (Parsol)
• Benzophenone
• Methoxycinnamate
• Para-aminobenzoic acid (PABA)

Your Makeup

Your dry, sensitive skin is likely to react with redness to allergens in makeup. While foundations are usually not a problem, blushers and eyeshadow can be.

Many brands of eyeshadow contain lead, cobalt, nickel and chromium, ingredients that can cause allergy in susceptible people. Shimmery shadows, blushers, and bronzers may contain sharp-edged particles like shells that can scratch and irritate dry, sensitive skin, as well as make the wrinkles look more prominent.

Cream eyeshadows and blushers are best, but if your cheeks are naturally pink, you can skip the blusher. (I do.) Powders, usually designed for oil control, are unnecessary and may make skin appear drier and more wrinkled. If you want coverage without using a heavy foundation, use tinted moisturisers with sunscreen. For very dry skin, apply it *over* your moisturiser. If your skin is only slightly dry, use the moisturiser on its own.

La Roche-Posay makes a colour cosmetic line free of most allergens for super sensitive dry types, such as those with eczema. Their lipsticks contain hydrating glycerine. You can find these products in pharmacies in France. (Great excuse for a trip.) Don't feel left out. We don't have them in the US either.

Foundations containing salicylic acid (BHA) to help improve acne are too drying for you. Stick to oil-containing foundations. Oil, contrary to popular belief, will not increase acne breakouts.

RECOMMENDED FOUNDATIONS

- £ Boots No7 Radiant Glow Foundation SPF 15
- £ Botanics Fresh Face Tinted Moisturiser
- ££ Bloom Foundation
- ££ Kevyn Aucoin The Dew Drop Foundation
- ££ Laura Mercier Moisturising Foundation
- ££ L'Occitane Tinted Day Care SPF 15
- ££ Tony and Tina Environmental Rescue Liquid Foundation
- ££ Trish McEvoy Protective Shield Tinted Moisturiser
- £££ La Prairie Skin Caviar Concealer Foundation SPF 15
- £££ Versace Fluid Moisture Foundation

Baumann's Choice: L'Occitane Tinted Day Care SPF 15 because you can never have too much sun protection. However, if you promise to wear a sunscreen underneath, I suggest Versace Fluid Moisture Foundation. It's very elegant.

RECOMMENDED CREAM EYE SHADOWS

- £ Almay Bright Eyes
- £ Revlon Illuminance Crème Shadow
- ££ Bliss Lidthicks
- ££ Bloom Eye Colour Cream
- ££ Bobbi Brown Cream Shadow Stick
- ££ Clinique Touch Tint for Eyes Cream Formula

££ Ruby and Millie Eye Colour Cream

££ Urban Decay Cream Eyeshadow

Baumann's Choice: Bliss Lidthicks with antioxidants

RECOMMENDED BLUSHERS

£ Avon Split Second Blush Stick

££ Aveda Uruku Cheek/Lip Cream

££ Bloom's Sheer Colour Cream

££ Bobbi Brown Cream Blush Stick

££ Estée Lauder BlushLights Creamy Cheek Colour

££ Jane Iredale Blush (powder blush with soothing minerals)

££ L'Occitane Colour Cream for Lips and Cheeks

£££ DuWop Velvety Cream Blush

Baumann's Choice: Aveda Uruku Cheek/Lip Cream because it has jojoba oil in it.

CONSULTING A DERMATOLOGIST

PRESCRIPTION SKIN CARE STRATEGIES

My prescription regimens are built around antibiotic medication to treat acne, and anti-inflammatory medication to treat facial redness and stinging. Although in general, DSNWs cannot tolerate retinoids, if acne is the primary manifestation of your skin sensitivity, and you have a low S/R score, you may be able to use a gentle retinoid such as Differin (see the instructions below).

If you suffer from eczema or atopic dermatitis, prescription drugs such as Elidel and Protopic can treat your skin when it's red and itching. Remember, properly moisturising your skin will help prevent eczema from worsening by rebuilding the skin barrier.

DAILY SKIN CARE

STAGE TWO: PRESCRIPTION REGIMEN

For acne:

AM	PM
Step 1: Wash with a sulphacetamide-containing cleanser	Step 1: Wash with a sulphacetamide cleanser
Step 2: Apply a prescription acne antibiotic medication	Step 2: Apply a prescription acne medication
Step 3: Apply a moisturiser with SPF and/or sunscreen	Step 3: Apply a night cream with antioxidants
Step 4: Apply a foundation with sunscreen (optional)	Step 4: Use a retinoid (optional for those with combination skin only; see instructions below)
	Step 5: Once or twice a week use a sulphur-containing mask

In the morning, wash your face with a cleanser containing sulphacetamide. Apply a prescription acne antibiotic, then a moisturiser with SPF. If you wish, finish with a foundation containing SPF.

In the evening, wash with a sulphacetamide cleanser, then apply prescription acne medication. Next, apply a night cream with antioxidants. If you do not have facial redness and flushing, and you have an O/D score of 17–26 or an S/R score of 25–33 (slightly dry or slightly sensitive), you may be able to use a gentle retinoid such as Differin. Start slowly, use it sparingly, and apply it on top of your night cream to prevent reactions.

Once or twice a week, use a mask containing sulphur.

How to Use a Retinoid

Most DSNWs cannot use retinoids, but if your main problem is acne rather than redness and stinging, you may tolerate it. On the days that you use a sulphur mask, apply the mask before using the retinoid. After washing the mask off, wait fifteen minutes before you apply the retinoid. Please go to 'Further Help for Dry, Sensitive Skin' for additional instructions on retinoid use.

STAGE TWO: PRESCRIPTION REGIMEN

For redness and stinging:

AM	PM
Step 1: Wash with a sulphacetamide-containing cleanser	Step 1: Wash with a sulphacetamide cleanser
Step 2: Apply a prescription anti-inflammatory medication	Step 2: Apply a prescription anti-inflammatory medication
Step 3: Apply a moisturiser with SPF and/or sunscreen	Step 3: Apply a night cream with antioxidants
Step 4: Apply a foundation with sunscreen (optional)	

In the morning, wash your face with a sulphacetamide cleanser, which helps reduce inflammation. To further calm your skin, you will next apply prescription anti-inflammatory medication, and then a moisturiser with SPF.

In the evening, wash with sulphacetamide cleanser. Apply anti-inflammatory medication, then a night cream containing antioxidants. This kind of night cream can help prevent wrinkles without irritating your skin.

Once your acne or redness clears up, you can return to the non-prescription, maintenance skin care regimen. Do not use retinoid or retinol-containing products, as they may be too irritating for you.

PRESCRIPTION PRODUCTS FOR YOUR SKIN

There are many excellent prescription topical antibiotics and sulphacetamide products, so ask your dermatologist which ones are right for you.

RECOMMENDED PRESCRIPTION MEDICATIONS FOR ACNE, AND TREATING AND PREVENTING WRINKLES

For use when there is no facial redness

- Aknemycin Plus (contains an antibiotic as well)
- Differin gel or cream

- Isotrex
- Isotrexin (contains an antiobiotic as well)
- Retin-A gel, lotion or cream
- Retinova

PROCEDURES FOR YOUR SKIN TYPE

Unfortunately there are no skin care procedures that can improve your dry, sensitive skin. If you suffer from frequent skin rashes in reaction to cosmetic products, your dermatologist can help you figure out what ingredients in these products are causing your rash by performing a series of patch tests. See Chapter Fifteen, 'Procedures for Your Skin Type', for information on patch testing.

Treatments for Wrinkles

Although using the right moisturiser can improve some of your fine wrinkles, for the rest of them you may want to consider using botulinum toxin or dermal fillers. Please see 'Further Help for Oily, Sensitive Skin' for details about Botox or Reloxin treatments and the methods for using Botox, Reloxin and dermal fillers for treating different kinds of wrinkles.

Light Treatments

Certain forms of light treatments, including non-ablative lasers, light emitting diodes, and Intense Pulsed Light, will probably be used in the future to prevent or treat wrinkles. Right now, though, the technology is not that effective for wrinkle treatment, though fine for other purposes. (I've seen people who've spent five to six thousand dollars on these treatments without seeing improvement in their wrinkles.)

However, light treatments *are* effective in treating some symptoms of rosacea. If you experience rosacea, please go to the light treatment section of 'Further Help for Oily, Sensitive Skin' for more information.

Light treatments are also good for acne treatment since blue light kills the bacteria known as P. acnes, thought to cause acne. Regular use of these light treatments can improve acne, studies show. A dermatologist administers the treatments, usually twice a week for four months, and after that, once a month until the problem clears. The regimen varies depending on the severity of the acne, and sometimes the dermatologist uses red rather than blue light.

What About Chemical Peels?

If redness and stinging is your problem, you don't need chemical peels, which contain ingredients that may make your skin more red and sensitive. Due to your impaired skin barrier, you can be burned by a vigorous peel. Stay away from these procedures. However, if you have acne without redness or stinging, you may benefit from chemical peels. My favourite chemical peel ingredients for acne are salicylic acid (BHA) and resorcinol.

ONGOING CARE FOR YOUR SKIN TYPE

Choose your products with care and moisturise regularly. Avoid the sun, quit smoking, and don't forget to eat your vegetables. For dietary and lifestyle recommendations, please consult 'Further Help for Dry, Sensitive Skin'.

CHAPTER FIFTEEN

Dry, Sensitive, Non-Pigmented and Tight: DSNT

THE PARCHED SKIN TYPE

'My skin is so-o-o dry, you'd think I was in a desert. My eyelids are flaking, my lips are cracked, and whatever skin cream I use burns; it makes my skin even worse.'

ABOUT YOUR SKIN

Scaling, flaking, reddened, rough and dull. If your questionnaire results show you to be a DSNT, your skin is literally thirsting for water. It's like that famous line from *The Rime of the Ancient Mariner:* 'Water, water, everywhere, nor any drop to drink.' You've tried everything. You followed the advice to keep well hydrated by consuming quarts of water per day, to no avail. You avoid caffeine because of its dehydrating effects. You know you need to moisturise, and in desperation, you try every product that comes along – but even the most costly creams can cause reactions in your sensitive skin.

Understanding your skin is the basis for making the right skin care choices. I must confess that I have this Skin Type. It isn't the easiest, and at least one of the reasons I've become so passionate about ingredients and products was to learn how to address my *own* skin challenges. So never fear, there is a Skin Type solution even for your fragile, dry skin.

DSNT CELEBRITY

Blonde actress Christina Applegate came to prominence on the Fox television show, *Married . . . with Children,* delighting audiences with her portrayal of the trampy daughter, Kelly Bundy. More recently, she's starred in the comedy *Anchorman,* showing her acting range in her portrayal of a cool and collected newswoman. Applegate's approachable appeal assures her popularity; she's the girl next door with a little oomph.

Applegate began her career as a baby in the arms of her actress mother, Nancy Priddy, another attractive, fair-haired, non-pigmented type. She went on to work as a child actor, until her star talent came to the fore. Applegate's beautiful pale and creamy skin is very obviously non-pigmented and tight. I am guessing that it may be dry and sensitive as well, since some photos of her show what might perhaps be a slight degree of redness and irritation. Makeup for film, television, and photo shoots can be irritating to people with dry, sensitive skin, and this skin tendency cannot always be so well camouflaged, since the cause and the cure are one and the same. Still, I applaud Applegate for not succumbing to the temptation of tanning. Her pale skin would be easy to ruin, but it's obvious she's taking the right steps.

OVERVIEW OF DSNT SKIN

Fair-skinned Caucasians who take good care of themselves and their skin most commonly have this type. Although its delicacy is much admired, caring for it can be a pain. You don't tan well. You'd do best to avoid the sun completely. Most DSNTs have figured out that excess sun is not a friend to supersensitive dry skin. Those who have not figured that out are paying the price, and it's likely that they would fall into the DSNW Skin Type, which is similar but wrinkled. At least you don't have to deal with preventing and addressing wrinkles. 'Aren't wrinkles inevitable?' many people wonder. No, they are not. Skin that never sees the sun does not wrinkle, so with the right behaviours wrinkles can be avoided, although the loss of fat in the face that occurs with aging cannot. Tight-skinned DSNs can congratulate themselves on good habits, like sun avoidance and smoking cessation. Many DSNTs also eat a healthy diet full of antioxidants (obtained from fruits and vegetables), which helps prevent wrinkles and maintain overall health.

Still, keeping your skin calm, hydrated and nonreactive at any age takes some work, along with careful product selection.

SKIN SENSITIVITY AND THE DSNT

Forty percent of the population has sensitive skin that reacts to products and ingredients with burning, stinging, itching and redness, and skin sensitivity is common everywhere. Since tracking down the exact culprit can be time-consuming, I recommend that you first eliminate common triggers by avoiding ingredients enumerated later in the product recommendation section of this chapter. If this does not produce results, you can always keep a food and product diary, writing down what you eat and what you use on your skin, so that you can track your reactions to potential allergens and ingredients. Ultimately, you can go to a dermatologist for patch testing, which will determine the precise allergen. But that process is less expensive if you have first narrowed the field.

Skin sensitivities and skin allergies are on the same spectrum; while you may not always be actively allergic to a particular skin care ingredient, unless that substance is soothing and desensitising, it can also damage your skin barrier and increase your overall skin sensitivity.

THE SKIN BARRIER

Key to managing your type is understanding the skin barrier. The skin's natural barrier is composed of cells (something like bricks) that are surrounded by fat (called lipids), which act as mortar. The fat molecules line up in a lipid bilayer (two rows of fat molecules) to form a three-dimensional structure. It functions like cling film, keeping water inside the layers of the skin, while keeping allergens, toxins and bacteria out.

People with resistant skin have strong skin barriers (like a solid brick wall) that maintain the skin integrity and keep skin care ingredients (and other substances) from gaining access to the deeper layers of the skin. For resistant types, I recommend stronger products, since gentler ingredients cannot readily penetrate its solid barrier. But you're on the other end of the spectrum.

With a weak skin barrier, substances pass through the barrier too readily, producing allergic or inflammatory reactions as the immune system recognises something foreign to the body and overreacts. Once the skin barrier is damaged, a cycle begins. Lack of protection leads to invasion of substances that cause inflammation; inflammation leads to itching and further breakdown of the barrier. As a result, the skin cannot hold on to water, and dehydration results. Dehydration triggers further inflammation, itching and dryness.

A whole host of insults can initiate or worsen the barrier breakdown. Skin care ingredients that are harsh or perfumed can cause inflammation and break down cells. While aromatherapy and fragrances, essential oils, and botanical ingredients are included in skin care products, DSNTs fared better when 'fragrance free' was the rage. Acetone in nail polish, chemicals used to treat fabric, dry-cleaning fluids, chemicals in building materials, carpets, furniture finishes, and industrial and auto pollutants can potentially cause problems. Even nickel in the diet or in contact with the skin can cause a skin rash if you happen to have a nickel allergy. Interestingly, the new European currency, the euro, has a high nickel content and is associated with an increase in nickel allergies.

Many DSNTs suffer from skin allergies. Many can't wear earrings that are not real gold or platinum, without getting a rash. This is often due to a nickel allergy. Watches and hooks on clothing or undergarments can cause rashes to develop. Red rashes may appear underneath a ring, but don't worry. It's not that your gold or platinum ring is phony. The more likely explanation is that when you wash your hands, soap detergent gets caught under the ring and irritates your skin.

DSNTs are sensitive to detergents and prone to dishpan hands more than any other type. Frequent hand washing may put massage therapists at higher risk of hand rashes and dryness. A recent study found that 15 to 23 percent of masseuses using aromatherapy oils got hand dermatitis.

People who come from families with allergies and asthma are more prone to the dryness leading to eczema. This may be due to an abnormality of an enzyme that helps maintain the structure of the skin.

In oily types, skin sensitivity will cause acne and flushing, while stinging, burning, and allergic reactions are less common because oil helps strengthen the skin barrier. However, those with a high score on the Sensitivity vs. Resistance scale will commonly experience allergies to many skin ingredients. Oily/dry combination types with sensitive skin will have more infrequent outbreaks, such as a few pimples every few months. In dry, sensitive types, dryness leading to eczema is the chief concern. The drier and the more sensitive your skin scored on the questionnaire, the higher your risk factor.

Maggie's Story

Maggie, a thirty-six-year-old yoga instructor of German ancestry, came to see me on her way back from a Caribbean yoga retreat. Skin dryness was her complaint. She also reported that she'd been feeling fatigued recently, and after a difficult relationship breakup, she'd had trouble sleeping.

'I eat a healthy diet and exercise regularly,' Maggie told me. 'But I feel like I'm falling apart. Even my fingernails are shredding.'

Maggie's nails were not her body's only dry spots. Her heels were cracked, her hands were pink and chapped, and her cheeks, eyelids and forehead were flaking. Fine lines were forming around her eyes. Stress can stimulate the body's inflammatory response, contributing to the cycle of inflammation and dryness. All of these symptoms made her look older than her age.

Maggie knew she had to moisturise but when she tried antiaging creams that contained fruit acids, her skin burned, stung and turned red, leaving blotches in their wake. The blotches dried out and flaked off several days later. Afterwards, her skin felt drier than before. The antiaging creams she used to correct the problem contained the wrong ingredients (irritating perfumes and fruit acids) and lacked the right ones (humectants and barrier-repairing oils, like evening primrose, borage seed, and omega-3 fatty acids). Her natural organic soap had detergents that stripped her skin's protective fats.

Maggie's vegan diet wasn't helping either, as she sorely needed essential fatty acids (EFAs) to help repair the skin barrier with plump lipids (fats) so that it could hold water and keep irritants out. The best sources of these EFAs are fatty fish, like salmon and mackerel, and cod liver oil supplements, all no-no's on Maggie's diet. Walnuts and flaxseeds are vegan sources of these fats but many people cannot convert them into the most useful chemical forms the body needs. Maggie had been eating these vegan omega-3 foods, I learned, but her persistent symptoms indicated that she was not able to adequately convert them from these sources. She did not feel comfortable consuming fish, which I recommended. So I suggested that she consider adding a high-quality cod liver oil supplement as a compromise. Vegan diets and low dietary cholesterol have been correlated to a susceptibility to dry skin and to eczema, some studies show. The supplements would supply the most critical missing ingredients.

Maggie was not that pleased with my suggestion, and I could see her dilemma. Although she was certainly entitled to her dietary philosophy, it seemed very likely that the food that she ate was not providing what her skin needed to flourish. Following the proper skin care regimen would help improve her skin's condition. But her body needed the right nutritional building blocks to create a healthy skin barrier.

I prescribed other skin care supplements, such as glucosamine, which helps the skin make more hyaluronic acid, a component of the skin that provides volume by helping it hold water. I also placed her on Biotin (a water soluble B vitamin) to help her nails.

Back home, Maggie let me know that she was following her new skin care regimen and had been taking the recommended supplements. She said that her energy and mood had lifted, and that her skin looked much better too. I never found out whether Maggie had decided to follow my suggestion and take the fish-based supplements, but I hoped that she had.

Like Maggie, with DSNT skin you may experience any of the following:

- Dryness
- Flaking
- Scaling
- Itching
- Blotches
- Redness
- Sensitivity to skin care ingredients
- Sensitivity to soaps and detergents
- Rashes under rings
- Rashes from jewellery that is not real gold or platinum
- Irritation and inflammation from pierced earrings
- Occasional pimples

Dry skin may be more than a skin-deep problem. It may be a symptom of hypothyroidism, a disease that is on the rise, affecting nineteen out of one thousand women and one out of one thousand men. In this disorder, the body does not produce enough thyroid hormone, causing the following symptoms: tiredness, depression, forgetfulness, dry, coarse hair, loss of hair on the last third of the eyebrow, puffy face and eyes, slow heartbeat, dry skin, cold intolerance, weight gain, heavy menstrual periods, constipation and brittle nails.

If you have any of the above-mentioned symptoms, please consult a physician to rule out the possibility that hypothyroidism may be the cause of your skin's dryness. Your doctor can order a blood test to determine if the body is producing enough thyroid hormone.

ENVIRONMENTAL AGENTS THAT CAN LEAD TO DRY SKIN

If you are experiencing extreme dryness or eczema, notice if any of these conditions could be contributing:

- Cold weather
- Dry climate

- Wind
- Prolonged exposure to hot water
- Detergents and soaps
- Friction from rough clothing
- Frequent air travel
- Air-conditioning
- Pollution

While many of these conditions are unavoidable, you can take protective action such as wearing extra moisturiser, covering your face in cold or windy conditions, and purchasing softer fabrics if you notice a problem.

Kevin, an outgoing forty-four-year-old from an Irish background, was the founder and president of a thriving company. He travelled a great deal for his work and liked to pack light, so he washed his face, body, and hair with the deodorant soap and shampoo the hotel supplied. It would never have crossed his mind to bring his own products when freebies were available. If his skin felt dry when he showered, he would take a little hotel-supplied body lotion and rub it over his face, and then rinse it off in the hot shower.

When dryness, flaking and redness began to appear, Kevin ignored them. In his view, men should not pay much attention to their skin. When his symptoms persisted, he began to dig around in the little jars of facial cream that his wife, Eileen, kept in a bathroom cabinet. He couldn't tell one from the other, so he tried one, and though it seemed to help temporarily, the itching and redness persisted and got worse. Over the next few weeks, as he tried different creams, his symptoms continued to worsen.

Finally, the redness and inflammation were so obvious that his wife scheduled an appointment for Kevin with me. Kevin was clearly a dry type, but his skin sensitivity had only become a problem due to a variety of environmental factors. Frequent air travel dried out Kevin's skin. To add insult to injury, Kevin went on to expose his weakened skin barrier to the harsh ingredients in the hotel soaps, shampoos, aftershave products, and moisturisers he used on his trips. Finally, allowing the problem to persist without addressing it prevented Kevin from catching it early before his skin barrier continued to deteriorate. He had begun to develop a dermatitis that resembled eczema.

To stop his itching and inflammation, I put him on a short-term prescription medication, Elidel, to soothe his irritated skin and prevent further damage. Then I began to educate Kevin about his real skin care needs. I recommended the regular use of a fragrance-free moisturiser with SPF and barrier repair ingredients, essential to moisturise and protect his skin from the sun. I strongly urged that he pack this product in his briefcase and reapply it every two hours during long flights. I told him what to look for in shopping for facial cleansing soap, shampoo, and aftershave products that would hydrate rather than attack his skin barrier. Detergent and foaming ingredients must be avoided. I gave him small travel-size product samples so that he could always bring them with him instead of winding up using harsh hotel products.

Under my care, Kevin was able to turn around these early signs of dermatitis and protect his dry, sensitive skin from the abuses of frequent travel and harmful ingredients. When he checked in with me six months later, he reluctantly admitted he was pleased his skin was now well cared for and trouble-free.

Airplane travel is a problem for everyone, but Dry Skin Types are the most affected. Whatever the outer conditions, our body's natural mechanisms work to maintain a constant level of water within every cell, and this includes skin cells too. These mechanisms evolved over thousands of years without the need to respond to flight at great speeds or at high altitudes, and without exposure to the cabin pressure, dryness, high altitude, sunlight, or other features of air travel. All these conditions challenge our water maintenance functions and cause dehydration. Travelling is stressful, and stress has been shown to impair the skin barrier. It takes three days for the skin to rebalance after travel. Quick turnaround trips are worse, and flying first class offers no protection from these negative impacts. That's why, when I travel, I put aside personal vanity and forgo makeup, opting instead to moisturise heavily and use a higher SPF sun protection product.

Soaking in hot water can also dry and potentially damage DSNT skin. Hot baths, steam rooms and facials are not for you. Instead take a quick shower using moderately warm water. Watch out for water quality. Hard or chemically treated water can be drying. Apply moisturiser after exiting the shower, while you're still damp, to trap residual water on the skin surface. Prolonged immersion (over an hour) in room-temperature water can disrupt the skin barrier.

Shampoos and conditioners that contact your face as you rinse should also be selected with care. Read labels to avoid the most common sensitising ingredients. Always rinse thoroughly after use. Bubbly shampoos pose the biggest risk, so avoid getting the shampoo on your face.

Even cleansing can further dry out DSNT skin unless you use a specially formulated cleanser. I'll point you towards the best products later in this chapter.

MOISTURISERS AND DSNT SKIN

Although your thirsty dry skin desperately needs moisturiser, in my opinion, your needs can be well served by products in the low-to-moderate price range. In most instances, the higher-end moisturisers are unnecessary unless you can afford them and happen to like their packaging. One well-known product, which receives a lot of magazine publicity, is often depicted as the Holy Grail of skin care that celebrities and makeup artists swear by. But in my view, its just the same old stuff with a little algae thrown in, bottled in a well-designed jar. To create super expensive products, most companies spend their dollars on advertising and package design to make you buy the product. Very little of the development cost is spent on goodies that actually wind up on your face. One friend of mine has the right idea. She buys supermarket products and pours them into the pretty bottles left over from her prior purchases of high-end brands. She gets the psychological boost the packaging affords along with the same skin care benefit. However, there are some high-end lines worth the price, and I'll guide you with my recommendations on when to splurge.

Although I recommend the use of retinol- and retinoid-containing products for those with oily or pigmented skin and for those prone to wrinkles, since you have non-pigmented, tight skin, they aren't necessary for you. Plus, despite their antiaging benefits, they can be drying and should be used selectively by only some of the Dry Types.

REPAIRING YOUR SKIN BARRIER

Now that I've alerted you to the problems caused by a weak barrier and the external conditions that may contribute to barrier damage, here comes the good news: what you can do to rebuild the barrier. Since it's composed of fatty acids, both the types of fats (and oils) that you eat and the types of fats (and oils) that you use on your skin can impact the barrier. Ingesting and using topically the right types of fats (and oils) is thought to be very important to maintain a healthy skin barrier and to repair a damaged one.

The three main components of a well-functioning skin barrier are cholesterol, fatty acids and ceramides, different types of fat molecules that must be present in the right ratio to form the correct three-dimensional structure to make the skin watertight.

Anything that disrupts any of these three types of fats either internally or externally can therefore undermine the structure of the skin barrier. Taking drugs that lower cholesterol levels worsens dry skin. Detergents, like sodium lauryl sulphate, strip fatty acids, leading to dry skin and irritation, research reveals. Sun exposure inhibits enzymes that help to make ceramides, resulting in dry skin.

While many skin care products contain one or more of the key fats needed for skin repair, the best products contain all three in the right ratio. In fact, replacing one alone may be counterproductive and may actually hurt the skin barrier. Several companies have researched how to develop skin barrier repair products. Unilever, the parent company of Dove, has extensively studied the skin's barrier and skin hydration, and even published a book on the topic called *Skin Moisturisation*. That's why the Dove facial line is designed to address your issues. Dove's dual product sequence provides all three components for dry skin repair. First, a cream cleanser deposits fatty acids on the skin; next, a moisturiser deposits cholesterol and ceramides. This is a rare instance where you really can believe the marketing hype to use two products together for best results. Another company called Osmotics also offers a barrier-repair moisturiser called Tri-Ceram, which, as the name implies, contains the three important barrier repair ingredients. NeoPharm, a Korean company that makes a skin care line called Atopalm, has taken it a step further. They have proven that their moisturiser is able to mimic the same three-dimensional structure that your native skin barrier has. All of these companies have shown that their products can improve dry, sensitive skin. I'm a big Dove fan myself, as my patients know.

In the next section of this chapter, I'll show you how to use the right kinds of products and ingredients to moisturise and rebuild your skin. If you have trouble finding any of the recommended products, visit www.DrBaumann.co.uk to learn where to locate hard to find products. Some of them will be sold at www.Baumannstore.co.uk.

Dr Baumann's Bottom Line: Prevent dryness by avoiding the detergents, soaps, harsh chemicals, and other environmental assaults that can undermine the solidity of your skin barrier. It's easier to prevent damage than to treat it once it occurs. Eat right, reduce stress, and take the right supplements. Use moisturisers that contain all three lipids needed to rebuild the barrier: cholesterol, fatty acids and ceramides. Address dryness, lessen sensitivity, and soothe irritation.

EVERYDAY CARE FOR YOUR SKIN

The goal of your skin care routine is to make your skin less dry and sensitive, using products that deliver ingredients that repair the skin barrier. All the products I'll recommend act to do one or more of the following:

- Prevent and treat skin dryness
- Prevent and treat skin redness
- Prevent and repair assaults to skin barrier

In addition, your daily regimen will help to address your other skin concerns by:

- Preventing and treating acne

As a DSNT, your needs are relatively simple. You need to avoid ingredients (such as alcohol) and products (such as foaming cleansers) that strip the necessary natural lipids from your skin. And second, use moisturisers with ingredients that help build and maintain your skin barrier. Finally, in 'Further Help for Dry, Sensitive Skin', you'll learn about the foods and supplements that will help your skin retain water.

For most DSNTs, I've created a Stage One, nonprescription regimen. As a rule, DSNTs don't need prescription medications, unless you suffer from eczema, acne or rosacea.

Your type has an increased risk of eczema (which usually occurs on the body, not the face). If you suffer from recurring red, dry, itching patches on your skin, see a dermatologist and get prescription medications to treat it.

If you have acne, I've provided a Stage Two prescription regimen to use with medications prescribed by a dermatologist.

DAILY SKIN CARE

STAGE ONE: NONPRESCRIPTION REGIMEN

AM	PM
Step 1: Wash with non-foaming creamy cleanser	Step 1: Wash with non-foaming creamy cleanser

Step 2: Apply anti-inflammatory serum	Step 2: Apply anti-inflammatory serum
Step 3: Spray soothing facial water	Step 3: Spray soothing facial water
Step 4: Apply eye cream (optional)	Step 4: Apply eye cream (optional)
Step 5: Immediately apply moisturiser with SPF or combination of moisturiser, sunscreen, and foundation for a total SPF of 15 or more	Step 5: Immediately apply night cream

In the morning, wash your face with a non-foaming creamy cleanser, then apply an anti-inflammatory serum. Next, spray facial water. Apply an eye cream, if desired, and finish with a moisturiser that contains SPF. Make sure to apply moisturising products while skin is still moist, to trap water in skin.

In the evening, wash with the same cleanser used in the morning and apply the same anti-inflammatory serum. Spray facial water, apply eye cream if you are using one, and apply a night cream.

Undertake this regimen for two weeks. If your skin does not improve, try another set of recommended products. If there is still no improvement after you have tried three sets of products, see a dermatologist.

Cleansers

Use only moisturising, non-foaming cleansers. Never use an ordinary soap.

RECOMMENDED CLEANSERS

£ Lutsine Gentle Cleansing Cream
£ Eucerin Gentle Cleansing Milk
£ Nivea Visage Gentle Cleansing Cream Wash
£ Olay Gentle Cleansing Milk
£ Stiefel Oilatum-AD Cleansing Lotion
££ Aesop Purifying Facial Cream Cleanser
££ Atopalm Facial Cleanser
££ Clinique Comforting Cream Cleanser
££ Elemis Rose Petal Cleanser

££ Jurlique Cleansing Lotion

££ La Roche-Posay Toleriane Derma-Cleanser

££ Organic Pharmacy Rose & Chamomile Cleansing Milk

££ Ren Calendula & Arctic Blackcurrant Milk Wash

£££ Christian Dior Prestige Cleansing Crème

£££ Guerlain Issima Flower Cleansing Cream

£££ La Prairie Purifying Cream Cleanser

Baumann's Choice: Stiefel Oilatum-AD Cleansing Lotion because it's very gentle.

Serums

Serums can confer powerful ingredients to help manage the inflammation that occurs with skin sensitivity. Most serums are too irritating for a DS Type, but I can recommend those below.

RECOMMENDED SERUMS

£ Olay Regenerist Daily Regenerating Serum

££ Clarins Skin Beauty Repair Concentrate

££ Dr Andrew Weil for Origins Plantidote Mega-Mushroom Face Serum

££ Elizabeth Arden Overnight Success-Skin Renewal Serum

££ Joey New York Calm and Correct Serum

££ La Roche-Posay Toleriane Facial Fluid

££ Laura Mercier Multi Vitamin Serum

££ Nars Brightening Serum (with aloe, antioxidants and macadamia nut oil)

£££ Jurlique Herbal Recovery Mist DS (Delicate/Sensitive)

Baumann's Choice: Clarins Skin Beauty Repair Concentrate with chamomile and licorice extract

Facial Water

DSNTs should never use toners, which are designed to strip much-needed fats out of the skin and may contain alcohol and other drying ingredients.

Instead, use a facial water. Spray it on your face immediately prior to applying an eye cream and moisturiser. The creams will help trap the water on the skin, giving the skin a reservoir to pull from. This is particularly helpful in low-humidity environments.

Facial waters come from thermal springs. They do not contain chemicals such as chlorine, which is added to our tap water to eliminate algae and other organisms. The constituents of the water vary according to the source. Vichy water contains sulphur, while the La Roche-Posay water contains selenium. This selenium-containing water has been shown to be effective in treating eczema. La Roche-Posay has a spa in France that treats thousands of eczema sufferers a year with their healing waters. Vichy also has a spa in France with renowned thermal springs with sulphur-containing water. Both selenium and sulphur can be anti-inflammatory.

RECOMMENDED FACIAL WATERS

- £ Evian Mineral Water Spray
- ££ Arbonne NutriMinC RE9 REstoring Mist Balancing Toner
- ££ Avène Thermal Water Spray
- ££ Chantecaille Pure Rosewater
- ££ Fresh Rose Marigold Tonic Water
- ££ La Roche-Posay Thermal Spring Water
- ££ Molton Brown Skin Boost 24 hour Moisture Mist
- ££ Shu Uemura Depsea Therapy
- ££ Vichy Thermal Spa Water
- £££ Jurlique Rosewater Freshener

Baumann's Choice: Thermal Spring Water by La Roche-Posay has selenium, which helps decrease inflammation. The Jurlique is a cult favourite in Australia.

Moisturisers

DSNTs need to moisturise as much as possible. The correct moisturisers will do more for your skin than anything else. Select different ones for morning and evening because the evening products may be too greasy for daytime, preventing your makeup from spreading well. If you use a daytime moisturiser that contains an SPF of 15, you won't need to apply an additional sunscreen. However, if your moisturiser contains less than that amount, you can use any combination of moisturiser, sunscreen and foundation with SPF to assure you attain that coverage.

RECOMMENDED DAYTIME MOISTURISERS

£ Boots No7 Uplifting Day Cream
£ Eucerin Lipo Balance Cream with Ceramide
£ Nivea Soft Intensive Moisturising Cream
££ Cutanix Dramatic Relief for Sensitive Facial Skin
££ Laura Mercier Mega Moisturiser with SPF 15
££ SkinCeuticals Daily Sun Defence SPF 20
££ Topix Glycolix Elite Sunscreen SPF 30
£££ Elemis Absolute Day Cream SPF 7
£££ Jurlique Day Care Face Cream
£££ L'Occitane Shea 24 hours Ultra Rich Face Cream
£££ Orlane Soleil Vitamins Face Cream SPF 30

Baumann's Choice: Cutanix Dramatic Relief for Sensitive Facial Skin. It contains quadrinone which has been shown to improve inflammation.

RECOMMENDED EVENING MOISTURISERS

£ Avène Eau Thermale Skin Recovery Cream
£ Eucerin Lipo Balance Cream with Ceramide
£ Nivea Soft Intensive Moisturising Cream
££ AtoPalm MLE Cream
££ Aesop Camellia Nut Facial Hydrating Cream
££ Burt's Bees Evening Primrose Overnight Crème
££ Clarins Multi-Active Night Cream
££ D.R. Harris Almond Oil Skinfood
££ Elizabeth Arden Good Night's Restoring Cream
££ Laura Mercier Night Nutrition Renewal Crème
£££ Crème de la Mer
£££ Jurlique Wrinkle Softener Beauty Cream
£££ Ren Calendula Omega 3/7 Hydra-Calm Moisturiser (not for acne)
£££ Sisley Botanical Moisturiser with Cucumber

Baumann's Choice: Atopalm MLE Cream (Not the face cream in the tube, the one in the jar with the red top.)

Eye Creams

Don't feel you have to use a separate eye cream. Using your nighttime moisturiser around the eye area is fine, unless you find it too heavy. Here are some suggestions for those who prefer a separate eye cream.

RECOMMENDED EYE CREAMS

- £ Olay Eye Contour Gel
- £ Olay Regenerist Eye Lifting Serum
- ££ Biotherm Biosensitive Soothing Eye Care
- ££ Bobbi Brown Hydrating Eye Cream
- ££ D.R. Harris Crystal Eye Gel
- ££ Korres Evening Primrose Eye Cream
- ££ Laura Mercier Night Nutrition Renewal Eye Crème
- £££ Jo Malone Apricot and Aloe Eye Gel
- £££ Lancôme Absolue Eye
- £££ L'Occitane Immortelle Eye Balm

Baumann's Choice: The best products contain Vitamin K, but I could not find any in the UK. The Olay products contain niacinamide so they are my first choice.

Exfoliation

DSNTs should not exfoliate unless they have a low S/R score of 30 or below. Those of you with higher S/R scores will likely develop facial redness and increased sensitivity if you try it. However, you can use a very light scrub with an emollient base once a week to help remove dry skin flakes. Just don't overdo it. My favourite product is the Clinique 7 Day Scrub Cream.

SHOPPING FOR PRODUCTS

Never use soaps – or any product – that contain detergents. How can you tell? First, notice the product's action. Though a small amount of foam is acceptable, if a cleanser, soap, shampoo, or bath product produces vigorous suds and bubbles, it contains detergent. Stay away from it.

Second, read ingredient lists and make sure you avoid all detergents and sensitising ingredients you find listed on the labels of skin care products and any other products that contact your skin, such as shampoos and other hair products, as well as bath and body products. Sodium lauryl sulphate is an irritating detergent commonly used in shampoos, conditioners, and other skin care products. Look out for it, and purchase brands that *don't* contain it. The lists on 376 will alert you to other ingredients you should avoid.

RECOMMENDED SKIN CARE INGREDIENTS

To prevent dark spots:

- Cocos nucifera (coconut extract), unless you have acne
- Cucumber
- Niacinamide
- Pycnogenol (a pine bark extract)
- Saxifraga sarmentosa extract (strawberry begonia)
- Soy

To improve dark spots:

- Arbutin
- Cucumber extract
- Glycyrrhiza glabra (licorice extract)

To prevent inflammation:

- Aloe vera
- Chamomile
- Colloidal oatmeal
- Cucumber
- Dexpanthenol (pro-vitamin B_5)
- Epilobium angustifolium (willow herb)
- Evening primrose oil
- Feverfew
- Perilla leaf extract
- Pycnogenol (a pine bark extract)
- Red algae
- Thyme
- Trifolium pretense (red clover)
- Quadrinone

To increase moisture:

- Borage seed oil
- Castor oil
- Ceramide
- Cholesterol
- Evening primrose oil
- Glycerin
- Jojoba oil
- Olive oil

- Cocoa butter (avoid if you have acne)
- Colloidal oatmeal
- Dexpanthenol (pro-vitamin B$_5$)
- Dimethicone
- Pumpkin seed oil
- Safflower oil
- Stearic acid and other fatty acids
- Sunflower oil

SKIN CARE INGREDIENTS TO AVOID

Due to irritating detergents:

- Dimethyl dodecyl amido betaine
- Lauryl sulphates
- Sodium dodecyl sulphate
- Sodium lauryl sulphate

Due to increasing acne or skin redness:

- Cinnamon oil
- Cocoa butter
- Cocos nucifera (coconut oil)
- Isopropyl isostearate
- Isopropyl myristate
- Peppermint oil

Due to problematic preservatives:

- Benzalkonium chloride
- Bronopol
- Chloroacetamide
- Chlorocresol
- Chlorohexidine
- Chloroquinaldol
- Diazolidinyl urea
- Dibromodicyanobutane (phenoxyethanol)
- Dichlorophen
- DMDM hydantoin
- Formaldehyde
- Glutaraldehyde
- Imidazolidinyl urea
- Kathon CG
- Parabens
- Phenylmercuric acetate
- Quaternium-15
- Sorbic acid
- Thimerosal
- Triclosan

Sun Protection for Your Skin

Although I recommend that you rely upon an SPF-containing moisturiser to keep well protected, you may also wish to reapply sunscreen regularly, choosing any of my selections.

RECOMMENDED SUNSCREENS

£ Nivea Sun Sensitive Lotion SPF 15, 30 and 50.
££ Bobbie Brown Extra SPF 25 Moisturising Balm
££ Dermalogica Sheer Moisture SPF 15
££ La Roche-Posay Fluide Extreme Anthelios SPF 60
££ L'Occitane Shea Ultra Moisturising Care SPF 15
£££ Clarins Hydration Plus Moisture Lotion SPF 15
£££ La Prairie Age Management Stimulus Complex SPF 25
£££ Lancôme Absolue Absolute Replenishing Cream SPF15

Baumann's Choice: Anthelios Fluide Extreme SPF 60 is my first choice. It comes in a cream form as well if you prefer a heavy sunscreen. You may need to order it on-line, or purchase it when you travel to France or Ireland.

SUNSCREEN INGREDIENTS TO AVOID

If you get skin rashes from sunscreen:

- Benzophenone
- Methoxycinnamate
- Padimate
- Para-aminobenzoic acid (PABA)

Your Makeup

In choosing makeup products, avoid any that contain the ingredients listed above. You should also stay away from shimmery shadows, since these products may contain pieces of shell that will irritate dry, sensitive skin. D and C red dyes in blusher and colour makeup can lead to acne, so if you tend to break out over the cheek area, make sure your cosmetics do not contain these dyes. There are many types of D and C red dyes but the xanthenes, mono-azoanilines, fluorans and indigoids are the most problematic.

RECOMMENDED FOUNDATIONS

£ Boots No7 Radiant Glow Foundation SPF 15
££ Bloom Foundation
££ Kevyn Aucoin Dew Drop Foundation
££ Laura Mercier Moisturising Foundation
££ L'Occitane Tinted Day Care SPF 15

££ Trish McEvoy Protective Shield Tinted Moisturiser
£££ Versace Fluid Moisture Foundation

Baumann's Choice: Laura Mercier Moisturising Foundation

RECOMMENDED CREAM EYESHADOWS

£ Almay Bright Eyes
£ Revlon Illuminance Creme Shadow
££ Bliss Lidthicks
££ Bloom Eye Colour Cream
££ Bobbi Brown Cream Shadow Stick
££ Clinique Touch Tint for Eyes Cream Formula
££ Urban Decay Cream Eyeshadow
££ Ruby and Millie Eye Colour Cream
££ SPACENK Creamy Eyeshadow

Baumann's Choice: SPACENK Creamy Eyeshadow can be found at a really cool store in London called Space NK.

RECOMMENDED BLUSHERS

£ Avon Split Second Blush Stick
££ Aveda Uruku Cheek/Lip Cream
££ Bobbi Brown Cream Blush Stick
££ Jane Iredale Blush (powder blusher with soothing minerals)
££ L'Occitane Colour Cream for Lips and Cheeks
££ Ruby and Millie Cheek Colour Cream
£££ DuWop Blush Therapy

Baumann's Choice: They are all good.

CONSULTING A DERMATOLOGIST

PRESCRIPTION SKIN CARE STRATEGIES

If you think you have eczema, see a dermatologist for prescription medications such as Elidel and Protopic, which can help. I've also provided a prescription regimen if you have acne or rosacea. Your goal is to treat it and prevent a recurrence without drying your skin. Studies actually show that just moisturising the skin will improve acne, so do not be afraid to moisturise. If your acne or rosacea does not improve on the nonprescription regimen, or if your acne is worse than six pimples a month, see your dermatologist for prescription medications.

If you have a higher S/R score (over 34), you are more likely to suffer from several subtypes of skin sensitivity. You may have acne, rosacea, or multiple skin allergies. Yours is milder than the severe acne seen with Oily Skin Types. Still, acne is tough to handle, since most acne products will either dry or irritate your skin. If you have only a few pimples, the nonprescription regimen may help. If not, see a dermatologist who will prescribe topical antibiotic medications and a cleanser with anti-inflammatory ingredients such as sulphacetamide. These prescription regimens will help both acne and rosacea without overdrying your sensitive skin. The dermatologist may give you tetracycline, an oral antibiotic, as well. Tetracycline may help decrease acne and rosacea through a mechanism different than merely killing bacteria; it also has anti-inflammatory properties. Acne and rosacea usually take eight weeks to improve.

As a DSNT, you should not use retinoids unless your dermatologist specifically recommends them.

DAILY SKIN CARE

STAGE TWO: PRESCRIPTION REGIMEN

For improving acne or rosacea:

AM	PM
Step 1: Wash with a prescription sulphacetamide cleanser	Step 1: Wash with a prescription sulphacetamide cleanser
Step 2: Apply antibiotic gel	Step 2: Apply antibiotic gel
Step 3: Spray soothing facial water	Step 3: Spray soothing facial water
Step 4: Immediately apply moisturiser with SPF, or combination of moisturiser, sunscreen, and foundation to achieve an SPF 15 coverage	Step 4: Immediately apply night cream

In the morning, wash with a medicated cleanser, and then apply antibiotic gel to your entire face. Next, spray soothing facial water and apply moisturiser with SPF. If you wish to apply eye cream, do so after Step 3. After your moisturiser, you can also use a facial foundation, if you wish.

In the evening, wash with cleanser, and apply antibiotic gel to your entire face. Next, spray soothing facial water and apply night cream.

PRESCRIPTION MEDICATIONS

There are many antibiotic gels and sulphacetamide cleansers, and you should discuss with your doctor which ones are best for you. Below I've listed just a few of your many options.

Sulphacetamide cleansers:

- Avar Cleanser
- Rosanil Cleanser
- Rosula Cleanser

The above-mentioned products are US name brands that may not be available in your country. Please ask your dermatologist for a substitution.

Antibiotic gels:

These products contain various combinations of sulphur, sulphacetamide, metronidazole and clindamycin. There are so many; I won't name them here as your dermatologist will choose one that is right for your particular needs.

PROCEDURES FOR YOUR SKIN TYPE

Your type does not need any skin care procedures. However, for some problems, you may wish to consult a dermatologist. For example, if your skin reacts to multiple skin care products, your dermatologist can patch test you to find out whether you are indeed allergic and, if so, precisely what you are allergic to. Patch testing involves taping small samples of several types of allergens on your back. You return to the doctor twenty-four hours later to see if any of the areas have developed redness, which indicates an allergic reaction. Sometimes several tests, using different allergens, are needed before you can find out what is causing your allergy.

Ongoing Care for Your Skin

Avoid harsh chemicals, environmental extremes, and anything that could undermine your skin barrier. Moisturise continually and spray water before moisturiser use. Make sure to incorporate essential fats into your diet, because repairing and maintaining a healthy skin barrier is your first priority.

Further Help for Dry, Sensitive Skin

In this section, you'll find follow-up information and instructions on product use and procedures for Dry, Sensitive Skin Types, as well as lifestyle recommendations, diet and supplements that can help your skin.

USING RETINOIDS

If retinoid use is recommended in your Skin Type chapter, here's some information about how to begin using it. For more information about how retinoids work, please consult 'Using Retinoids' in 'Further Help for Oily, Resistant Skin'.

For dry, sensitive types, retinoids must be started very slowly. At first, use only a pea-size amount of retinoid once a week, applying it *on top of* your night cream, and avoiding the eye area. After two weeks of use, apply the retinoid twice a week. After another two weeks, apply it every other night. You may then increase the frequency to every night, if you can tolerate it. If your skin becomes highly irritated at any point, stop, wait a week, and begin again. If you develop redness or excessive scaling, use a lesser amount that you are able to tolerate. You may never be able to use the retinoid more than twice a week. If so, that is fine, it will still benefit you. Retinoids should not be used by pregnant or lactating women, or by those who plan to become pregnant in the near future.

LIFESTYLE RECOMMENDATIONS FOR DRY, SENSITIVE SKIN

Keeping your skin hydrated is essential. Humid climates are easier on your skin. Put a humidifier in your house. It's a myth that drinking more water will help hydrate your skin. However, the water you use to bathe and rinse yourself *is* important.

Washing yourself with hard water (which contains increased amounts of calcium) can contribute to dryness and redness, studies show. Reverse osmosis water filters will help convert hard water to soft water, so you might want to consider such a purchase. Water temperature also matters. Studies have shown that very hot water temperatures, such as 40 degrees celsius, can dry the skin out and lead to redness.

If you like, you can immerse your entire body at one of the many spas around the world that offer gentle hydrotherapy – and I mean 'gentle'. Scalding temperatures, intense treatments, running from hot saunas into a wintry snow is for hardy souls with hardy skin, not for you. Even bubble bath and perfumed bath oils and massage products can be irritating.

Whenever you go for relaxing treatments, make your choices with care. Be ultra alert in selecting spa and beauty treatments. Exfoliation massages, loofahs, facials, and steam rooms can all strip oils from your skin. They are not for you. Aromatherapy massages may be counterproductive, depending upon the oils used. The acetones in nail polishes and removers can be irritating. That spa pedicure may not be so relaxing if it causes a flare-up.

All Dry, Sensitive Skin Types benefit from thalassotherapy skin and body treatments, including body wraps, baths, mud packs, and jet sprays that use seaweed and seawater to hydrate and heal the skin. However, it's important to limit immersion in the water to less than one hour so as not to impair the skin barrier. Very popular throughout Europe, thalassotherapy treatments are used for relaxation, stress management, muscle and skin restoration, and to fight cellulite. Many tour companies offer destination spa packages. If your chequebook can handle it, you can travel to spas specialising in these treatments. Otherwise, certain seaweed-based products for home purchase can also be effective in hydrating dry, sensitive skin. Just make sure to read the ingredient list to make sure they do not contain anything you might find irritating.

Massage is great for eczema. A study performed at the University of Miami showed that children with eczema who were treated with moist-urisers and massaged improved more compared to those who were not massaged and were treated with moisturiser alone. Another study compared massage using essential oils versus massage without essential oils, revealing that both groups improved, likely due to the massage. Because essential oils may lead to an allergic reaction, they should be used with caution.

PROTECTING THE SKIN BARRIER

Damage to the skin barrier results from a combination of genetic predis-position and exposure to sensitising chemicals and other substances. That's why avoiding irritants is as important as using products that help. In skin care, the most common irritants are perfumes and preservatives. Although many products are labelled as 'fragrance free', that's really a misnomer. Nearly all products contain some fragrance to mask their odour; so-called fragrance-free products just contain less than regular ones.

What's more, the fragrances used in many products (even pricey perfumes) are synthetic. For sensitive individuals, the chemical brew can be a problem. Nowadays many natural fragrances are extracted using harsh solvents rather than old-fashioned distillation methods, in which fewer chemicals come into contact with the essential oil of the flower, so unless you can determine the extraction method, be cautious. That's one reason why many individuals react to the essential oils used in aromatherapy massages and products. Studies show that massage therapists have more contact dermatitis due to exposure to these extracts.

Preservatives including formaldehyde, parabens, and others commonly used in skin, hair and beauty products can also provoke allergic reactions, according to several studies. Although they are needed to maintain product shelf life, and only minute amounts are present in any given product, many different kinds of products contain these same preservatives, including skin care products, make-up, medications, antiperspirants, toothpaste, and foods. In addition, many of these products are used on a daily basis. As a result, the overall exposure to these ingredients is higher than would occur if only a single product were to be used.

Up until now no studies have investigated the cumulative impact of repeated exposures to preservatives in a variety of products and ingredients. For the majority of people, these preservatives are a boon, not a problem. However, some Dry, Sensitive Skin Types may be among the minority who have a problem. I recommend that you carefully read labels for all products that come into contact with your skin internally or externally to assure that they don't contain the listed ingredients that you must avoid.

SIX-STEP PLAN TO ELIMINATE SENSITISERS AND ALLERGENS

In addition, many other kinds of chemicals we're exposed to every day can induce inflammation in susceptible individuals. As a Dry, Sensitive Skin

Type, you are more at risk for reactions, especially if you are already experiencing extreme dryness or eczema symptoms.

If you have these symptoms, first of all, you must take active steps to rebuild your barrier. While you are doing that, help yourself out by going through this progressive plan to identify and, where possible, eliminate sensitising ingredients. Whether what you experience is merely a sensitivity or a bona fide allergic reaction, anything that causes inflammation will further degrade your barrier. So give your skin a chance to heal by protecting it from things that may cause a reaction.

1. Eliminate problem ingredients in skin care and perfumes. (Consult my recommendations and lists of ingredients to avoid.)
2. Eliminate problem ingredients in soaps; shampoo, bath, body care, dental, shaving, and conditioning products; and medications. Avoid products that foam or contain detergents. Always rinse thoroughly after cleansing and shampooing. Protect your skin with moisturiser.
3. Avoid direct contact with dish and laundry detergents, household cleansing products, paints, strippers, furniture polishes, and other products containing harsh chemicals. Wear gloves, moisturise, or avoid altogether. Studies show that residual detergent remaining in laundered clothing may be a prime contributor to eczema. Rinse your clothing well.
4. Notice whether fabrics in clothing, furniture, or bedding are irritating your skin due to their rough texture or chemicals treating them. Remove any offenders.
5. Pay attention to contact allergies from jewellery, cutlery and coins or other metals containing nickel, a common allergen. (It's present in the euro!)
6. Check out water quality and avoid hard water, chlorinated water, excessively hot water, or long soaks in baths, showers, or hot tubs, which can strip oils from your skin.

Later, when your skin barrier has been restored to health, you may very likely be able to withstand these common irritants and practises, but during the healing process, notice what bothers you and avoid contact with it to give your skin a chance to rebuild. If you still have problems, ask your dermatologist about patch testing, which can help you determine exactly what you're allergic to.

ADDRESSING STRESS

One further factor I've yet to mention is the role of stress in your skin problems. Stress hormones trigger inflammation, and inflammation increases skin reactivity, dryness, and (in pigmented types) pigmentation leading to dark spots. That's why addressing stress, or in some cases, becoming aware of things that you find stressful, is another key to caring for your skin. Make sure to get a good night's sleep. Insomnia may increase your incidence of allergic reaction because of the effects of sleep deprivation on the immune system.

Remember that your ideal activity must be calming and soothing. I mention this because reactive people sometimes need to learn *how* to calm down.

Liz, a classic type A personality, who worked in the high-pressure, competitive environment of the stock exchange, came in for a follow-up visit. 'I tried relaxing like you said, and I'm totally wiped out,' she reported. I asked her what she did, and it turned out that in trying out some of my suggested relaxation options, her selections had been a little off the mark. For example, when she decided to try a yoga class, instead of a restorative class, she wound up in a heated room jammed with sweating students who performed extreme postures as the teacher shouted into a microphone. Not exactly an anti-inflammatory environment! Instead of getting a relaxing massage, she received a weight-loss massage from a Japanese masseur who pounded her back with a wooden mallet. Again, contraindicated. Do I need to tell you that her idea of a relaxing walk in nature was rock climbing? And her way of relaxing with a pet was to run round the reservoir with her black Lab, Cutlass. All of this was fun, and it was great exercise; but it wasn't exactly relaxing – that is, until Liz dropped into bed exhausted and drained at the end of her two weekends of relaxation.

There is nothing wrong with invigorating activities like these, and some people thrive on them. But if you need to rest, restore, and soothe away stress, choose differently. Practising relaxation will help to lower the levels of the stress hormones that can cause problems.

DIET FOR DRY, SENSITIVE SKIN

Eating the right foods (and avoiding the wrong ones) can help prevent wrinkling and minimise the signs of aging, according to several studies.

Following a so-called Mediterranean diet, featuring ample vegetables, legumes, and olive oil (and eating them together), may be helpful because the oil may help your body absorb and benefit from fat-soluble antioxidant vitamins and phytochemicals, such as vitamin E, lycopene and isoflavones. Organic produce contains a higher level of beneficial antioxidants than conventionally raised fruits and vegetables.

With dry skin issues like yours, it's important to get the right types of fats into your diet. But what are the right types of fats? Understandably, many people are confused. For example, increased intake of saturated fat and monounsaturated fat in the diet has been associated with a decrease in skin hydration. Yet, other studies reveal that people on cholesterol-lowering drugs are at higher risk for dry skin disorders, most likely because cholesterol is a key component of the skin barrier. So consuming some saturated fats, but not too many, seems to be best.

Countless studies show that an omega-3 fat deficiency is associated with dry skin and skin problems like eczema. That's why it's important to consume adequate amounts of these (yes, they are) essential fats, to be found in fatty fish, fish oils, flaxseeds, flaxseed oil, and a few other food sources. Don't confuse them with their cousins, the omega-6 polyunsaturated vegetable oils (including corn, canola and safflower), formerly hailed as healthy for the heart. Here's why: a study published in the *American Journal of Clinical Nutrition* (2001 by Bernard Henrig) points to an overly high ratio of omega-6 to omega-3 fats as a key contributor to cardiovascular illness. In other words, most people need to eat *more* omega-3s and *less* omega-6 oils. (For omega-3 food and supplement recommendations, read on in this section.)

The dairy products you eat (and avoid) can also make a difference in skin aging. Butter, full-fat milk, margarine, and sweets should be minimised, while yogurt, cheese, and reduced-fat milk are neutral in their aging effects. The epidermis (upper layer of the skin) is composed of 25 percent monounsaturated fatty acids. In the cell membranes, both monosaturated fats and saturated fats resist oxidation, a key process in cellular aging. Omega-6 polyunsaturated oils, on the other hand, contribute to the production of free radicals, the by-products of oxidation, the aging process which antioxidant vegetables help tame. This would increase both wrinkling and the risk of developing skin and other cancers, including melanoma.

Therefore, it's beneficial to eat more olive oil (a monounsaturate) while avoiding omega-6 polyunsaturated oils, such as corn, canola, safflower, soy and others. Trans fats, present in margarine, most baked goods, fried foods, processed foods, and sweets, are oxidised polyunsaturates, making them even more detrimental. In studies, they have been shown to displace beneficial omega-3 fats in the cellular and hormonal pathways. Freeing the omega-3s to do their job will help the body absorb lipids needed in the skin cells and improve the action of hormones. Since skin aging is caused by hormonal shifts that occur naturally in the aging process, it's best to eliminate the polyunsaturates and trans fats that disrupt the absorption of fats you need for your skin and hormones.

Fish oils and fish are sources of omega-3 polyunsaturated fatty acids, which can increase the lipid content of your cells. These fats have been associated with improvement in psoriasis and other severe dry skin conditions. However, the mercury content in fish is of concern, particularly to pregnant women, nursing mothers, and young children, so supplements may be the safest way of obtaining these fats vital to skin health.

A second important factor in treating dry, sensitive, and wrinkled skin is increasing dietary antioxidants, obtained from fruits and vegetables, such as spinach, kale, collard greens, turnips, romaine lettuce, broccoli, leeks, corn, red peppers, peas and mustard greens. Egg yolks and oranges contain the antioxidant lutein.

Overall, your diet should include:

- A wide variety of whole plant foods
- Fats from whole foods – nuts, seeds, olives and avocados
- Monounsaturated fats, such as olive or nut oils
- Good sources of omega-3 oils, but never heat them. Take them in capsule form or use them in salad dressings.
- Moderate your use of omega-6 oils (corn, safflower, canola and soy oils)
- Limit your intake of processed foods and deep-fried foods, which are high in trans-fats omega-6 fatty acids. Trans fats, also called hydrogenated fats, are present in fried foods; fast foods; and most chips, cookies, sweets and baked goods sold by national food suppliers. They may interfere with the hormonal pathways needed for healthy fat metabolism and preventing inflammation.
- Consume sources of omega-3 fats daily, including a source of essential fatty acids (EFA) and dihydroxyacetone (DHA). (See 'Further Help for Oily, Sensitive Types' for supplement recommendations.)

SUPPLEMENTS

To help prevent wrinkles and skin cancer, you can take antioxidant supplements. Ultraceuticals Ultra Active Age Defiance has vitamins C, and E, as well as zinc, selenium and natural Fish Oil – a powerhouse combination for wrinkle prevention, addressing sun damage, and dry skin. *Polypodium leucotomos,* or fern, extract is found in a product called Heliocare, which can help to lessen sun damage, according to recent studies. Organic Pharmacy Super Antioxidant Capsules is my favourite UK supplement. It contains alpha lipoic acid, DMAE, L Glutathione, Co Q10, Grapeseed, and Pycnogenol. Please go to www.DrBaumann.co.uk and let me know if you can find a similar product at a lower cost.

Chinese herbal medicine can successfully treat eczema in European patients, as shown using double-blind, placebo-controlled, and short-term treatment in both children and adults (study by Sheehan et al. working with Luo, a Chinese herbalist in London). The herbs used in this study consisted of at least ten plant extracts: *Potentilla chinensis, Tribulus terrestris, Rehmannia glutinosa, Lophatherum gracile, Clematis armandii, Ledebouriella seseloides, Dictamnus dasycarpus, Paenia lactiflora, Schizonepeta tenuifolia,* and *Glycyrrhiza glabra.* If you live in a major city where there is a Chinatown, you may wish to seek out a Chinese pharmacist or herbalist.

PART FIVE

Skin Care for Dry, Resistant Skin

CHAPTER SIXTEEN

Dry, Resistant, Pigmented and Wrinkled: DRPW

THE NEGLECTED SKIN TYPE

'I never paid much attention to my skin because I never had any skin problems. I never bothered with skin care products because I didn't need to. Now that I'm seeing wrinkles and spots forming, I guess it's just too late.'

ABOUT YOUR SKIN

I love DRPWs because there is so much that I can do to help your skin. And my DRPW patients are grateful for what cosmetic dermatology can offer. Younger DRPWs rarely consult a dermatologist, so I usually see this type once the signs of aging have appeared.

With DRPW skin, wrinkles are the chief complaint. Your skin may feel tight, rough to the touch, and even sore, especially in drying environmental conditions, such as on a plane. In the winter, when indoor heating is used, your skin gets even more dehydrated, making the wrinkles look worse. Your skin may catch on wool and other rough clothing. You may also notice wrinkles on your hands.

Older DRPWs come into my office, desperate to address the skin wrinkling, and they feel a lot of regret. Although genes certainly play a role in everyone's skin condition, for DRPWs, decades of neglect, or even mistreatment, of their skin is most frequently the source of their skin problems. Many say that if they knew then what they know now, they would have done it differently. That's why I want to alert DRPWs young and old to take steps now to protect your skin and prevent wrinkles.

You are the type that goes for a day of fun on the beach without sun protection, who sails or skis without moisturising against the harsh winds or blasting cold. You head out without a hat, figuring your easy-to-tan skin can handle anything. Many of you prefer to be active, rather than take the time to mess around with beauty stuff.

On a daily basis, you may rarely wear sunscreen, use any old moisturiser, and wash with drying soaps. You wouldn't wear foundation to save your life. You shrug off antiaging treatments. You can't be bothered. Most of you fail to protect your skin, and your dry skin can't take the abuse. As early as your early thirties, and increasingly as you get older, the signs of aging appear and accelerate. At first, you try to ignore the wrinkles, pretending they don't matter. Soon you can't ignore them, but you still don't like to admit that your obvious skin problems *are* problems. Once you admit that they upset you, you believe that it's too late. 'I just have to grin and bear it,' one DRPW patient shrugged and told me. Overnight, the carefree go-for-it girl or guy becomes the resigned, prematurely aging woman or man. Skin problems sneak up on you, and once they manifest, many of you just give up.

But you *can* do something about it, whatever your age. If you are an older DRPW, don't give up, I can help even you. And if you are a younger DRPW, take heed and act now to prevent the worst downsides of your type.

DRPW CELEBRITY

Stunning red-haired actress Julianne Moore is a class act. A talented actress and icon of glamour, this beauty is also a devoted wife and mother. She's received four Oscar nominations, tributes to her ability to transform herself into a wide range of characters, from the desperate housewife in *The Hours* to the tragic adulteress in *The End of the Affair,* from the wistful romantic in *Vanya on 42nd Street* to the determined heiress in *The Big Lebowski.* Her selection of diverse roles in interesting films is a testament to a subtle and perceptive nature, perhaps nurtured by her social worker mother. Moore's ability to inhabit and radiate the feminine ideal, while at the same time evoking the yearning, fulfilment, and disappointment of romance, is unparalleled.

Although I've never personally examined Moore's skin, and therefore cannot unquestionably determine her Skin Type, my guess is that she's a DRPW. Her face rarely appears shiny, blemished, or red in photos defining her as a Dry, Resistant Type, while her red hair and freckles unquestionably reveal that her skin is pigmented. I'm indicating that she may be a Wrinkled Type (even though her skin looks tight and fabulous in her early forties) due to her genetics. But it's probable that Moore has done a lot to protect her skin and change her skin's destiny. Plus, the questionnaire measures the tendency to wrinkle and not the current extent of wrinkling.

People with her porcelain pale skin, freckles and red hair are vulnerable to sun exposure and the attendant wrinkling. Innately, her skin would not age that well without a number of protective skin care habits. I see no signs that surgery is responsible for her youthful appearance in her fifh decade. I would guess that some of her relatives haven't fared as well as she has.

The excellent condition of her skin is a testament to the power of prevention. It looks as though Moore wears sunscreen religiously; I've never seen her tanned in any photo or role. Her maturity and wisdom, revealed in interviews, may also have led Moore to a healthy diet, rich in wrinkle-fighting antioxidants. Hopefully, she'll pass on the same healthy skin habits to her kids. Though a Wrinkled Type by birth, Moore has taken charge to assure that the beauty that her many fans admire shines on.

Coincidentally, Moore may share this Skin Type with Anglo-Irish actor Pierce Brosnan, renowned as Remington Steele, and later, James Bond, who starred with Moore in the film, *Laws of Attraction*.

THE HARSH REALITY OF DRPW SKIN

During their teens and twenties, DRPWs have great skin. Unlike oily types, you experience no acne. Unlike sensitive types, you have no problems using skin care products and ingredients. As far as pigment goes, there are two types of DRPWs: the fair-skinned and freckled who don't tan well, like Moore, and the people who can easily achieve the Hawaiian Tropic Tan. If you're in the latter group, you may often fail to use sunscreen regularly. Fair-skinned DRPWs may have frequently burned trying to achieve that unobtainable tan, attaining instead only freckles and peeling skin.

For women, the first problems crop up in their twenties or thirties, the age when many get pregnant or take birth control pills. Dark spots and dark under-eye circles may result. In your early thirties, you may develop lines around your eyes and between your eyebrows. DRPWs often develop both lines underneath the eyes just below the lower lids and under-eye dark circles. Your skin's dryness makes the wrinkles even more noticeable. Moisturisers are absorbed quickly, providing only minimal hydration. With age (and menopause), skin dryness and wrinkles worsen.

Though some DRPWs abuse their skin through sunning, smoking, and poor dietary habits, you (along with many other DRPWs) may not have abused your skin, but are trying to overcome a genetic tendency to wrinkle. Your best chance is to do everything possible to tip the scales in your favour. A little sun here, a cigarette occasionally at a party, an occasional indulgence in junk food may not be the worst thing in the world for many types, but you cannot afford it. In a high-risk group, you must do everything right to limit visible aging. Follow my preventive strategies whenever possible.

DRPWs have some of the most dreaded skin issues. Wrinkles, sags, premature aging, dryness, dark spots, flaking and peeling skin result from years of disregard. By the time you reach your late forties and fifties, your skin's wrinkling and dryness may make you feel like giving up on your skin in frustration.

At any age, knowing how to protect, hydrate and moisturise your skin is key. For those of you who are starting early in the game – congratulations. If you use sunscreen, include antioxidants (obtained via foods, supplements and topical products), and learn how to protect and moisturise, chances are excellent that you can moderate your skin's tendency to wrinkle.

For older DRPWs, there's still much that can be done. After all, chances are you have another twenty to forty years left to live with your skin, so it's never too late to begin.

SUNTANNING

Many people with this Skin Type (or its close cousin, the DRPT Skin Type) may have a medium skin tone and tan well, like George Clooney and Teri Hatcher. I have numerous DRPW Spanish, Italian, Greek, Latin-American, Portuguese, Brazilian, Indian, Chinese and Thai patients. DRPWs with a lighter skin colour will often have freckles, like Julianne Moore, and may have many fine wrinkles.

I see a lot of DRPWs in my Florida practise: fishermen, tennis players and golfers of both sexes and all nationalities troop into the clinic since they know that there's a lot that cosmetic dermatology can offer. Pigmented, Wrinkled Types who tan well are sadly most likely to ignore warnings about sun exposure until it's too late.

Sun exposure worsens dry skin, and you are one of the types most vulnerable to sun-induced aging. The UV rays inhibit skin enzymes that produce key components in your skin, and thus damage your skin's ability to hold on to water. That's why sunburned skin flakes and peels off, and this damage can lead to ongoing dryness and flaking. Sun exposure also decreases the skin's hyaluronic acid (HA) content. HA is a chain of sugars that draws water into the skin and plumps it up, giving it volume. Sun-damaged skin tends to have less volume to it due in part to a loss of HA. Sun stimulates the cells to produce melanin, the skin pigment that makes dark spots and freckles.

Some dry, resistant types can feel the sun's drying effect and naturally avoid sun exposure. However, they are more likely to test as tight types, especially if they've avoided the sun their entire lives. I, too, have dry skin, and always protect my skin, a habit I learned from my mum, who is a DSNT like me. My mother was a smoker for many years and could have easily wound up a non-pigmented, wrinkled type rather than a non-pigmented, tight type except that she didn't care for the sun because her non-pigmented skin burned. To me, she's a clear example of how even a single lifestyle factor can change your type.

Sunscreen use is essential to protect against wrinkles and dark spots. Apply it to your face and to the backs of your hands. Purchase a sunscreen that blocks both UVB (which give you a tan) *and* UVA rays (more insidious because they penetrate more deeply into the skin, initiating a collagen breakdown cascade that will ultimately produce wrinkles). The first sun-screens were problematic because they only blocked UVB rays, encouraging people to stay in the sun longer, believing they were protected. Tanning beds, which use UVA rays, are worse for your skin than going to the beach. Avoid them at all costs.

Instead follow the example of Asian women, who hardly worry about skin wrinkling because they follow culturally ingrained skin protective habits. Speaking at conferences in the Far East, I've had frequent opportunities to visit Japan, where many women walk under sun umbrellas when they go out in the sun. It looks so feminine and romantic, unlike our culture where people bare their leathery bodies on the beach. Whatever happened to parasols? Let's bring them back into style.

YOUR MELANOMA RISK

Although you are less likely to get non-melanoma skin cancer than non-pigmented types, light-skinned DRPWs are at greatest risk for developing melanoma skin cancers, which are curable when detected early. Make sure to get annual dermatology checkups, especially if you have frequently sunburned. Light treatments offered by a dermatologist can easily remove any worrisome spots that could develop into non-melanoma skin cancers but it's still important to know your risk factors and get an annual skin cancer exam to look for melanoma lesions.

If you're a DRPW with several of the following factors, you are at higher risk of developing melanoma:

- Light skin
- Sunburn easily
- History of one or more severe sunburns
- Many freckles
- Family members with history of melanoma

While all light-skinned DRPWs should pay heed, any of the above factors will increase your risk. In addition, if you have red hair, your risk *further* increases. Here's why: the MC1R gene is involved in red hair, freckle and melanoma formation, research reveals. Bottom line? Freckles are not just a cosmetic concern. They may be an early warning sign of the potential for future skin cancers. A landmark study published in the *Journal of the American Medical Association* showed that children who used sunscreen developed fewer freckles. While some consider freckles 'cute', their presence may indicate an increased melanoma risk. Any mole that grows suddenly; changes in size, shape, or colour; or bleeds should be seen by a dermatologist immediately. In addition to checking your skin frequently, wear protective clothing and sunscreen when possible. Please consult 'The A, B, C and D of Melanoma' in Chapter Nine for a complete description of what to look out for.

The lip area is most prone to skin cancer because the lips do not secrete sebum, which contains a high concentration of vitamin E, an antioxidant that protects against aging and cancer. That's why some formulations of ChapStick and lip balm contain vitamin E as a protectant. Health food stores also sell vitamin E oil, which, though too oily for most skin areas, can be used on the lips.

A Mother-Daughter Story

Brenda, a fifty-six-year-old widow with flaming red hair, had been a typical fun-loving DRPW in youth. She now had many fine lines, deep wrinkles, freckles, dark spots, and surgical scars from the removal of skin cancers, thanks to far more sun than her freckled and wrinkle-prone skin could handle.

She stopped using Retin-A years before when her doctor informed her that the topical cream and suntanning didn't mix. However, I told Brenda that a new study says that retinoids protect the skin from the sun by inhibiting the formation of collagenase, an enzyme that destroys collagen. They also have an antioxidant effect. However, retinoids do allow UVA and UVB to penetrate more deeply into the skin, which is why they must always be used in conjunction with sunscreen.

Because in youth Brenda had not prevented aging, now she was spending large sums on multiple cosmetic treatments to turn back the clock, such as Intense Pulsed Laser (IPL) treatments for her dark spots, and Botox injections for her forehead and frown lines. Finally, to fill in her lines and replace her skin's volume loss, Brenda received Hylaform Plus injections.

Even though Brenda could easily afford these treatments, there were still limitations to what I could do for her, so she decided to turn her attention to her daughter, Annie.

Annie had inherited her mother's dark auburn hair and DRPW skin – and her father's trust fund. When it concerned Annie, it was hard to say whether Brenda was more overwrought about threadbare Casanovas or sun damage.

'She has my skin,' Brenda announced tragically when she first dragged Annie into my office. Annie rolled her eyes. Aging is not a primary concern when you are nineteen, gorgeous, rich, and have a highly dramatic, over-protective mother – but it should be.

By seeing both ends of the time line, I could validate Brenda's concerns. As the years passed, Annie's clear face could well end up like her mum's unless we intervened now.

When I examined Annie and evaluated her responses to the questionnaire, it was evident that Annie did indeed have the same DRPW skin as her mother. Annie had already begun to develop dark spots on the bridge of her nose and her chest. When I looked at her skin under a special UV light, I could see the presence of sun damage.

I put her on a daily regimen: she would first use a glycolic acid cleanser, which helps hydrate the skin and removes the top layer of dead cells, giving the skin a smoother texture. Following cleansing, she would use a lactic acid moisturiser, which also increases hydration by removing dead cells, helping Annie win the battle against dryness.

Both the glycolic and lactic acids would increase the penetration of the stronger age prevention ingredients Annie's skin needed. These were anti-oxidants (delivered via a sunscreen) to prevent wrinkles, and retinols or retinoids (delivered via a nighttime moisturiser) to prevent wrinkles and dark spots. At night, Annie used a cream cleanser, followed by Renova, a retinoid offered in a very hydrating formulation, which is ideal for dry skin. I warned Annie that if she had any plans to become pregnant, she should discontinue retinoid use as soon as she began trying to get pregnant, or at the very latest, when she became pregnant. Finally, Annie was to use a moisturiser rich in fatty acids, cholesterol and ceramides, as well as an eye cream containing antioxidants to protect the eye area.

Starting young with an antiaging program was like taking out insurance on Annie's skin. Even though her daily programme involved multiple steps, Annie followed it consistently. While I would not recommend as complex a programme for all Skin Types with dry, wrinkle-prone skin, it's well worth it to do everything possible to preserve and protect skin while you're young and possibly avoid expensive procedures after the damage has been done.

A CLOSE-UP LOOK AT YOUR SKIN

Like Annie and Brenda, with DRPW skin you may experience any of the following:

- Dry flaking skin
- Itching
- Thin skin with easy tearing of the skin if you are over fifty
- Easy bruising of the skin
- Dark spots on face, chest, arms and hands
- Wrinkles beginning around the eyes
- Wrinkles on the forehead and between the eyebrows
- Wrinkled hands
- Higher risk of melanoma skin cancer

Aged skin is more likely to be dry. In addition, dry skin is more susceptible to skin aging for several reasons. First, skin enzymes that repair skin damage function less efficiently in skin with a lower water content. Second, dry types produce less sebum, an oily substance that contains large amounts of vitamin E, a skin protective antioxidant that combats aging and skin cancer. Third, the cell cycle (which produces new skin cells) slows down, causing dead skin cells to pile up in little hills and valleys. Though not visible to the naked eyes, these make the skin appear rough. Finally, when oestrogen levels decline with perimenopause and menopause, the skin becomes drier.

TREATING WRINKLES

Yours is an underserved Skin Type. You experiment with various skin care products, but nothing seems to make a difference. In general, over-the-counter products are not strong enough because companies don't offer products with higher concentrations of effective ingredients, because they can't regulate who purchases their products. They compromise and offer lower-strength products that anyone can safely use without side effects. But don't worry, I am trying to get some companies to develop products for this type.

It's my hope that as Skin Typing becomes better known and people learn their type, manufacturers will be able to safely produce products specifically geared towards the different types. Also, now that China and India have become important cosmetic markets, many companies are working to develop skin care for these groups, many of whom are DRPTs and DRPWs. Will these new product lines contain sufficient levels of active ingredients to meet your needs? That remains to be seen.

In any case, until more powerful over-the-counter products are offered, you can use stronger prescription products. Your skin can deal with them. However, you must commit to consistent sunscreen use to protect your skin, because retinoid prescription medication may allow increased penetration of the sun's harmful sun rays. Despite this, in my opinion, it's the most valuable product for DRPW skin because it prevents wrinkles and dark spots, and even helps to eliminate existing dark spots and some fine wrinkles. Buy the cheapest cleansers and sunscreens, because your resistant skin does not require babying. Instead, save your money for prescription medications like retinoids that really do the job.

Retinols and DRPWs

To prevent or minimise the wrinkles to which this type is prone, many DRPWs use retinol in over-the-counter cosmetics or Retin-A in prescription formulations. They both work the same way, by increasing cell renewal and preventing the breakdown in collagen, which is a key contributor to skin aging.

Which is right for you? Here are the pros and cons.

On the one hand, most nonprescription retinol-containing products are not sufficiently concentrated to completely address all your spots or wrinkles. Retinol is very unstable. If in the manufacturing or packaging process it's exposed to air or light, it will be rendered ineffective. The packaging itself must keep the product protected from light, which is why aluminium tubes are frequently used. A retinol product offered in a clear jar or bottle is inactive. That's why my product recommendations list creams that I know are produced and packaged in the right way. If you are starting young and have not yet begun to see wrinkles (or if your wrinkles are just beginning to show), they may help. However, you may find that they are not strong enough and that you need to graduate to prescription-strength products, especially if you have many visible wrinkles already.

Many DRPWs have trouble with prescription-strength products because they cannot tolerate the dryness and flaking that result from the full-strength retinoids. That's why I'll guide you in introducing retinoid use in a way your dry skin can tolerate.

Still, for you I maintain that a retinoid prescription product will give the best value. Most antiaging creams will either not contain sufficient quantities of active ingredients or, if they are potent enough, they will most likely be expensive (over £100) because of the high cost of these ingredients. A £90 prescription of Avage cream would do more for you. The prescriptions usually last for one year. At the dermatologist visit, be sure to ask for an all-over skin cancer check. You are at a risk for melanoma and this visit could also save your life.

Gina, a popular scuba instructor at a local resort, had the lively personality, dark eyes, and medium-toned skin typical of her Sicilian ancestry. Also typical was her readiness to speak her mind about just about anything.

A divorcée, Gina had a trim, toned physique that allowed her to look great in form-fitting clothes designed for women half her age. But her DRPW skin (and her greying hair) made Gina look every day of her forty-three years, and then some. Snacking on power bars, guzzling diet drinks, teenage smoking, and a suntanned youth had endowed Gina with abundant wrinkles without the beneficial antioxidants to protect her. Yes, she got some lycopene from her grandmother's tomato sauce, but how often did she visit her grandmother?

When she came in to see me, Gina was agitated about her appearance because, to her, aging was the enemy for one simple reason: each line and wrinkle blocked the way to Mr Right.

'I know he's out there,' she informed me during her skin exam. My job, should I choose to accept it, was to remove any facial obstacle to marital bliss – a tall order.

Before the birth of her son, Gina had briefly tried Retin-A but had discontinued its use when she wanted to start a family. In her late thirties, as wrinkles and lines formed, she had decided to give it another go and had obtained a prescription from a dermatologist. But she hated the way it made her skin feel and became convinced that retinoids were not for her.

'My skin moulted like a snake's,' she complained.

I prevailed upon Gina to give retinoids another try, but this time follow my instructions for introducing them slowly. She agreed, and to her surprise, she was able to tolerate them and derive their benefits.

When I next saw Gina, about six months later, some of the wrinkles which had so concerned her had already begun to disappear. I reminded her that the longer she used the retinoid, the better it would work. It was preventing future wrinkles as well as getting rid of the ones she had now. 'I wish you could prevent grey hairs,' she retorted and laughed as she tossed her newly brown locks on her way out of the office.

Wrinkle Prevention

In addition to using retinoids, antioxidants are another vital ingredient in your antiwrinkle campaign because they block the harmful effects of free radicals. Free radicals are oxygen molecules that have an odd number of electrons. They like to have an even number, so they 'steal' electrons from vital skin components such as DNA and cell membrane lipids. Losing the electron damages the DNA or cell membrane lipids, leading to skin cancers and aging.

Although antioxidant green tea has been proven beneficial to the skin, many products contain such low amounts that they are near to worthless. Green tea turns brown when used in large amounts; as a result, companies often only put in small quantities. The products I'll recommend that are brown contain higher quantities of green tea. Don't let the brown colour worry you. Think about the benefit to your skin.

L-ascorbic acid, or vitamin C, is another important antioxidant in the skin. Studies have shown that it both prevents the breakdown of collagen *and* increases collagen production. However, vitamin C comes in many forms, and not all of them are helpful. Vitamin C esters attached to a fatty acid are poorly absorbed into the skin when applied topically, so products that contain this form of vitamin C are not that effective, while certain other forms of vitamin C, such as L-ascorbic acid, penetrate the skin more readily. That's why I'll be recommending vitamin C-containing products that really work.

To combat dryness, topical oestrogen creams and soy-containing products are an option for female postmenopausal DRPWs who do not opt for hormone replacement therapy. Fortunately, there are also many new technologies that can help treat the problems common to this type.

If wrinkles have already appeared, you need it all. And if you feel distressed at having to go to such lengths to retain a youthful appearance, consider this: thankfully, you are not a sensitive type, which means that your resistant skin can handle the strong stuff.

Dr Baumann's Bottom Line: Spend the money to see a dermatologist. It will save you money in the long run. If you go to a spa, forget the facial treatments and get a massage. They can't do anything strong enough to help you – but I can.

EVERYDAY CARE FOR YOUR SKIN TYPE

The goal of your skin care routine is to address wrinkles, dark spots, and dryness with products that deliver lightening, moisturising and antiwrinkle ingredients. All the products I'll recommend act to do one or both of the following:

- Prevent and treat wrinkles
- Prevent and treat dark spots

In addition, your daily regimen will also help to address your other skin concerns by:

- Preventing and treating dryness

Your daily regimen is based on protecting, hydrating and moisturising your dry skin. But since your skin is resistant, you need strong ingredients to treat your wrinkles and dark spots.

I've provided two nonprescription regimens for you, the first for when you have no dark spots and the second for when you do. I know that many of you will first want to try the nonprescription dark spots regimen.

Nevertheless, in my opinion, you'd do best to jump to my prescription regimens, which deliver the strong ingredients you need to protect your skin from aging as well as treat wrinkles and dark spots. I've provided two of these as well, one for times when dark spots are present and the other for when they're not. If you can afford it, go straight to your dermatologist, who can prescribe the strong products that may really work for you.

DAILY SKIN CARE

STAGE ONE: NONPRESCRIPTION REGIMEN

For when you have no spots:

AM	PM
Step 1: Wash with cleanser	Step 1: Wash with cleanser
Step 2: Apply eye cream	Step 2: Use an exfoliator
Step 3: Apply antiaging serum to face, neck and chest	Step 3: Apply eye cream
Step 4: Apply moisturiser with sunscreen to face, neck and chest	Step 4: Apply a retinol-containing moisturiser
Step 5: Apply foundation (optional)	Step 5: Apply a moisturiser

In the morning, wash with cleanser, then apply eye cream. Next, apply an antiaging serum to your face, neck and chest. Apply moisturiser and/or sunscreen, and then finish with foundation if you wish to use one. Assure you attain an SPF of 15 or more from the products you use.

In the evening, wash with a cleanser. Then, once a week, use microdermabrasion or an exfoliating scrub as your second step. Look for options and instructions under 'Exfoliation'. Next, apply eye cream, and then a night cream containing retinol. Finish with a moisturiser.

STAGE ONE: NONPRESCRIPTION REGIMEN

To get rid of dark spots:

AM	PM
Step 1: Wash with cleanser	Step 1: Wash with cleanser
Step 2: Apply eye cream	Step 2: Use an exfoliator
Step 3: Apply lightening serum or gel to dark spots	Step 3: Apply eye cream

Step 4: Apply moisturiser with
      sunscreen

Step 5: Apply foundation
      (optional)

Step 4: Apply lightening serum or
      gel to dark spots

Step 5: Apply moisturiser
      containing retinol

Step 6: Apply night cream

In the morning, wash with cleanser, then apply eye cream. Next, apply lightening serum or gel to your dark spots. Then apply moisturiser with SPF to your face, neck and chest. Finally, apply foundation if you choose. Make sure your product selection provides a minimum SPF of 15.

In the evening, wash with a cleanser. Then, use an exfoliating scrub or microdermabrasion kit one to four times a week (see instructions under 'Exfoliation' below). Apply eye cream, then apply a lightening serum or gel to your dark spots. Next, apply a moisturiser containing retinol. Finish with a night cream.

There's one more option you can try to get rid of resistant dark spots before seeing your dermatologist. It's the Alpha Beta Daily Face Peel by Dr Dennis Gross, which you can find at www.mdskincare.com or www.Baumannstore.co.uk. I would prefer that you see a dermatologist, but this is the next best thing. Use it once daily as the second step of the regimen. (In that case, Step 2 would become Step 3, and so on.) If after one week, you experience no redness or irritation, you can use it twice a day.

Cleansers

DRPWs benefit from cleansers containing ingredients like glycolic acid that hydrate, exfoliate and moisturise the skin, as well as antioxidants that help prevent wrinkles. The UK has different regulations than the US on the use of glycolic acid,, so you may be able to find stronger products, suited to your resistant skin, in the US. However, recent research suggests that alpha hydroxy acids (AHA) may make the skin more sensitive to sunlight. So if you are out in the sun a lot and tend to be lax about sunscreen use, you may not want to use a glycolic acid cleanser. In that case, my next choice is Topix Replenix Fortified Cleanser, which contains antioxidants such as vitamins A, C and E, green tea and white tea.

RECOMMENDED CLEANSING PRODUCTS

£ Gly Derm Gentle Cleanser (has glycolic acid 2%)

££ DDF Glycolic Exfoliating Wash 7%

££ Jan Marini Bioglycolic Facial Cleanser

££ MD Forté Facial Cleanser II (has glycolic acid 15%)

££ MD Forté Facial Cleanser III (has glycolic acid 20%)

££ Topix Replenix Fortified Cleanser

££ Vichy Rich Detoxifying Cleansing Cream

£££ MD Formulations Facial Cleanser

£££ Rodan & Fields Reverse Wash (with lactic acid)

Baumann's Choice: MD Forté Facial Cleanser III because it has 20 percent glycolic acid, a high percentage that allows ingredients in eye creams and moisturisers to penetrate better. You can find it at www.Baumannstore.co.uk.

Serums and Emulsions

These products should contain antioxidants or skin lighteners to treat dark spots. I never thought I would find a vitamin C product that I could recommend until recent advances resulted in the development of La Roche-Posay Active C and others that are perfect for your Skin Type. The vitamin C reduces pigment and increases collagen production to improve and treat wrinkles.

RECOMMENDED SERUMS AND EMULSIONS

££ La Roche-Posay Active C

££ Laura Mercier Multi Vitamin Serum

££ Philosophy Save Me (with retinol and vitamin C)

££ Replenix Retinol Smoothing Serum

££ Vichy Reti-C

£££ SkinCeuticals C + AHA serum

£££ SkinCeuticals C E Ferulic

Baumann's Choice: La Roche-Posay Active C or one of the SkinCeuticals products. Here you need to splurge to get the best product; formulating vitamin C properly is expensive.

Moisturisers

Your moisturiser and eye cream should contain hydrating, lightening and antioxidant ingredients. In addition, your daytime moisturiser should contain sunscreen.

RECOMMENDED DAYTIME MOISTURISERS

- £ Neutrogena Ultimate Moisture Day Cream (with soy)
- £ Nivea Antiwrinkle Q10 Plus Day Cream
- £ Olay Regenerist Replenishing Cream
- £ Roc Retin-Ox Anti-wrinkle serum–max.
- ££ Elizabeth Arden Ceramide Plump Perfect Moisture Cream SPF 30
- ££ Laura Mercier Mega Moisturiser with SPF 15
- ££ L'Occitane Face and Body Balm SPF 30
- ££ Pevonia Glycocides Cream
- ££ Vichy Nutrilogie 1 SPF 15 Sunscreen Lotion
- £££ Bobbi Brown Extra SPF 25 Moisturising Balm
- £££ La Prairie Cellular Moisturiser Face

Baumann's Choice: Roc Retin-Ox Anti-wrinkle serum–max. This has retinol. Make sure you buy the max and not the light because it's stronger.

RECOMMENDED NIGHT CREAMS

- £ Neutrogena Visibly Young Night Cream
- £ Nivea Antiwrinkle Q10 Plus Night Cream
- £ Olay Regenerist Replenishing Cream
- ££ Elizabeth Arden Ceramide Moisture Network Night Cream
- ££ Kiehl's Lycopene Facial Moisturising Cream
- ££ Laura Mercier Night Nutrition Renewal Crème
- ££ L'Occitane Shea Butter Ultra Moisturising Night Care
- ££ Origins Look Alive Vitality Moisture Cream
- ££ Topix Citrix 20% (vitamin C)
- ££ Z. Bigatti Re-Storation Enlighten Skin Tone Provider
- £££ Crème de la Mer
- £££ Ella Baché Age Defence Night Cream
- £££ Sekkisei Cream Excellent

Baumann's Choice: Kiehl's Lycopene Facial Moisturising Cream, with lycopene to prevent wrinkles.

RECOMMENDED EVENING MOISTURISERS
CONTAINING RETINOL

£ Roc Retin-Ox Correxion Intensive Nourishing Anti-wrinkle Care
££ Philosophy Help Me face cream with retinol
££ Sothy's Retinol 15
££ Topix Replenix Retinol Smoothing Serum 3x
£££ Clarins Renew Plus Night Lotion
£££ Estée Lauder Diminish Anti-Wrinkle Retinal Treatment
£££ Jan Marini Factor A Plus Lotion
£££ Lancôme Resurface
£££ Prescriptives Skin Renewal Cream
£££ SkinCeuticals Retinol 0.5 or 1%

Baumann's Choice: Roc Retin-Ox Correxion Intensive Nourishing Anti-wrinkle Care

RECOMMENDED EYE CREAMS

£ Aveda Pure Vital Moisture Eye Cream
£ Nivea Visage CoEnzyme Q_{10} Plus Wrinkle Control Eye Cream with SPF 4
£ Olay Regenerist Eye Lifting Serum
££ Dermalogica Intense Eye Repair
££ Elizabeth Arden Ceramide Plump Perfect Eye Moisture Cream SPF 15
££ Korres Eye Bright Firming Eye Cream
££ La Roche-Posay Active-C Eyes
££ Laura Mercier Eyedration Eye Cream
££ Origins Eye Doctor
££ Relastin Eye Cream
£££ Erno Lazlo Ocu-pHel Emollient Eye Cream
£££ SkinCeuticals C + AHA exfoliating antioxidant treatment

Baumann's Choice: Active-C Eyes by La Roche-Posay

Exfoliation

To exfoliate when you're on a nonprescription regimen, use a scrub or microdermabrasion kit once, then wait a week to see how you tolerate it. If your skin does not become red or feel tender, use the kit two times the next week. After two weeks you can move to three times a week. Very resistant skin may even be able to tolerate microdermabrasion creams or scrubs four times a week, but in most cases this will be too irritating.

As an alternative to home care, you can go to a spa for an exfoliation treatment. Be sure your spa services professional uses an exfoliator with antioxidant ingredients.

If you're on the prescription regimen you don't need to exfoliate, since you'll be using prescription retinoids, which will exfoliate for you.

RECOMMENDED MICRODERMABRASION OR EXFOLIATION KITS

- £ Aapri Apricot Scrub
- £ Avon Sweet Finish Sugar Scrub
- £ L'Oréal ReFinish Micro-Dermabrasion Kit (but use a moisturiser on my list rather than the one in the kit)
- ££ Ahava Gentle Mud Exfoliator
- ££ Clinique 7 Day Scrub Cream
- ££ Neova Microdermabrasion Scrub
- ££ Philosophy Resurface
- £££ Dr Brandt Microdermabrasion in a Jar

Baumann's Choice: Clinique 7 Day Scrub Cream, which I use myself. I love the texture and it also provides some moisture.

SHOPPING FOR PRODUCTS

With resistant skin, should you wish to, you can widen your selection from the products I specifically recommend. Look for products that contain the recommended ingredients and where those you should avoid are minimal. If you find a favourite product that contains these ingredients but is not on my list of recommendations, please go to www.DrBaumann.co.uk and share it with me.

RECOMMENDED SKIN CARE INGREDIENTS

To prevent wrinkles:

- Basil
- Caffeine
- Camilla sinensis (green tea, white tea)
- Coenzyme Q_{10} (ubiquinone)
- Copper peptide
- Curcumin (tetrahydracurcumin or turmeric)
- Ferulic acid
- Feverfew
- Ginger
- Ginseng
- Grape seed extract
- Idebenone
- Lutein
- Lycopene
- Punica granatum (pomegranate)
- Pycnogenol (a pine bark extract)
- Rosemary
- Silymarin
- Vitamin C
- Vitamin E
- Yucca

To improve the appearance of wrinkles:

- Alpha hydroxy acids (glycolic acid, lactic acid)
- DMAE
- Retinol
- Vitamin C (asorbic acid)

To moisturise:

- Aloe vera
- Borage seed oil
- Ceramide
- Cholesterol
- Cocoa butter
- Colloidal oatmeal
- Dexpanthenol (pro-vitamin B_5)
- Dimethicone
- Evening primrose oil
- Glycerin
- Glycolic acid
- Jojoba oil
- Lactic acid
- Linoleic acid
- Niacinamide
- Olive oil
- Safflower oil
- Shea butter

To prevent dark spots:

- Cocos nucifera (coconut extract)
- Pycnogenol (a pine bark extract)

- Cucumber
- Niacinamide
- Saxifraga sarmentosa extract (strawberry begonia)

To improve dark spots:

- Arbutin
- Vitamin C (ascorbic acid)
- Cucumber extract
- Glycyrrhiza glabra (licorice extract)
- Kojic acid
- Magnesium ascorbyl phosphate
- Mulberry extract
- Tyrostat

SKIN CARE INGREDIENTS TO AVOID:

- Alcohol
- Detergents that foam vigorously

Alcohol, often used as an ingredient in skin care, can increase dryness. However, not every kind of alcohol is a problem. A glycol is a beneficial alcohol that increases the penetration of other ingredients. But alcohol that has a low molecular weight, such as ethanol, denatured alcohol, ethyl alcohol, methanol, benzyl alcohol, isopropyl alcohol and SD alcohol, should be avoided.

Sun Protection for Your Skin

Whenever you're in the sun for longer than fifteen minutes, you need extra protection, over and above your everyday SPF. So at those times of longer exposure, layer on a sunscreen that is SPF 45 or more. For DRPWs, I suggest cream or lotion sunscreens. If your skin is very dry, use cream; if it's only slightly dry, use lotion. Fortunately for you, there are no sunscreen ingredients you need to avoid.

Studies show most people apply only a quarter of the amount of sunscreen that they need. If a high price will make you unwilling to apply a large amount, avoid expensive sunscreens: you need to use about a 10p-size dollop on each exposed area, your face, neck, hands and chest. Make sure the combined SPF of all products you use during the day, such as moisturiser, sunscreen, and foundation, will provide an SPF of at least 15.

RECOMMENDED SUN PROTECTION PRODUCTS

£ Boots No7 Sun Protection Energising Facial Suncare SPF 15

£ Hawaiian Tropic Baby Faces Sunblock SPF 60+

£ Nivea Sun Face Sunscreen SPF 30

££ Garnier Ambre Solaire Ultra Protect Face Cream SPF 50

££ La Roche-Posay Anthelios Fluide Extreme SPF 60 (available in Ireland)

££ SkinCeuticals Ultimate UV Defence SPF 30

£££ Darphin Sun Block SPF 30

£££ Decléor Écran Très Haute Protection SPF 40

£££ Orlane B21 Soleil Vitamines Face Cream SPF 15

Baumann's Choice: SkinCeuticals Ultimate UV Defence SPF 30 with antioxidants as well as sunscreen or SkinCeuticals Sport UV Defence SPF 45 if you want a sweatproof sunscreen.

Your Makeup

Wait a few minutes after applying sunscreen to apply foundation or other cosmetic products. This gives your sunscreen time to soak in. If you have very dry skin, look for cream eyeshadows and blushers. A nice cream eyeshadow for your type is Laura Mercier Metallic Creme Eye Colour. Avoid powders, which will make your skin look drier.

RECOMMENDED FOUNDATIONS

£ Boots No7 Radiant Glow Foundation SPF 15

£ Max Factor Pan-Stick Ultra-Creamy Makeup

£ Revlon Age Defying MakeUp SPF 15

££ Awake Skin Renovation Foundation

££ Bloom Foundation

££ Chantecaille Real Skin Foundation SPF 30 for Dry Skin

££ Laura Mercier Tinted Moisturiser

££ Vichy Aera Teint Silky Cream Foundation

£££ La Prairie Cellular Treatment Foundation

£££ Versace Fluid Moisture Foundation

Baumann's Choice: Revlon Age Defying MakeUp SPF 15; I prefer a foundation with sunscreen.

CONSULTING A DERMATOLOGIST

PRESCRIPTION SKIN CARE STRATEGIES

The first prescription regimen below uses both a prescription retinoid and a prescription bleaching cream to get rid of dark spots. The second regimen uses retinoids in a cream formulation to prevent and treat wrinkles.

When you are on a prescription regimen, you don't need to use facial scrubs or at-home microdermabrasion kits.

DAILY SKIN CARE

STAGE TWO: PRESCRIPTION REGIMEN

To get rid of dark spots:

AM	PM
Step 1: Wash with an over-the-counter cleanser that contains glycolic or lactic acid	Step 1: Wash with an over-the-counter cleanser that contains glycolic or lactic acid
Step 2: Apply prescription bleaching cream to dark spots	Step 2: Apply prescription bleaching cream to dark spots
Step 3: Apply moisturiser with antioxidants	Step 3: Apply a nighttime moisturiser
Step 4: Apply sunscreen	Step 4: Apply a prescription retinoid
Step 5: Apply foundation (optional)	

In the morning, wash your face with a cleanser containing glycolic or lactic acid, selected from my nonprescription recommendations. Next, apply a prescription bleaching cream to your dark spots. If you wish to use an eye cream, you can do so between Steps 2 and 3, but it's optional. Next, apply a moisturiser that contains antioxidants, then put on your sunscreen (if your moisturiser or foundation do not provide a minimal coverage of SPF 15). Finally, apply foundation if you wish. You can also mix a sunscreen in with either your moisturiser or foundation, and apply them together.

In the evening, wash your face with the same cleanser used in the morning. Apply a prescription bleaching cream to your dark spots, and then a nighttime moisturiser. Finally, apply a prescription retinoid to your face, neck and chest according to the instructions in 'Further Help for Dry, Resistant Skin'.

PRESCRIPTION REGIMEN

For when you have no dark spots:

AM	PM
Step 1: Wash with an over-the-counter cleanser that contains glycolic or lactic acid	Step 1: Wash with an over-the-counter cleanser that contains glycolic or lactic acid
Step 2: Apply antiaging serum to the entire face	Step 2: Apply eye cream
Step 3: Apply moisturiser with antioxidants	Step 3: Apply moisturising night cream
Step 4: Apply sunscreen	Step 4: Apply prescription retinoid
Step 5: Apply foundation	

In the morning, wash your face with a glycolic or lactic acid-containing cleanser. Next, apply an antiaging serum to your entire face, then apply a moisturiser that contains antioxidants, followed by a sunscreen (if your moisturiser or foundation does not provide a minimal coverage of SPF 15). Finally, apply foundation if you choose to wear it. You can also mix a sunscreen in with either your moisturiser or foundation, and apply them together.

In the evening, wash with the same cleanser you used in the morning. Then apply an eye cream and a moisturising night cream, followed by a prescription retinoid according to the instructions in 'Further Help for Dry, Resistant Skin'.

In some cases, unless otherwise noted, the products I'll recommend next are US name brands that may not be available in your country. Please ask your dermatologist to help you find a substitution.

RECOMMENDED PRESCRIPTION PRODUCTS

To combat dark spots:

- Alustra
- Claripel
- Eldoquin Forte
- Epi-Quin Micro
- Lustra
- Solaquin Forte
- Tri-Luma

Baumann's Choice: Hydroquinone, the main ingredient in these products, is not allowed in the UK. Please ask your dermatologiat for recommendations that are available in your country.

For wrinkles:

- Aknemycin Plus (has an antibiotic as well)
- Differin gel or cream
- Isotrex
- Isotrexin (has an antiobiotic as well)
- Retin-A gel, lotion or cream
- Retinova

Baumann's Choice: Any of these are good. Look for a cream form rather than a gel.

PROCEDURES FOR YOUR SKIN TYPE

In my experience, most DRPWs with medium to dark skin tones can best treat their dark spots with prescription topical products and chemical peels. Lasers and light treatments cannot be used on dark skin, since these procedures can lead to inflammation and worsening, or development, of dark spots. People with resistant, pigmented skin are at an advantage over SP types, because they can use stronger ingredients without fear of sensitivity, and these stronger ingredients may work faster. Still, you should expect to wait about four to six weeks to see improvement.

DRPWs with light skin have the added option of skin procedures such as laser and light therapy to lighten the dark spots without causing inflammation that leads to more dark spots. Please see 'Further Help for Dry, Resistant Skin'.

For wrinkle treatment, both lighter- and darker-skinned DRPWs can benefit from botulinum toxin injections and dermal fillers. Please see 'Further Help for Oily, Resistant Skin' for detailed information about these procedures.

Lighter-skinned DRPWs also have the option of dermabrasion, a resurfacing treatment for lines around the mouth. This method requires an experienced physician. For more details on the procedure and finding physicians who can perform it, see 'Dermabrasion' in the procedures section of Chapter Ten.

ONGOING CARE FOR YOUR SKIN

Protect – and moisturise without delay – every day. Pay attention to prevention now and eat an antioxidant-rich diet. Although aging well is one of your chief challenges, many new technologies can help address your problems. See a dermatologist. You'll never regret it.

CHAPTER SEVENTEEN

Dry, Resistant, Pigmented and Tight: DRPT

THE GLOBAL SKIN TYPE

'Beauty is a state of mind. But attitude alone is not enough. I like to take care of myself, so of course, I take care of my skin. Why not make the best of what Mother Nature gave you?'

ABOUT YOUR SKIN

If your questionnaire results revealed you as a DRPT, you share this Skin Type with many beautiful women from every place on this planet. Italian icons, like Sophia Loren; Asian stunners, like Lucy Liu; gorgeous women of colour, like Halle Berry; and striking Spanish beauties like Penelope Cruz all have that golden-toned DRPT skin. Although not every DRPT will be blessed with their gorgeous, rich skin colour, nearly every ethnic group can have this Skin Type. Though less common among Caucasians of northern European background, this Skin Type can occur among all groups, making it one of the most universal.

Your smooth, ageless skin is the envy of other types who struggle with wrinkles. You're rarely troubled with oiliness and outbreaks, and pass through your teens and twenties unconcerned. Though your skin may grow slightly drier as you age, this can be easily addressed since your resistant skin can readily handle products that other types must avoid.

Although light- and medium-toned DRPTs tan quite well due to their moderate to high pigment levels, tanning can cause wrinkles, dark spots, and melasma, and is best avoided. Most of you have got the message to shun excess sun exposure. Along with good genes and a healthy diet, that's why you enjoy the blessings of tight skin.

Constant moisture will help preserve your skin's youthful qualities. Be vigilant to protect your skin from the elements and use non-drying products.

Tight skin results from a combination of lifestyle factors and genes, and for the majority of DRPTs, good genes play a major part. In medium- to dark-skin-toned people, resistant, highly pigmented skin tends to wrinkle less. It has more resilience and lifelong elasticity than lighter-toned skin. For lighter-skinned people who scored as DRPTs, lifestyle factors play a bigger role in maintaining your skin tightness. Using moisturisers, avoiding the sun, eating antioxidant-filled fruits and vegetables, never smoking, protecting your skin from drying environments like chlorine pools, hot rooms, cold winds, drying climes, steam baths, and even facials are key to maintaining your dry, tight skin.

DRPT CELEBRITY

Actress Lucy Liu brings talent, beauty, and high energy to her roles in film and television. She first came to attention as a cast member of the hit TV series *Ally McBeal* and attained film stardom as part of the dynamic trio in *Charlie's Angels*. The daughter of Chinese immigrants living in New York City, Liu both embraces her cultural origins (by studying Chinese culture, language and martial arts) and transcends them (by playing parts that are not ethnically designated as Asian).

My guess, though I can't prove it, is that Liu is a DRPT, which is one of the two most common Skin Types among people of Asian descent (the other common type is DSPT). With hours under movie lights wearing makeup, I can't rule out that Liu may have developed some skin sensitivity. However, with no sign of it, I'd judge her as a Resistant Skin Type. What we can see are her freckles, clear signs of pigmentation. Liu needs more sun protection as sun exposure can increase pigmentation and result in freckling and dark spots.

Liu skis, rock climbs, and rides horses. With her physically active lifestyle (not to mention the leaps, fights and skirmishes she enacted during the filming of *Charlie's Angels* and *Kill Bill*), she might possibly be at risk for one of the DRPT's key problems. In the aftermath of cuts, bruises and scrapes, pigmentation results in dark spots that take a while to heal. While not seen in Liu's films and photos, it may be because Hollywood makeup artists have covered them with a base foundation. Or perhaps Liu is under a dermatologist's care. Whatever the case, I hope Liu is now taking steps to protect her beautiful tight skin with sunscreen. Bridging two cultures with daring and aplomb, Liu is a true twenty-first-century heroine with a beauty that's worth preserving.

PIGMENTATION AND YOUR SKIN

While this Skin Type is common among people with medium and darker skin tones, some DRPTs do have light skin with many skin areas showing signs of pigmentation, such as dark spots, freckles, melasma or sunspots. If you're an Irish redhead with a tendency to freckle, don't retake the test; this can be your type as well. What you all have in common is the tendency to pigment. Redheads may have trouble getting a tan but they easily freckle. Darker-skinned DRPTs tan easily but are more susceptible to dark spots.

Many people consider freckles attractive, but there are a wide variety of other ways that higher pigment levels show up, and they aren't so pretty. Pigmentation and skin dryness may interact to give you rough, dark, dry patches over the knees and elbows. No amount of scrubbing with soap and water will remove these 'dirty' looking areas.

Dark raised bumps may appear on the backs of your arms and on the sides of your thighs. Called keratosis pilaris, these unsightly bumps, which are about the size of a pinpoint, are produced by friction and skin dryness. Your parents or siblings likely have them too, as they can run in families.

You're also susceptible to developing dark spots on your face, especially when you are pregnant, on oral contraceptives, or hormone replacement therapy, as higher oestrogen levels make melanocytes produce more melanin (skin pigment). For both men and women, sun exposure can instigate freckles or sunspots anywhere on the body. When these appear on the hands, they're called liver spots.

Dark patches can result from skin traumas, such as cuts, ingrown hairs or pimples, as well as heat exposure. In low humidity and cold, your dry skin gets even drier, especially on your arms and legs. When exceptionally dry, your skin may itch. Dry skin worsens with age, which is why preserving skin moisture and hydration is crucial.

Dark spots, patches, and melasma all result from high pigment levels. Dryness, rough fabrics, or any form of heat, irritation or inflammation will stimulate their formation.

Light-skinned DRPTs can benefit from dermatological procedures to treat dark spots, while medium-dark- and Asian-skinned people should follow my product recommendations for dark skin.

Finally, thick, velvety-looking dark patches that appear *under* the arms could be a skin disorder called acanthosis nigricans, which is most common in overweight people. The skin-lightening ingredients I'll offer will not treat this condition. Instead, see your physician, who may recommend that you lose weight.

Rosa's Story

With medium-toned skin, dark hair and almond-shaped eyes, Rosa was a thirty-five-year-old former beauty show contestant. She always took good care of her skin by wearing sunscreen and avoiding the sun because she knew that her light-toned skin conferred an increased risk of skin cancer.

One day, Rosa noticed a 'peach fuzz' of dark hair on her upper lip. Although she didn't realise it, the hair growth resulted from hormones in her birth control pills. Certain types of synthetically produced hormones, called progestins and present in some birth control pills, can fit into receptors in hair follicles to stimulate hair growth. Unaware of this, Rosa had her new peach fuzz removed via a hot wax treatment at a beauty salon. Afterwards, she noticed a dark shadow darkening the skin over her upper lip. To make matters worse, when the fuzz grew back, the dark shadow made the fuzz even more noticeable.

Fed up, Rosa decided to address her problem and came see me to schedule a hair removal laser treatment. After Rosa filled out the Baumann Skin Type Questionnaire, it revealed her as a DRPT. With that knowledge, I questioned her and it soon became clear what had happened.

While her particular brand of birth control pills caused the hair growth on her upper lip, hot waxing only made matters worse because the heat and trauma stimulated the production of skin pigment. The end result was a form of melasma. Rosa's upper lip had become a war zone with escalating hormonal expression and pigment production.

To undo the damage, we had to de-escalate by reversing the steps that led to her condition and address her needs in better ways. First of all, changing the birth control pill formulation can frequently resolve the problem. Some brands help eliminate facial hair, and different people react differently to different medications. Rosa went to her gynaecologist, who prescribed a newer brand, which contained a form of progestin less likely to lead to hair growth.

Rosa needed a method of hair removal that did not use intense heat. I recommended laser hair removal that employs a cooling device such as a spray or a cool gel to lower skin temperature during treatment.

In addition, I advised she use a sunscreen containing ingredients that block UVA rays that lead to dark spots. For use every morning on the dark areas, I prescribed a prescription skin lightener and daily sunscreen use. Two weeks after changing oral contraceptives and using the new regimen, her 'dark shadow' disappeared. After three laser treatments, each about four weeks apart, the hair over her lip was barely visible. Plus, with her new pills, Rosa wouldn't have to fear a regrowth.

A CLOSE-UP LOOK AT YOUR SKIN

Like Rosa, with DRPT skin you may experience:

- Dry skin
- Rough patches over the knees and elbows that appear darker than the rest of your skin
- Freckles or sunspots
- Dark patches on cheeks (such as melasma, or mask of pregnancy)
- Dark eye circles, giving you a raccoon-like appearance
- Dark areas in site of previous injury or inflammation, such as a cut, pimple or scrape
- Itching skin
- Flaking skin
- Chemical peels or other treatments worsen dark spots

Under-eye circles are quite common, caused by decreased (or congested) blood flow, which is thought to result in the deposit under the eyes of a substance called hemisiderin, which also appears in bruised skin, causing the purplish colour. Beneficial eye creams will include vitamin K or arnica, which address dark circles by speeding up the rate at which the purplish cast clears.

Over time, some DRPT skin issues worsen while others improve. Women experience a lessening of melasma when oestrogen levels drop due to mid-life changes. On the other hand, freckles and sun spots increase with age, as does drying, which often worsens after menopause.

ASIAN DRPTS

From my extensive travels to the Far East and many discussions with colleagues from different countries there, I've learned about the different approach to skin care practised in that part of the world. Asian consumers are really into skin care, and many international companies, like L'Oréal and Shiseido, market product lines especially devoted to Asian skin. Koreans are very interested in the advanced dermatology procedures in which I specialise, and a number of prominent Korean doctors have visited or served as guest fellows at my clinic. The textbook I authored is translated into Korean, and there are a number of high-end Korean skin care lines devoted to DRPTs.

Although many Asians complain of oily skin, when I measure their surface skin oil, they most often are dry types, revealing that it's hard for people to accurately assess their own skin. The majority of Asians are pigmented types, and fall into the DRPT and DSPT categories. Asians are less concerned with wrinkling than with dark-spot treatment, a major emphasis in product offerings for the Asian market. For some reason, Asians are also more vulnerable to developing pigmentation problems after long-term use of hydroquinone, a skin lightener used in the US That's why in Asia and elsewhere, other ingredients, such as kojic acid, are used to lighten skin. Although in the US and Australia, dermatologists can offer patients hydroquinone-containing products, elsewhere kojic acid, azelaic acid, and other bleaching agents are used instead.

Highlights of an Asian Beauty Ritual

In the Far East, the approach to cleansing is radically different from that practised by Americans. Most Asians would not dream of using soap or soapy cleansers on their dry skin, because as part of their cultural beauty wisdom, they know that such products strip the oils from the skin. Although American companies have developed products that act like cleansers but do not contain harsh detergents in order to satisfy the American preference for cleansers, Asians don't use them. They prefer to cleanse with oil, a makeup remover, water-based gel, and finish with a cream.

The next step is called 'the caring step', in which they supply a special treatment to their skin. This could be a cosmetic water to increase hydration or what is called a 'white perfecter', a kind of depigmentation agent used to lessen dark spots, melasma, or other skin discolourations.

Following that, they might apply a treatment serum and would next treat acne, afterwards using a product to treat or prevent wrinkles. They would finish their ritual by applying moisturiser and a special eye cream.

Asians are religious in their sun avoidance and use of sunscreen to protect the clarity of their complexions. They might use an SPF of 50 or more on a daily basis and shun the sun, using hats, parasols and sun protective clothing. Many Asian women also use foundation and face powder, and there are a wide range of different hues to meet their needs. Although Caucasian skin can usually be matched by eight different foundation shades, it takes over forty shades to match the wide range of Asian skin tones.

Because of these many beauty products, Asians are exposed to many ingredients, and are therefore more likely to develop reactions which could potentially degrade the skin barrier and increase skin sensitivity, which is why many also fall into the DSPT Skin Type.

With age, there is a tendency for Asian skin to become more yellow in colour, which occurs when one kind of skin pigment called eumelanin converts to pheomelanin, a second type where the yellow tone predominates. Yet another reason why many Asian women rely upon foundation. Many of the skin care techniques that have evolved in the different Asian countries will benefit people of Asian ethnicity who reside in the West, as well as other DRPTs, which is why I've included some of these techniques in the DRPT's Daily Skin Care Regimens.

BLACK DRPTS

DRPTs with dark-toned skin are prone to develop 'ashiness', which is a grey appearance caused by flaking skin lighter in colour than the dark-toned skin showing through underneath. Common to many dry-skinned people of colour, this skin problem can be easily treated with a moisturiser, though there are many marketed directly for it as well.

Dark spots in response to injury trouble many dark-skinned DRPTs because skin pigmentation developed at the site of injury may last much longer than the injury itself. Black patients frequently fear that these dark spots are permanent scars, but they are neither permanent nor scars. However, you may have a harder time getting rid of the dark spots than light-skin-toned DRPTs. Light treatments (commonly used to treat them) are not useful for you because the light can affect your overall skin colour pigment as well as the spot you want to remove. Instead, you'll have to rely on the products I recommend. When my black and Asian patients are upset because they cannot avail themselves of these procedures, I remind them that their cancer risk is much lower than it is for light-skin-toned DRPTs. It's a trade-off.

Christina's Story

C hristina, a divorced single mum with two teenagers, was a high school guidance counsellor, and an avid football-player on weekends. She got knocked about a fair amount while playing – that was part of the fun! High energy and enthusiastic, Christina enjoyed the attention that she received from the guys on the team.

But a combination of skin dryness and pigmentation created a problem that wasn't so attractive. The soap she used when she showered after the game at the sports centre was drying out her skin. She had dark patches on her elbows and knees, along with many nicks, scrapes and cuts from the game.

She came in to see me because all those tiny injuries added up and were making an unsightly mess of her arms and legs. Due to Christina's skin pigmentation, every cut and scrape left a record on her arms and legs, and they weren't disappearing anytime soon. It was hard to find a foundation shade that matched Christina's skin tone well enough to cover them. 'I'm all scraped up,' she complained when she came to my office. 'Is there anything you can do about it?'

I recommended that Christina undertake a series of chemical peels and use prescription skin lighteners to help fade the spots. We could not change Christina's tendency to develop dark spots with injury. But at least we could fade them faster when they appeared. I recommended a moisturiser Christina could use to address the dryness on her elbows and knees.

In addition, I advised Christina to wear sunscreen during her games or whenever she went out because the sun would increase the skin pigment that caused her dark spots as well as weaken her immune system's response to these minor injuries. As a dark-skin-toned woman, Christina believed she was not at risk for sunburn and, as a result, rarely wore sunscreen. When she'd tried it before, the white-coloured product gave her dark skin a purplish cast. I was able to make recommendations that work well for people with dark skin, such as tinted sunscreen products or those with micronised zinc. I told her that contrary to popular belief, dark skin can both burn and suffer sun damage. Christina was delighted to find a product that blended well with her dark skin and began to use it regularly.

When Christina checked back with me three months later, our programme was working, and though she played as vigorously as before, her arms and legs looked better – even in tank tops and short shorts.

Like Christina, with dark-toned DRPT skin you may experience any of the following:

- Dry skin
- Rough patches over the knees and elbows that appear darker than the rest of your skin
- Dark patches on the cheeks (such as melasma, or mask of pregnancy)
- Dark areas in site of previous injury or inflammation, such as a cut, pimple, scrape
- Itching skin
- Ashiness
- Flaking skin
- Chemical peels or other treatments worsen dark spots

If your skin measures very dry on the questionnaire, you may develop dryness, dandruff, and peeling all over your face and head as well. For people of colour, often dryness is worsened by harsh hair products. Unlike those with sensitive skin, resistant types do not always develop reactions (such as rashes or itching) to these ingredients, but you still can find them very drying. While hair care products are outside the scope of this book, if you notice that you're developing extreme dryness and dandruff, I would suggest that you seek out milder products, avoiding shampoos and conditioners that contain detergents, and steer clear of hair straighteners, hair growth products, hair dyes, and professional treatments with harsh chemicals. You might also consider spacing out your hair appointments to minimise exposure.

YOUR MELANOMA RISK

Light-skinned DRPTs are at risk for developing melanoma skin cancers. Light treatments offered by a dermatologist can easily remove any worrisome spots that could develop into cancers, but it's still important to know your risk factors and get an annual skin cancer exam.

If you're a DRPT with any of the following factors, you are at higher risk of developing melanoma:

- Light skin
- Light-coloured hair
- Sunburn easily
- History of one or more severe sunburns
- Many freckles
- Family members with history of melanoma

While all light-skinned DRPTs should pay heed, any of the above factors will increase your risk. In addition, if you have red hair, your risk *further* increases. Here's why: the MC1R gene is involved in red hair, freckle and melanoma formation, research reveals. Bottom line? Freckles are not just a cosmetic concern. They may be an early warning sign of the potential for future skin cancers. If you fall into this category, you should be seen by a dermatologist at least annually, especially if you have a history of frequent sunburns. Please consult 'The A, B, C and D of Melanoma' in Chapter Nine for a complete description of what to look out for.

The lip area is most prone to skin cancer because the lips do not secrete sebum, an oil that contains a high concentration of vitamin E, an antioxidant that protects against aging and cancer. That is why many new formulations of ChapSticks and lip balms contain vitamin E to act as a protectant. Health food stores also sell bottles of vitamin E oil. Though it's far too oily for most skin areas, it can be used on the lips with no problem.

YOUR NEED FOR MOISTURE

Moisturising is vital to counteract skin dryness. But applying oil in and of itself is not enough. Your goal is to trap water in the skin. That's why I recommend spraying facial water *before* moisturiser application. I'll recommend specific products later in this chapter. Make sure that you apply your moisturiser immediately after spraying the water. If you allow your skin to dry first, it will only increase skin dryness. At the minimum, you should always use a moisturiser with an SPF factor to prevent sun exposure leading to pigmentation. Allow your skin to absorb the product for five minutes before applying your makeup. This will prevent streaking. Foundations can also provide additional moisture and sun protection. Whether or not you opt for a foundation, you may also apply an additional moisturiser, if needed, both morning and evening.

Because your skin is resistant, you need products with ingredients that penetrate the skin, such as retinol and vitamin K, which are contained in many of my recommendations. Products containing alcohol are too drying for you. Study ingredient lists to ensure that any products you are considering purchasing do not contain alcohol among the first seven ingredients. Glycerine, used in many creams, lotions and soaps, helps to hydrate the skin, so you can look for products that contain it. You'll find information about moisturising in the next section of this chapter.

Dr Baumann's Bottom Line: My moisturiser recommendations will help your dry skin and reduce the itching and ashiness that often accompany it. Make sure to wear sunscreen to protect your skin and decrease pigmentation.

EVERYDAY CARE FOR YOUR SKIN TYPE

The goal of your skin care routine is to address dryness and pigmentation, with products that deliver hydrating, moisturising, and skin lightening ingredients. All the products I'll recommend act to do one or both of the following:

- Prevent and treat dryness
- Prevent and treat dark spots

In addition, your daily regimen will also help to address your other skin concerns by:

- Preventing skin cancer

Antioxidants (like vitamins C and E, as well as green tea) can both lessen inflammation leading to dark spots and stave off aging, while retinol has antiaging benefits and can also help to lighten dark spots.

All DRPTs will benefit from my daily skin care regimen. If after two months of use, you find that you need more help in addressing skin pigmentation issues, graduate to my prescription regimen later in this chapter.

DAILY SKIN CARE

STAGE ONE: NONPRESCRIPTION REGIMEN

AM	PM
Step 1: Wash with cleanser	Step 1: Wash with cleanser
Step 2: If dark spots are a concern, apply a skin lightener	Step 2: Apply lightener if you have dark spots (optional)

Step 3: Spray facial water	Step 3: Spray facial water
Step 4: Apply eye cream (optional)	Step 4: Apply eye cream (optional)
Step 5: Apply moisturiser with SPF	Step 5: Apply night cream
Step 6: Apply foundation with SPF (optional) or use a combination of moisturiser, sunscreen and foundation to assure a minimum SP of 15.	

In the morning, wash your face with a cleanser. If you have dark spots, apply a skin lightener directly to the spots. Next, spray facial water over your entire face and neck, and then, if you wish, apply eye cream. After that, apply a moisturiser that contains SPF. Finally, apply foundation if you wear it.

In the evening, wash with cleanser, and apply a lightener to your dark spots. Next, spray facial water over your entire face and neck, and afterwards use eye cream if you wish. Last, apply a night cream.

Cleansers

DRPTs should avoid heavily foaming cleansers since they are drying. Cleansers with glycolic acid help your resistant skin absorb other beneficial ingredients delivered in the regimen. They also help brighten your complexion. Glycerin soaps are great for DRPTs, since glycerin is very hydrating. Use any of the many brands available.

RECOMMENDED CLEANSING PRODUCTS

- £ Anthony Logistics Glycerin Cleansing Bar Citrus Blend (for men)
- £ Cetaphil Liquid Cleanser
- £ Eucerin Gentle Cleansing Milk
- £ Glycerine soap (any brand that is natural)
- ££ Aesop Fabulous Face Cleanser
- ££ Aveda All Sensitive Cleanser
- ££ Biotherm Biosource Softening Cleansing Milk for Dry Skin
- ££ DDF Brightening Cleanser

££ Donell Super-Skin Lightening Cleanser
££ Gly Derm Gentle Cleanser 2% (has glycolic acid)
££ Jan Marini Bioglycolic Facial Cleanser
££ L'Occitane Olive Harvest Olive Daily Face Cleanser
££ MD Forté Facial Cleanser III (has glycolic acid)
££ MD Formulations Facial Cleanser (has glycolic acid)

Baumann's Choice: DDF Brightening Cleanser has many botanical lighteners and glycolic acid.

Skin Lighteners

Use a skin lightening gel when you have dark spots. If the products listed below are ineffective, visit a dermatologist to get stronger prescription products.

RECOMMENDED SKIN LIGHTENERS

££ NeoStrata Bionic Skin Lightening Cream SPF 15
££ Peter Thomas Roth Potent Skin Lightening Lotion Complex
££ Philosophy A Pigment of Your Imagination
£££ DDF Fade Gel Corrector Swabs
£££ Dr Brandt Lightening Gel
£££ L'Occitane Immortelle Brightening Serum
£££ Pevonia Lightening Gel
£££ SkinCeuticals Phyto +
£££ TYK White Glow Retinol, Kojic, Mag-C Absolute Skin Brightener

Baumann's Choice: SkinCeuticals Phyto + because it's the easiest to find in the UK. Go to DrBaumann.co.uk to learn where to find the other products or tell me your favourite products in this category.

Facial Waters

Facial waters come from thermal springs and are free of chemicals such as chlorine that are added to our tap water to prevent contamination with algae and other organisms.

Spray water on your face and neck right before applying an eye cream and moisturiser. The moisturiser and eye cream will help trap the water on the skin, giving the skin a reservoir to pull from. This is important when the humidity is low.

RECOMMENDED FACIAL WATERS

£ Evian Mineral Water Spray
££ Avène Thermal Water Spray
££ Chantecaille Pure Rosewater
££ Fresh Rose Marigold Tonic Water
££ La Roche-Posay Thermal Spring Water
££ Shu Uemura Depsea Therapy
££ Vichy Thermal Spa Water
£££ Jurlique Rosewater Freshener

Baumann's Choice: Jurlique Rosewater Freshener because it smells amazing!

Moisturisers

These moisturisers will help your dry skin and reduce the itching and ashiness that accompany it. In addition, your daytime moisturiser options all contain sun protective factors to help minimise dark spots while preventing skin cancers.

RECOMMENDED MORNING MOISTURISERS

£ Neutrogena Ultimate Moisture Day Cream
£ Olay Complete Defence Daily UV Moisturiser SPF 30
££ Avon Anew Luminosity Ultra SPF 15
££ Korres Watercress 24 Hour Moisturiser with SPF 6
££ L'Occitane Shea 24 Hours Ultra Rich Face Cream
££ Topix Citrix 15% Cream (no SPF, so use with a sunscreen and/or SPF containing foundation)
££ Vichy Thermal S2 SPF 14
£££ Pevonia Glycocides Cream
£££ SkinCeuticals Daily Moisture (no SPF, so use with a sunscreen or foundation to assure a minimum SPF of 15)

Baumann's Choice: Neutrogena Ultimate Moisture Day Cream because it has 'active soy' that helps prevent dark spots.

RECOMMENDED EVENING MOISTURISERS

£ Neutrogena Ultimate Moisture Night Cream
£ Olay Total Effects 7x Visible Anti-Aging Vitamin Complex
££ Atopalm MLE Cream
££ Ella Baché Age Defence Night Cream
££ Sekkisei Cream Excellent
££ Thalgo Absolute Hydration
££ Vichy Nutrilogie 2
£££ L'Occitane Immortelle Face Cream Mask
£££ RéVive Moisturising Renewal Cream with AHA
£££ Sisley Botanical Moisturiser with Cucumber
£££ Z. Bigatti Re-Storation Enlighten Skin Tone Provider

Baumann's Choice: Atopalm MLE Cream from Korea. You can get it at www.Baumannstore.co.uk. If you have dark spots then I recommend Neutrogena Ultimate Moisture Night Cream because it has active soy.

RECOMMENDED EYE CREAMS

£ Neutrogena Visibly Young Eye Cream
£ Olay Regenerist Eye Lifting Serum
££ DDF Nutrient K Plus
££ Ella Baché Eye Lift Gel
££ Laura Mercier Eyedration
££ MD Skincare Lift & Lighten Eye Cream
££ Peter Thomas Roth AHA/Kojic Under Eye Brightener
£££ La Prairie Cellular Eye Moisturiser
£££ Sisley Eye and Lip Contour Cream

Baumann's Choice: DDF Nutrient K Plus (with vitamin K and horse chestnut)

Body Moisturisers

Although, in general, body products are outside the scope of this book, your dry skin needs treatment so badly that for you I am making an exception. Heavy creams such as Cetaphil cream and oils such as baby oil are generally not desirable for use on the face because they often feel too greasy. However, you might use one as a night cream, and you can use them on your body. I travel internationally a lot, and I use heavy, greasy creams on the aeroplane, but I am mortified when I run into someone I know. I usually have on my Gap sweats, no makeup, and a greasy face. Not exactly how I want to be seen!

RECOMMENDED HEAVY CREAMS
FOR BODY MOISTURE

£ Cetaphil Cream
£ Crabtree & Evelyn Rosewater Glycerine Body Cream
£ Nivea Cream
£ Oilatum Cream
££ Del-Ray Dermatologicals Rea Lo 30 Urea Cream
££ Elizabeth Arden Green Tea Body Butter
££ Ferndale Nouriva Repair Moisturising Cream
££ La Roche-Posay Lipikar Baume
££ Quintessence Dual Action Moisturising Lotion
£££ Laura Mercier Crème Brûlée Soufflé Body Crème

Baumann's Choice: Laura Mercier Crème Brûlée Soufflé Body Crème because it smells amazing. I use Cetaphil three times a day and the Laura Mercier on special occasions.

SHOPPING FOR PRODUCTS

It's a good idea when purchasing skin care products to read labels carefully. Some ingredients will enhance a product's hydrating potential, while others will make your skin drier. If you have a favourite product that contains these ingredients but is not on the list, please enter it at www.DrBaumann.co.uk.

RECOMMENDED SKIN CARE INGREDIENTS

To moisturise and hydrate skin:

- Ajuga turkestanica
- Aloe vera
- Borage seed oil
- Dimethicone
- Evening primrose oil
- Glycerin

- Canola oil
- Ceramide
- Cholesterol
- Cocoa butter (avoid if you have acne)
- Colloidal oatmeal
- Dexpanthenol (pro-vitamin B₅)
- Jojoba oil
- Lanolin
- Macadamia nut oil
- Olive oil
- Rose hip seed oil
- Safflower oil
- Shea butter

To get rid of dark spots:

- Arbutin
- Bearberry
- Cocos nucifera (coconut fruit juice)
- Cucumber extract
- Epilobium angustifolium (willow herb)
- Gallic acid
- Glycyrrhiza glabra (licorice extract)
- Hydroquinone
- Kojic acid
- Mulberry
- Niacinamide
- Resorcinol
- Retinol
- Salicylic acid (beta hydroxy acid or BHA)
- Saxifraga sarmentosa extract (strawberry begonia)
- Vitamin C (ascorbic acid)

SKIN CARE INGREDIENTS TO AVOID

Due to drying:

- Alcohol listed among first seven ingredients
- Cleansers that foam vigorously
- Fragrance

Due to worsening melasma:

- Estradiol
- Oestrogen
- Genistein

Sun Protection for Your Skin

Your morning moisturiser should contain sunscreen; make sure that your moisturiser, sunscreen and foundation (whether you use one or more of these products) provide you with a minimum coverage of SPF 15 for normal daily wear. However, if you plan to be in the sun for more than fifteen minutes, apply one of the sunscreen products listed below *over* your moisturiser and under any makeup foundation or powder. (Even if you do this, you should also use a foundation with SPF – you cannot get too much SPF, even if you have dark skin.)

The best sunscreens for you are cream formulations. If you find them too greasy, cover the sunscreen with an SPF-containing powder such as Maybelline Pure Stay Powder SPF 15 or Jane Iredale's Amazing Base Loose Minerals SPF 20.

If you have darker skin, you may not like sunscreens containing zinc oxide and titanium dioxide unless they are tinted with colour, because they appear so white on the skin. Look for tinted products or those containing micronized zinc (often called Z-cote), an ingredient in SkinCeuticals Ultimate UV Defence SPF 30, which provides protection without the white appearance.

RECOMMENDED SUN PROTECTION PRODUCTS

£ Boots No7 Sun Protection Energising Facial Suncare SPF 15
£ Nivea Sun Face Sunscreen SPF 30
£ Olay Complete UV Defence Moisturiser
£ Vichy Capital Soleil Sun Block Fluid SPF60
££ Clarins Sun Wrinkle Control Cream SPF30
££ Dermalogica Sheer Moisture SPF 15
££ Garnier Ambre Solaire Ultra Protect Face Cream SPF 50
££ La Roche-Posay Anthelios Fluide Extreme SPF 60 (In Ireland)
££ L'Occitane Shea Ultra Moisturising Care SPF 15
££ Philosophy A Pigment of Your Imagination SPF 18
££ Topix Glycolix Elite Sunscreen SPF 30
£££ Lancôme Absolue Absolute Replenishing Cream SPF15
£££ SkinCeuticals Ultimate UV Defence SPF 30 (contains Z-Cote)

Baumann's Choice: Vichy Capital Soleil Sun Block Fluid SPF60 because it's a good price for such a high SPF.

Your Makeup

Studies show that vitamin K and substances such as horse chestnut that aid circulation may improve dark circles under the eyes. One eye product containing both vitamin K and horse chestnut is DDF Nutrient K Plus.

Concealers

You can use a concealer to cover both dark circles under your eyes and dark spots. The concealers listed below offer a good colour selection for those with darker skin tones and are also hydrating rather than drying.

RECOMMENDED CONCEALERS

£ Revlon Age Defying Concealer
£ Max Factor Erace Concealer Stick
££ Bloom Concealer
££ Clarins Concealer Plus Corrector
££ Dermablend Reflections Concealer
££ Elizabeth Arden Flawless Finish Sponge-on Cream Makeup
££ Laura Mercier Secret Concealer
££ MAC Select Cover Up
££ Victoria's Secret Cream Concealer
£££ Armani Skin Retouch
£££ Estée Lauder Re-Nutriv Custom Concealer Duo

Baumann's Choice: All of these are good. Select whichever one is a good match for your skin colour.

CONSULTING A DERMATOLOGIST

If you feel that pigmentation is a problem for you, you may wish to graduate to prescription products and procedures. Many DRPTs have only minor skin pigment issues, while some really struggle with persistent dark spots, melasma or excessive freckles. It's your call into which category you fall.

PRESCRIPTION SKIN CARE STRATEGIES

My Stage Two regimen for DRPTs focuses on using stronger, non-retinoid prescription products to treat dark spots. Although retinoids are also effective in treating dark spots, they are drying, so unless wrinkles are also a concern, it's not my first choice for your dry skin.

DAILY SKIN CARE

STAGE TWO: PRESCRIPTION REGIMEN

AM	PM
Step 1: Wash with cleanser	Step 1: Wash with cleanser
Step 2: If dark spots are a concern, apply a prescription skin lightener	Step 2: Apply a prescription skin lightener
Step 3: Spray facial water	Step 3: Spray facial water
Step 4: Apply moisturiser with SPF	Step 4: Immediately apply night cream
Step 5: Apply foundation with SPF (optional)	

In the morning, wash with cleanser, then apply a prescription skin lightener. You can apply the product directly to dark spots when you have them; or if they are an ongoing problem, you can apply it to your entire face. Next, spray facial water and apply a moisturiser that contains SPF. Last, apply a foundation containing SPF, assuring a combined SPF 15 coverage.

In the evening, wash your face with a cleanser, then apply a prescription skin lightener. Spray facial water, then immediately apply a night cream.

Eye cream use is optional, but if you choose to use one of the non-prescription eye creams, you can apply it right before you apply your moisturiser.

PRESCRIPTION MEDICATIONS

Many of the prescription skin lighteners in this regimen contain the lightener hydroquinone. Prescription products contain 4 percent or more hydroquinone, while over-the-counter products contain 2 percent hydroquinone or less.

RECOMMENDED PRESCRIPTION PRODUCTS

- Claripel
- Eldopaque Forte
- Eldoquin Forte
- EpiQuin Micro
- Glyquin
- Lustra
- Melanex
- Nuquin HP
- Solaquin Forte

These US brand names may not be available in your country, but your dermatologist can recommend similar products.

PROCEDURES FOR YOUR SKIN TYPE

Light-skinned DRPTs can consult a dermatologist for the possible use of lasers, Intense Pulsed Light, and chemical peels to treat their dark spots. Many dermatologists choose to use a combination of these procedures, along with topical bleaching and sunscreen agents. If you have light skin and light hair with lots of freckles, or a history of sunburns, any of these treatments are good for you. You should also see a dermatologist annually to check for skin cancer.

People with darker skin need more careful treatment because any kind of injury or inflammation to the skin can worsen dark spots rather than minimise or eliminate them. For you, a slow approach is best. Most dermatologists choose a regimen of topical prescription medications and chemical peels. If you have dark skin, make sure your dermatologist specializes in treating skin of colour and only uses the gentlest procedures.

If you're Asian, your skin appears light-toned, but tends to react similarly to dark-toned skin. Therefore, Asian skin should also be treated very carefully to avoid inflammation and trauma that could worsen the dark spots. So if you are Asian or have a medium skin tone, follow the recommendations for dark skin.

Light Treatments

Light-skin-toned DRPTs can benefit from light therapy. This procedure lightens dark spots without causing inflammation that leads to more dark spots. Light treatments can also help get rid of redness and blood vessels. For more information on these procedures and how they can help, please consult 'Further Help for Oily, Sensitive Skin'. Again, light treatments are not recommended for Asian or dark-skin-toned DRPTs.

Chemical Peels

People with darker skin tones or those who do not want (or cannot afford) light treatments can benefit from chemical peels containing glycolic acid, resorcinol, and other depigmenting ingredients. The Jessner's peel is a good choice for this Skin Type.

These peels range from £50 to £100 per peel and a series of five to eight is normal.

ONGOING CARE FOR YOUR SKIN

Sun protection and moisturising are equally important. Use sunscreen religiously to prevent pigmentation and skin cancer. Unless you have very dark skin, don't forget to get annual checkups to safeguard you from skin cancer, especially if you are a light-skinned or freckled DRPT.

CHAPTER EIGHTEEN

Dry, Resistant, Non-Pigmented and Wrinkled: DRNW

THE MAJORITY SKIN TYPE

'I've always had good skin but overnight it's become very dry. Whenever I look in the mirror, I notice new wrinkles. How can I look as young as I feel?'

ABOUT YOUR SKIN

The DRNW Skin Type is shared by many Americans. In youth, DRNWs enjoy great skin, with fewer breakouts than the Oily Types; little skin irritation, giving you a wider range of product choices than the sensitive types; and minimal pigmentation to produce the discolouration, dark spots, and freckles that sometimes bother pigmented types. Up until the age of twenty-five, your skin is easy, and most of you don't pay much heed to skin care.

Most people with this Skin Type have light-toned skin and northern European ancestors, with Scandinavian, English, Irish, Scottish, German, Russian, Polish, and other Slavic ethnicities. This delicate pale skin, untouched by freckles or skin discolouration, can be much admired, but it's more fragile than pigmented skin and, unless it's properly cared for, doesn't age that well. This comes as an unpleasant surprise in the second half of life. Currently, baby boomers are reaching this stage, and there's been an explosion of interest in antiaging, skin care, and advanced skin procedures. Is there a connection between the two occurrences? You bet.

Yours is an *over-served* type. Boomers are not the only group interested in these services; adults below the age of forty want to preserve their youthful looks as well. As a result, a plethora of products and services are suddenly appearing in the marketplace, in clinics, and in spas. And while many of them are marketed to DRNWs, unless they are formulated to address your specific combination of the four factors, they may be useless, no matter how pricey they are. How to separate the wheat from the chaff? How to know which products and services are truly effective and which are pretty packaging and marketing hype?

Well, that's my job.

DRNW CELEBRITY

Beloved actress Lucille Ball was a household name before she became a breakthrough star in a new medium in her forties. Lucy was the first in many departments. She was indisputably the First Lady of Comedy. She was one of the first to see and develop the potential of television, starring in and producing the most popular television show of the 1950s, *I Love Lucy*, as well as mounting (via her production company) a couple of other shows that didn't do too badly, *Mission: Impossible* and *Star Trek*. And she was the first woman studio head (of Desilu).

With her flawless pale skin, light blue eyes, and clear complexion, Lucy was a non-pigmented type. She was not a true redhead. Given all the years under lights in makeup and exposed to hair dyes, I'm guessing she was a dry, resistant type, since there's little evidence of the breakouts, redness, or rashes that would result from oiliness and skin sensitivity. Although I've never seen her tanned, photos in later years reveal her as a wrinkled type, probably due to a combination of genetics and smoking. Yes, Lucy's famous throaty laugh resulted from a long-term habit.

Coming of age in the Depression era made Lucy a hard worker. Playing small parts in forty-three forgettable films led her to be dubbed 'the Queen of the B-movies'. But her career really took off after hairstylist Sidney Guilaroff dyed her hair orange, asserting that 'the hair may be brown, but the soul's on fire'. The new hair colour became her signature, and from that point on, Lucy became and remained a star. Her success was hard-won. Like many women, Lucy did not believe that she was beautiful. In a 1938 magazine interview called 'Secrets of an Ugly Duckling', Lucy revealed how far she felt she deviated from the beauty ideal of that time. 'Nearly everything was wrong with me,' she complained, 'My eyebrows grew too low, I'd formed the habit of letting my upper eyelids sag, I had a mouth like a fish . . .'

While many of these so-called deficiencies could be corrected today through plastic surgery, Lucy overcame them through a combination of controlling her facial muscles, artful makeup, fortitude and laughter. Her eyebrows were shaved off and pencilled in where desired. Sagging eyelids were countered by her wide-eyed, raised eyebrow expression. If she'd been born perfect, who knows if she would have turned to comedy? But thankfully, in spite of her self-perceived beauty problems, she did.

Two contemporary comediennes are the heiresses of Lucy's outrageous, self-deprecating humour – and they too very likely have DRNW skin. I'm talking about Edina and Patsy, the undaunted heroines of my favourite BBC comedy, *Absolutely Fabulous*. Even if you take my advice and avoid the sun, if your lifestyle mimics Patsy's (especially her smoking), you'll increase the chance of wrinkles forming later in life.

AN OUNCE OF PREVENTION

For DRNWs like Lucy, in the springtime of life, your skin seems deceptively easy. While other teens fight breakouts, you bask in compliments on your clear, even complexion. Over time, you may experience some dryness, but using any moisturiser brings relief without side effects or reactions. Unlike Sensitive Skin Types (who must avoid irritating ingredients) and Oily Types (who can't bear oil-based sun products), your dry, resistant skin can tolerate most any sunscreen – if you remember to use it.

In youth, your skin is low maintenance, so you neglect simple preventatives to assure great skin throughout life. Or you unknowingly abuse your skin, which leads to accelerated aging. And that's why later, in their forties and fifties, the DRNWs come trooping into my office, wanting a last-minute fix.

I urge you, take heed now, because using the right approaches and avoiding the wrong habits will make a big difference long-term. Since young DRNWs, with their 'Why worry?' skin, will probably be the least likely to buy this book, give a copy to your DRNW friend, relative, or loved one. You'll be doing her or him a big favour.

Karen's Story

K aren, a forty-six-year-old housewife and the mother of three, came from a Scotch-Irish background. When mid-life wrinkling caught up with her pale skin, her sister persuaded her to come in for a consult with me. It was Karen's first dermatology visit.

She'd always had good skin and never worried about skin care or sun exposure, even though she lived in the sunny South. Plus, her diet was not the best. With three athletic sons consuming vast quantities of food, Karen succumbed to their constant begging for fast food, junk food, and fizzy drinks ''cause it's easier.' She and her husband ate a similar diet. From fast food burgers and fries to TV dinners to snacking on chips, tacos, and diet soda, there was never a vegetable in sight. The only fruit that came near her was the artificial flavour in a Snapple. As a result of this poor-quality diet, Karen struggled with her weight, gaining and losing an extra forty pounds many times.

Karen's diet was a problem, first, because she lacked antioxidants (obtainable from fruits and vegetables) that help prevent wrinkles. Second, instead of being supplied with the right kinds of fats (such as omega-3s, which provide the building blocks that help preserve skin moisture), her cells were bombarded with trans fats, highly processed fats present in many fast foods, processed foods, baked goods, crisps and sweets. They can, if consumed in excess, displace needed fats in the cell membranes. Karen was counting on her good genes, but they only go so far. Eventually, Karen's poor lifestyle habits caught up with her and she began to see lots of wrinkles.

Karen began going through menopause shortly after she hit forty. At that time, her doctor had prescribed the medication Prempro, which she took until a government study revealed that its long-term use significantly increased the chances of invasive breast cancer, blood clots and heart attacks.

Karen decided to stop taking the medication. However, instead of easing off the medication gradually under medical guidance to allow her body to adjust, Karen went off it abruptly. She then began to experience a mild depression, along with occasional hot flushes. But Karen grew more concerned when she looked in the mirror and perceived that her face suddenly aged 'overnight'.

Since lowered oestrogen levels can result in skin thinning and wrinkling, I placed her on a topical oestrogen cream called Estrace. Although this medicine is prescribed for vaginal use, several studies have shown that topical oestrogen applied to the face can help to increase skin hydration, thickness, and collagen content, without being absorbed into the bloodstream and causing systemic effects.

In addition, Karen opted for Botox injections to minimise her frown lines and the crow's-feet around her eyes. I filled in the lines around her mouth with a dermal filler known as Captique.

When Karen returned for her tri-annual injections, she was thrilled at the texture and hydration of her skin. Many of her friends were so impressed that they wanted to use topical oestrogen creams too. I reminded Karen that her friends should first consult their physicians before using any prescription medications.

A CLOSE-UP LOOK AT YOUR SKIN

Like Karen, with DRNW skin you may experience any of the following:

- Ease in using sunscreens
- Trouble tanning
- Streaking with self-tanners
- Minimal skin problems in youth, with little or no acne, eczema, skin allergies, or problems with cosmetics or moisturisers
- Crepiness appears around your eyes in your early thirties
- Accelerated wrinkling from mid-thirties on
- Increased dryness and wrinkling in your forties and fifties

Starting young with both sun protection and wrinkle prevention can make a huge difference in how your skin ages. If you follow my instructions, you can wind up looking like a DRNT, especially with the lifestyle factors I'll offer you. Luckily, DRNWs tolerate sunscreens well. Although Oily Types complain that sunscreens feel greasy, DRNWs don't mind it because your dry wrinkle-prone skin needs oil. Instead of tanning, use self-tanners, which provide a safe tanned look, but always use a separate sunscreen as well. Since self-tanners often streak on dry skin, follow my special instructions and recommendations for self-tanner use and products in Chapter Ten, 'Self-Tanners'. You'll find products that can work for your type in the products section of Chapter Nineteen, following my sunscreen recommendations.

DRNW skin is also more prone to non-melanoma skin cancer, because of several factors:

- Fair-toned skin
- Easily sunburned and hard-to-tan skin
- History of excess sun exposure
- History of smoking
- Diet does not contain enough fruits and vegetables (antioxidants)

According to some estimates, 60 percent of people over the age of forty who meet the above criteria may have at least one incidence of a pre-malignant condition called actinic keratosis. Sixty percent of non-melanoma skin cancers arise from this condition. That's why it's important to know the signs and get checked by a dermatologist annually.

How to Recognise a Non-Melanoma Skin Cancer

A squamous cell carcinoma (SCC) may appear as red, scaling patches that form scabs in sun-exposed areas such as the face, ears, chest, arms, legs and back. They don't heal but may be covered by a hard white scale that resembles a wart. Any spot that fits this description and persists for one month or more should be seen by a dermatologist.

A basal cell carcinoma (BCC) may appear as a white, shiny bump, luminous like a pearl. It may have either a central ridge with a little hole or depression, or tiny blood vessels visible in the border. It can also look like a crater or scar that suddenly appears although there has been no prior trauma. Sometimes the border is 'ruffled' or heaped up around the central crater.

Enlarged facial oil glands can be easily confused with basal cell carcinoma, since they are both yellowish bumps. Make sure to check out anything suspicious with a dermatologist.

KEY GUIDELINES FOR YOUR SKIN

Hydration, or keeping moisture in the skin, preserves skin's youthful freshness, so dry types must take special care to hydrate. Drinking lots of water, though possibly helpful for other reasons, will not help skin dehydration. Water is held in the skin by certain lipids, or fats, which is why I'll recommend that you consume healthy omega-3 fats in the dietary recommendations later in 'Further Help for Dry, Resistant Skin'. Skin damage and aging occur through the formation of free radicals, renegade molecules that break down the basic skin biochemicals that maintain skin structure and safeguard hydration. Free radicals promote the dissolution of collagen, hyaluronic acid, and elastin, the three cornerstones of youthful skin. Antioxidants quench free radicals to protect these vital skin chemicals.

Antioxidants can be obtained from foods and supplements, and via topical skin products. DRNWs under the age of thirty should seek out skin products that contain antioxidants like vitamins C and E, green tea, coenzyme Q_{10}, and lycopene (often found in moisturisers appropriate for this type, such as Kiehl's Lycopene Facial Moisturising Cream). In your thirties, I suggest starting a prescription retinoid – with the caution that pregnant women and nursing mothers, as well as those who plan to become pregnant, should defer retinoid use from the time you plan to become pregnant until after you've finished breastfeeding. At the first sign of wrinkles, add an alpha hydroxy acid or polyhydroxy acid to your regimen. You can find my recommendations later in this chapter. DRNWs of all ages should use a daily sunscreen.

Menopause can be a hard time for DRNW women. Falling oestrogen levels can dry out – and thin out – your skin. In fact, studies have shown a sharp decline in skin thickness in women after the fifth decade of life. Most declines in skin collagen, a key factor in skin thickness, occur during the first few years after menopause, with a 30 percent decline in the first five years, and an average decline of 2.1 percent per postmenopausal year thereafter over a period of twenty years. Hormone replacement therapy or the use of topical oestrogen reverse this process, many studies show. However, given other concerns about HRT, this is a decision you will want to make with your primary care physician.

DOS AND DON'TS FOR AGING GRACEFULLY

If you want to age gracefully, there are two big don'ts. First, don't allow your non-pigmented skin to burn. Second, don't smoke. Baking your skin may seem harmless, but waking up in your thirties and forties to numerous wrinkles is a common – and avoidable – DRNW fate. Beware the sun, and use sunscreen daily. The worst-case scenario is when DRNWs (most of whom have trouble tanning) subject themselves to tanning beds or the application of baby oil while lying down to tan on aluminum foil. For DRNWs, both of these buy now–pay later habits set you up for premature wrinkling. For more on tanning beds, see Chapter Ten, 'Indoor Tanning',

Your biggest do? Moisturise. Keeping your skin well hydrated supports key enzymes that prevent aging. Hyaluronic acid is one of the three key skin components. The other two are collagen and elastin. Wrinkles are caused by their loss, and that's why most antiaging creams will aim to increase one or more of these three. Alpha hydroxy acids (such as glycolic acid and lactic acid) will help hydrate the skin and improve the skin's texture, making it appear more radiant. According to one study, glycolic acid can increase collagen and hyaluronic acid production, which may be one of the reasons it improves the appearance of wrinkled skin. Vitamin C also increases collagen production, studies show. Retinoids increase collagen production and elastin production as well as preventing the breakdown of collagen.

CHOOSING THE RIGHT MOISTURISER

There are thousands of moisturisers, antiaging creams, and treatments to prevent wrinkling, and they are all targeted to you. Unlike your close Skin Type cousins, the DRPWs, who are underserved, you're one of the largest market segments. Companies are trying to help you – and going after your dollar. The upside? You have so many options. The downside? You have so many options, but no way of knowing what really works. That's why it's important to learn what kinds of products and ingredients are of real benefit.

You can get temporary relief from dryness and wrinkles with many different products as many moisturisers hydrate and plump up the skin, making fine lines disappear for anywhere from an hour to two days.

But I'll let you in on a little trade secret. Companies asserting their product reduces wrinkles in a certain number of days often base these claims on in-house studies, designed so that the participants use no moisturiser for a week prior to the study. As a result, dry types will develop tiny dry lines especially around the eyes, visible in photos taken at their first visit, where the 'baseline' condition of their skin is documented prior to use of the product. Then they use the study cream and what do you know? Those fine lines appear minimised after a few days of moisturising.

While no over-the-counter creams have been convincingly proven to improve wrinkles long-term, your dry skin requires regular moisturising, so why not minimize the appearance of wrinkles as well? Your resistant skin can tolerate a higher concentration of active ingredients than some other types. However, not everything you put on your face can be absorbed and utilised as you intend.

For example, some antiaging skin care products contain hyaluronic acid, which lubricates the skin cells. When HA levels decrease with age, the skin dries out, loses volume, and becomes more likely to form wrinkles, which is why delivering HA would help combat skin aging. Although often found in skin care products, when applied topically, HA cannot penetrate into the skin because the molecule is too large. That's why companies developed an injectable form of HA available via fillers, which plump the wrinkles and restore lost volume to the skin for four to six months. Examples of these HA-containing fillers are Captique, Hylaform, Juvéderm and Restylane.

Taking supplements of glucosamine may increase HA production, some studies suggest. Since HA is broken down by free radicals, taking antioxidant supplements (like vitamins C and E) or eating a diet high in antioxidant-rich fruits and vegetables may help prevent your skin from losing HA.

L-ascorbic acid, or vitamin C, is an important antioxidant that prevents the breakdown of collagen and increases collagen production. However, vitamin C comes in many forms, and not all are helpful. Vitamin C esters attached to a fatty acid are poorly absorbed topically, so creams with it are not that effective. L-ascorbic acid (another form of vitamin C) penetrates better. Vitamin C ester (or regular vitamin C) is more readily absorbed via oral supplements. What's more, in topical products, vitamin C has a poor shelf life. If not packaged and stored properly, it will lose its activity. To help you get the right type of vitamin C, in the right packaging, I've removed the guesswork and identified products with active ingredients and protective packaging.

THE FUTURE OF SKIN CARE

Skin product companies are actively researching substances and products to turn back the clock. Growth factors, similar to hormones, increase the rate at which cells in the body grow. Some scientists are trying to use them to help new skin grow more rapidly and maintain skin's youth. However, since certain growth factors may increase the growth rate of undesirable cells, more research is needed to assure their safety and to find out which growth hormones are 'desirable' and which are not. Although some products currently available do use them, I am not recommending them, because it's not clear if they penetrate the skin.

Skin Medica makes a product called TNS Recovery Complex that contains growth factors produced by fibroblast cells, which also make collagen and hyaluronic acid. This growth factor-rich product is a funny pinkish colour and does not smell great, but it may stimulate your fibroblasts to make more collagen. Studies are evaluating this unique facial product.

TGF beta is a growth factor that increases collagen production. It is found in several face creams, such as Cell Rejuvenation Serum by Topix. I believe that TGF beta and other growth factors will become more important in aging prevention as more is learned about how they work.

EVERYDAY CARE FOR YOUR SKIN TYPE

You will age more gracefully if you are proactive in maintaining and protecting your skin in youth. And it's never too late to start. With medical advances happening every day, who knows what the average life span will be? Take action now so you can continue looking your best, even if you live to be 150.

The goal of your skin care routine is to address dryness and wrinkles with products that deliver antioxidants, moisturisers and retinoids. All the products I'll recommend act to do one or both of the following:

- Prevent and treat dryness
- Prevent and treat wrinkles

In addition, your daily regimen will also help to address your other skin concerns by:

- Preventing premature skin aging

I've provided two regimens, one prescription and one nonprescription. You can choose either one, depending on your age and budget. If you are in your twenties, you will only need the nonprescription regimen. If you're over thirty, use a nighttime moisturiser that contains a retinol or antioxidants. You can stay on the regimen indefinitely.

However, in my opinion, if you're over thirty, you'd do even better to follow my prescription regimen, which includes a prescription retinoid to prevent development of wrinkles.

DAILY SKIN CARE

STAGE ONE: NONPRESCRIPTION REGIMEN

AM	PM
Step 1: Wash with cleanser containing glycolic acid	Step 1: Wash with cleanser containing glycolic acid
Step 2: Apply antioxidant serum	Step 2: Apply antioxidant serum
Step 3: Spray facial water	Step 3: Spray facial water
Step 4: Apply eye cream	Step 4: Apply eye cream
Step 5: Apply moisturiser with SPF, assuring that your combination of moisturiser and sunscreen provides a minimum SPF of 15	Step 5: Apply night cream

In the morning, wash your face with cleanser, then apply an antioxidant serum. Spray facial water on your face and neck, then immediately apply eye cream and a moisturiser containing sunscreen.

In the evening, wash with the same cleanser, then apply antioxidant serum. Then spray facial water, next apply eye cream and nighttime moisturiser. If you are over thirty, choose a night cream with retinol, alpha hydroxy acids, or vitamin C.

Cleansers

Never wash your face with soap or shampoo, as any products that foam contain detergent that is much too drying for your skin. Instead use cleansers that contain alpha hydroxy acids, such as glycolic acid and lactic acid, which help hydrate the skin and increase collagen production. In addition, they remove the top layer of dead skin cells so that beneficial ingredients can penetrate. In this regimen, after cleansing, you'll be using antioxidant serums, which will act more powerfully when they follow these AHAs. Some of my recommendations don't contain AHAs for those who prefer not to use them. They can make you sun sensitive so those of you who don't wear sunscreen may choose a non-AHA cleanser.

RECOMMENDED CLEANSERS

£ Gly Derm Gentle Cleanser (with glycolic acid 2%)
££ DDF Glycolic Exfoliating Wash 7%
££ Estée Lauder Rich Results Hydrating Cleanser
££ Eve Lom Cleanser
££ Fresh Rice Face Wash
££ Jan Marini Bioglycolic Facial Cleanser
££ MD Forté Facial Cleanser II (with glycolic acid 15%)
££ MD Forté Facial Cleanser III (with glycolic acid 20%)
££ Topix Replenix Fortified Cleanser
££ Vichy Rich Detoxifying Cleansing Cream
£££ Dior Prestige Cleansing Creme
£££ Dr Hauschka Cleansing Milk
£££ Jurlique Face Wash Cream
£££ N.V. Perricone M.D. Olive Oil Polyphenols Gentle Cleanser
    with DMAE

Baumann's Choice: MD Forté Facial Cleanser III (with glycolic acid 20%)

Antioxidant Serums

Serums are a good way to deliver the concentrated antioxidants your type needs for wrinkle treatment and prevention. My choice here, SkinCeuticals C + E, has the right vitamin C at the right pH and is packaged properly. The research on this product is stellar. It's expensive, but its benefits give you a reason to splurge. If you plan to have sun exposure against my advice, you should choose the SkinCeuticals C and E Ferulic serum, which may help prevent some of the sun's damage to your skin.

RECOMMENDED ANTIOXIDANT SERUMS

- ££ Dr Andrew Weil for Origins Plantidote Mega Mushroom Serum
- ££ Laura Mercier Multi Vitamin Serum
- ££ MD Formulations Moisture Defence Antioxidant Serum
- ££ Topix Replenix Cream CF (caffeine enhanced)
- ££ Vichy Aera Teint Silky Cream Foundation
- £££ Elizabeth Arden Prevage Anti-aging Treatment
- £££ SkinCeuticals C + E
- £££ SkinCeuticals C E Ferulic

Baumann's Choice: SkinCeuticals C E Ferulic

Facial Water

DRNWs should avoid toners, which often contain drying alcohol. Instead, use a facial water. Spray it on your face immediately before you apply moisturiser. The moisturiser helps trap the water on the skin, giving the skin a reservoir to pull from. Note that although you may like the 'soothing' ingredients in the more expensive of these products, you don't actually need them.

RECOMMENDED FACIAL WATERS

- £ Evian Mineral Water Spray
- ££ Avène Thermal Water Spray
- ££ Chantecaille Pure Rosewater

££ La Roche-Posay Thermal Spring Water
££ Molton Brown Skin Boost 24 Hour Moisture Mist
££ Organic Pharmacy Rose Facial Spritz
££ Shu Uemura Depsea Therapy
££ Vichy Thermal Spa Water
£££ Jurlique Rosewater Spray

Baumann's Choice: Evian, because it's the cheapest and easiest to find. Jurlique smells the best.

Moisturisers

If you are under thirty, look for moisturisers containing antioxidants. If you are older, you will need heavier moisturisers. Those over thirty should also look for a nighttime moisturiser that contains retinol.

In some situations you may want to use a lighter moisturiser. Before a big evening event, I suggest using a facial scrub followed by a hydrating mask (see the 'Exfoliation' and 'Masks' sections of this chapter). Once the mask is removed, apply a thin layer of light moisturiser followed by your evening makeup. (Not too much moisturiser. You do not want to look shiny.) Your face will look fresh and flake free. One good option is Caudalie Vinopulp C80 cream. Lacking sunscreen, it's not good for daytime use, and it's too light for nighttime use, but it works in this case.

RECOMMENDED DAYTIME MOISTURISERS

£   Neutrogena Visibly Young Day Cream
£   Nivea Antiwrinkle Q10 Plus Day Cream
£   Roc Retin-Ox Correxion Intensive Nourishing Anti-wrinkle Care
££ Elizabeth Arden First Defence Anti-oxidant Cream SPF 15
££ Estée Lauder Daywear Plus Multi Protection Anti-Oxidant Creme SPF 15 for Dry Skin
££ Exuviance Essential Multi Defence Day Creme SPF 15
££ Laura Mercier Mega Moisturiser with SPF 15
££ L'Occitane Face and Body Balm SPF 30
££ Vichy Nutrilogie 1 SPF 15 sunscreen
£££ Bobbi Brown Extra SPF 25 Moisturising Balm
£££ La Prairie Cellular Moisturiser for the Face

Baumann's Choice: Neutrogena Visibly Young Day Cream because it contains copper pepitde which may improve wrinkles.

RECOMMENDED NIGHTTIME MOISTURISERS

- £ Burt's Bees Carrot Nutritive Night Crème
- £ Eucerin Lipo Balance Cream with Ceramide
- £ Nivea Antiwrinkle Q10 Plus Night Cream
- £ Rachel Perry Ginseng-Collagen Wrinkle Treatment with MSM & Bioflavonoids
- ££ Atopalm MLE Cream (in the jar, not in the tube called 'face cream')
- ££ Exuviance Evening Restorative Complex
- ££ Forticelle Elastin Fortifying Facial Complex
- ££ Kiehl's Lycopene Facial Moisturising Cream
- ££ Laura Mercier Night Nutrition Renewal Crème (for very dry to dehydrated skin)
- ££ Shu Uemura Depsea Therapy Moisture Recovery Cream
- ££ Topix Replenix Cream
- ££ Weleda Iris Night Cream
- £££ Dior Facial Energy-Move
- £££ Sisley Paris Comfort Extreme Night Skin Care
- £££ Z. Bigatti Re-Storation Skin Treatment

Baumann's Choice: Topix Replenix Cream – don't worry, it looks brown due to the large concentration of green tea. I also like Nivea Antiwrinkle Q10 Plus Night Cream because it contains coenzyme Q10 which helps prevent wrinkles.

RECOMMENDED EVENING MOISTURISERS WITH RETINOL

- £ Roc Retin-Ox Correxion Intensive Nourising Anti-wrinkle Care
- ££ Philosophy Help Me Face Cream
- ££ Sothy's Retinol 15
- ££ Topix Replenix Retinol Smoothing Serum 3x
- £££ Clarins Renew Plus Night Lotion
- £££ Estée Lauder Diminish Anti-Wrinkle Retinal Treatment
- £££ Jan Marini Factor A Plus Lotion
- £££ Lancôme Resurface

£££ Prescriptives Skin Renewal Cream

£££ Skinceuticals Retinol 0.5 or 1%

Baumann's Choice: Prescription products are stronger but among the over-the-counter products, the Roc offers the best value.

RECOMMENDED EYE CREAMS

£ Neutrogena Visibly Young Eye Cream

£ Nivea Visage Coenzyme Q_{10} Plus Wrinkle Control Eye Cream

££ Caudalie Grape-Seed Eye Contour Cream

££ Laura Mercier Night Nutrition Renewal Eye Crème

££ Relastin Eye Cream

£££ Dr Brandt Lineless Eye Cream

£££ Jurlique Eye Gel

£££ La Prairie Cellular Moisturiser for the Eye

£££ Natura Bisse Glyco-Eye Contour Exfoliator

£££ Pevonia Evolutive Eye Cream

£££ SkinCeuticals Eye Balm

Baumann's Choice: Relastin Eye Cream has been shown to tighten the lower eye lids, reducing fine lines. It's very new and hard to find so go to www.DrBaumann.co.uk to learn where you can purchase it.

Moisture Emergency

During travel, when engaged in winter sports, in dry climates, or other extreme dry conditions, dry types may have what I call a 'moisture emergency', when more intensive moisturising is required. If your skin is excessively dry, cracked, or in need of moisture, you can use these heavier products, which can also be applied to your feet, hands or body. Although a little greasy, they're formulated for problematic dryness and definitely come in handy from time to time. Since they are right in between prescription medications and regular moisturisers, you may have to ask your pharmacist for them, as they are not usually displayed with regular moisture creams.

RECOMMENDED HEAVY MOISTURISERS
FOR FACE OR BODY

£ Cetaphil Moisturising Cream (better for body than face)

£ Crabtree and Evelyn Lavendar Body Cream

£ Oilatum

££ Atopalm MLE Cream

££ Clinique Happy Body Butter

££ Elizabeth Arden Eight Hour Cream Skin Protectant

££ Ferndale Nouriva Repair Moisturising Cream by Ferndale

££ Kiehl's Crème de Corps

££ LBR Lipo cream by Ferndale

££ L'Occitane Vanilla Parfait Body Cream

££ Origins Ginger Souffle Whipped body cream

££ Osmotics Tri-Ceram

£££ Korres Bitter Almond Body Oil

£££ Laura Mercier Souffle Body Crème

£££ Pevonia Body Moisturiser with AHA

Baumann's Choice: Atopalm is the least greasy and best for facial use. Cetaphil is my favourite for body use on a daily basis. I save the more expensive ones for special occasions.

Exfoliation

You should exfoliate once or twice a week, unless you are on retinoids. When using a retinoid, you don't need to exfoliate unless you'd like to remove superficial scaling caused by the retinoid. In that case, you can exfoliate once a week.

RECOMMENDED SCRUBS

£ Burt's Bees Citrus Facial Scrub

£ Nivea for Men Deep Cleaning Face Scrub

£ St Ives Swiss Formula Invigorating Apricot Scrub

££ Clinique 7 Day Scrub Cream

££ Elemis Skin Buff

££ Laura Mercier Face Polish

££ L'Occitane Shea Butter Gentle Face Buff

££ Philosophy The Greatest Love Microdermabrasion Scrub
£££ Dr Brandt Microdermabrasion in a Jar
£££ Fresh Sugar Face Polish

Baumann's Choice: Clinique 7 Day Scrub Cream. I love the texture and the moisture it leaves behind.

Masks

Once or twice a week, you might like to use a hydrating mask. My choice here is the least expensive product, because I would rather see you spend your money on a prescription retinoid and an expensive serum. Masks are not that important, anyway; they don't stay on your face very long.

If you are not trying to save money, use the Caudalie mask. It has grape seed extract, which will give your skin some wrinkle prevention, and it's very luxurious.

RECOMMENDED MASKS

£ Bath and Body Works Le Couvent des Minimes Honey & Shea Face & Neck Comforting Masque
£ Bath and Body Works Pure Simplicity Olive Nourishing Face Mask
£ Montagne Jeunesse Stage 1 Zen Flower Sensitive Mask with ceramides
££ Laura Mercier Intensive Moisture Mask
££ L'Occitane Immortelle Cream Mask
£££ Caudalie Moisturising Cream Mask
£££ Lancôme Hydra-Intense Masque
£££ La Prairie Cellular Hydralift Firming Mask

Baumann's Choice: Bath and Body Works Le Couvent des Minimes Honey & Shea Face & Neck Comforting Masque. Why spend more?

SHOPPING FOR PRODUCTS

When you purchase products, be sure to read ingredient labels carefully. With your resistant skin, the only ingredients you need to avoid are the detergents in cleansers and shampoos. But you can also look for ingredients that help treat dryness and prevent wrinkles. If you have favourite products that contain these ingredients but are not on my lists, please share them with me at www.DrBaumann.co.uk.

RECOMMENDED SKIN CARE INGREDIENTS

To prevent wrinkles:

- Basil
- Caffeine
- Camilla sinensis (green tea, white tea)
- Carrot extract
- Coenzyme Q_{10} (ubiquinone)
- Copper peptide
- Curcumin (tetra-hydracurcumin or turmeric)
- Ferulic acid
- Feverfew
- Genistein (soy)
- Ginger
- Ginseng
- Grape seed extract
- Idebenone
- Lutein
- Lycopene
- Phytol
- Punica granatum (pomegranate)
- Pycnogenol (a pine bark extract)
- Rosemary
- Silymarin
- Yucca

To improve the appearance of wrinkles:

- Alpha hydroxy acids
- Citric acid
- Gluconolactone
- Glycolic acid
- Lactic acid
- Phytic acid
- Polyhydroxy acids
- Retinol

To hydrate and moisturise skin:

- Ajuga turkestanica
- Aloe vera
- Apricot kernel oil
- Borage seed oil
- Canola oil
- Ceramide
- Cholesterol
- Cocoa butter
- Colloidal oatmeal
- Dexpanthenol (pro-vitamin B_5)
- Dimethicone
- Evening primrose oil
- Glycerin
- Jojoba oil
- Macadamia nut oil
- Olive oil
- Safflower oil
- Shea butter

Sun Protection for Your Skin

It's essential that you wear sunscreen every day. If you don't expect more than fifteen minutes of exposure, you can use a daytime moisturiser or foundation that contains SPF. But if you plan to be in the sun for more than fifteen minutes, layer another sunscreen on top of your moisturiser and under your foundation. Make sure that whether you use one or multiple products, you obtain a minimum coverage of SPF 15. For more than one hour of sun exposure, reapply sunscreen every hour and use an SPF of at least 30. When you swim, use a waterproof sunscreen and reapply after immersion.

Creams are best for your type. Use a broad-spectrum sunscreen that covers both UVA and UVB.

RECOMMENDED SUN PROTECTION PRODUCTS

- £ Hawaiian Tropic Baby Faces Sunblock SPF 60+
- £ Nivea Sun Face Sunscreen SPF 30
- ££ Avon Hydrofirming Bio6 Day Cream SPF 15
- ££ Dermalogica Solar Defence Booster SPF 30
- ££ Elizabeth Arden First Defence Anti-oxidant Cream SPF 15
- ££ La Roche-Posay Anthelios Fluide Extreme SPF 60 cream (available in France and Ireland)
- ££ Prescriptives Insulation Anti-Oxidant Vitamin Cream SPF 15
- £££ Lancôme Rénergie Intense Lift SPF 15
- £££ Orlane B21 Soleil Vitamines Face Cream SPF 30

Baumann's Choice: Elizabeth Arden First Defence Anti-oxidant Cream SPF 15 also provides antioxidant protection against free radical environmental damage.

Your Makeup

In choosing a foundation be sure to use one that contains oil. An oil-free foundation is not right for your dry skin. When possible, use a foundation that contains SPF.

RECOMMENDED FOUNDATIONS

- £ Almay Time-Off Age Smoothing Makeup SPF 12
- £ Boots No7 Radiant Glow Foundation SPF 15
- £ Revlon Age Defying Makeup
- ££ Dr Hauschka Translucent Makeup
- ££ Elizabeth Arden Ceramide Plump Perfect Makeup SPF 15
- ££ Laura Mercier Moisturising Foundation
- ££ Vichy Aera Teint Silky Cream Foundation
- £££ Chantecaille Real Skin Foundation SPF 30 for dry skin
- £££ Diane von Furstenberg Beauty Skin Tint SPF 15

Baumann's Choice: I prefer any foundation for dry skin that has sunscreen.

CONSULTING A DERMATOLOGIST

PRESCRIPTION SKIN CARE STRATEGIES

If your bank balance will allow it, it would be best to begin following this prescription regimen once you are in your thirties, so that you can use a retinoid to prevent wrinkles. You may also want to go for Botox or hydroxy acid peels as soon as you detect lines in your face. However, as mentioned earlier, defer both retinoid use and Botox until after pregnancy and nursing or even if you plan to become pregnant in the near future.

DAILY SKIN CARE

STAGE TWO: PRESCRIPTION REGIMEN	
AM	PM
Step 1: Wash with cleanser	Step 1: Wash with cleanser

Step 2: Apply antioxidant serum

Step 3: Spray facial water

Step 4: Apply eye cream (optional)

Step 5: Apply moisturiser with
SPF, assuring that with
moisturiser, sunscreen and/or
foundation you obtain a
minimum SPF of 15

Step 2: Apply eye cream (optional)

Step 3: Apply prescription retinoid

Step 4: Apply night cream

In the morning, wash your face with cleanser, then apply antioxidant serum. Spray facial water, and immediately apply eye cream and a moisturiser containing sunscreen.

In the evening, wash with cleanser, then put on eye cream if you'd like to use one. Next, apply a prescription retinoid (see instructions in 'Further Help for Dry, Resistant Skin' for the first phase of retinoid use). Last, apply nighttime moisturiser.

PRESCRIPTION MEDICATIONS FOR WRINKLES

- Aknemycin Plus (contains an antibiotic as well)
- Differin gel or cream
- Isotrex
- Isotrexin (contains an antiobiotic as well)
- Retin-A gel, lotion or cream
- Retinova

Baumann's Choice: I recommend any of these products, which are best for you in a cream form containing as high a percentage of active ingredients as your skin can tolerate.

PROCEDURES FOR YOUR SKIN TYPE

Botox/Reloxin

Along with prescription medications, botulinum toxin injections and dermal fillers are mainstays for treating wrinkles for your Skin Type. Please see 'Further Help for Oily, Sensitive Skin' for details on the Botox/Reloxin procedures and on methods for treating different kinds of wrinkles.

Other Options

For light-skinned DRNWs, dermabrasion will help treat deep wrinkles. In addition, there is a new technique called Thermage that treats sagging skin. You can learn more about these and other upcoming procedures appropriate for wrinkle treatment in 'Further Help for Oily, Resistant Skin'.

ONGOING CARE FOR YOUR SKIN

Avoid the sun and stop smoking to preserve your skin. Plus, use retinols and retinoids to reverse sun damage and the signs of aging. Eat an anti-oxidant-rich diet. If your bank balance will permit, go for procedures that will bring real results. Your resistant, non-pigmented skin will help protect you from the side effects that other Skin Types develop after these procedures. The latest technology is there for you.

CHAPTER NINETEEN

Dry, Resistant, Non-Pigmented and Tight: DRNT

THE EASYGOING SKIN TYPE

'Why spend a lot of time hassling about skin care? Life is just too short. I think beauty comes from inside anyway. I just do what's easiest and devote my energy to other things.'

ABOUT YOUR SKIN

Congratulations. You won the Skin Type lottery. You have dream skin. You've probably never been near a dermatologist's office. In your teens and twenties, you were the envy of all your friends because you had the best skin – minimal acne, no oiliness, few freckles. Perhaps you suffered from occasional dry skin patches, but this was no big deal. If you are older, you may have noticed that your skin has become drier, but you can control dryness with most moisturisers. If you're older than forty-five, and not taking hormones, your skin's dryness may have worsened due to the loss of oestrogen. But you still look pretty good, and people often guess your age at five to ten years younger than you actually are.

When it comes to skin care, the DRNT's motto is 'Feel good, look good.' You don't realise how lucky you are to have low-maintenance DRNT skin. When others compliment your skin, you have no idea what they mean. It's just skin, isn't it? You're particularly lucky if you have a darker skin tone because you have the benefits of darker skin without the dark spots and patches that sometimes plague a related but pigmented skin type, the DRPT.

You're more concerned with how you feel than with how you look. Although you don't differentiate skin care from overall self-care, you do treat yourself right by eating a healthy diet and getting plenty of rest and exercise. Many people with this Skin Type value quality of life and make choices that maintain it.

A W/T score always results from a combination of genes and lifestyle choices. A light-skinned, dry, non-pigmented type is prone to sun damage, and if you'd persisted in tanning your non-tannable skin (or repeatedly burned and tanned), then you'd most likely be a DRNW rather than a DRNT. If you have dark skin, the melanin in your skin helps protect you from wrinkles and skin cancer. Other factors also help keep you a T Skin Type, such as having T ancestors, eating a lot of antioxidant-filled fruits and vegetables, ceasing smoking, avoiding secondhand smoke, and maintaining a steady slender weight, rather than going through yo-yo weight gain and loss, which stretches the skin. Stress contributes to the body's inflammatory response, one factor in skin sensitivity. Like everyone, you experience stress, but you've found ways to cope.

DRNT CELEBRITY

Cool, calm and collected, leading lady Gwyneth Paltrow is both second-generation Hollywood royalty and an Oscar winner in her own right. Her creamy, pale, tight, unblemished skin typifies the classic DRNT beauty. With films like *Shakespeare in Love, The Talented Mr Ripley, Sylvia* and *Proof,* Gwyneth is a pacesetter for glamour and style, who also sets the pace in her own life – recently, it's been downtime for baby. Following the birth in May 2004 of her daughter, Apple (with musician husband, Chris Martin), Gwyneth took time out for motherhood while remaining front and centre in the public eye. Asked by Oprah Winfrey what her next role would be, new mum Paltrow replied, 'I don't know and I don't care.' Few stars are as self-possessed and sure of their values. Or perhaps she's just confident that film offers will continue to flood in. Given the way paparazzi follow her every move, she's probably right.

Paltrow owes her fabulous skin to genes only in part. She has long espoused a healthy lifestyle, as do many DRNTs. She practises yoga, eats a macrobiotic diet, and has received Ayurvedic and Chinese medical treatments – although she confessed that while pregnant she had unholy urges for grilled cheese sandwiches and french fries.

Although most DRNTs have light skin, certain moderate- to dark-skin-toned celebrities may also be DRNTs, such as Sandra Bullock, Beyoncé, and Diana Rigg, who I guess share this favourable Skin Type.

DRNTS AND LIFESTYLE CHOICES

How do DRNTs luck out in the Skin Type lottery? Like Paltrow, they often preserve their skin through good habits, such as eating a skin-healthy diet and taking beneficial supplements like omega-3 fats. Many try relaxation therapies, like Reiki or massage, or go to spas. Pampering their dry skin, health-conscious DRNTs often avoid sun exposure or use protective sunscreens. Unlike sensitive types, who are irritated by many sunscreen ingredients, DRNTs can use anything from Coppertone to Aubrey's to a high-end brand. As a result, it's easier to use sunscreen consistently to protect from the sun's harsh rays. Moderating stress through exercise, like walking or yoga, or lifestyle behaviours, like meditation or keeping a diary, helps them maintain balance in this challenging modern world. While some greet stress by going into overdrive, DRNTs tend to slow down, set priorities, and set boundaries – just like Paltrow, who has called a halt to the London photographers dogging her every step.

DRNTS AND SKIN COLOUR

The majority of DRNTs have light to medium skin tones, while dark-skin-toned DRNTs are in the minority. Most people with dark skin are pigmented types because they have higher pigment levels overall than light-skin-toned people. However, the questionnaire differentiates between overall pigment levels and pigment problems, such as melasma or dark spots. Therefore, dark-toned DRNTs will be free of the dark spots that trouble many people of colour. They owe their smooth, even skin to a combination of lucky genes and sun avoidance. Dark-skinned DRNTs typically have different sun habits than the majority of people of colour. Most dark-skinned people assume that they don't need sunscreen but sun exposure can increase pigmentation, resulting in an uneven complexion. In contrast to other people of colour, I've noticed that dark-skinned DRNTs *do* use sunscreen or they avoid the sun. As a result, like the stunning fashion model Iman, they have exceptionally even complexions. What good fortune. Moreover, although light-skin-toned DRNTs are at higher risk for skin cancer, dark-skin-toned DRNTs are protected by their overall pigment levels – the best of all possible worlds.

Elizabeth's Story

E lizabeth, age eighteen, came in with her mum, Veronica, who was concerned because Elizabeth, a blonde with light blue eyes, was insisting on regular tanning bed visits to tan her hard-to-tan skin. In youth, Veronica herself had tanned frequently and now had the scars, literally, to show for it. Since excess sun exposure increases the risk of developing skin cancer, she did not want Elizabeth to make the same mistake.

Elizabeth felt that her mother was overreacting. She wanted some colour on her legs and arms. 'I look fluorescent white and it embarrasses me,' she admitted. She had already tried self-tanners without success. 'They all streak on me, leaving orange lines on my legs. Believe me, I've tried every product on the market,' she told me.

DRNTs (and all dry types) find it tough to attain an even tan with self-tanners. To overcome that problem, here's a tip: first, exfoliate with a scrub or exfoliation product to smooth away dry skin flakes. Next, choose a self-tanner with antioxidant ingredients for a less orange look.

Elizabeth followed my basic guidelines and product suggestions, and I was glad that she got the message. The DRNT predisposition to skin cancers, exacerbated by excess tanning and sun exposure, cannot be ignored.

When I saw Elizabeth six months later, she told me that she was having great results with the facial scrub followed by a self-tanner that I had recommended. (She used Clarins' Gentle Exfoliating Refiner, a scrub, followed by Clarins' Radiance-Plus Self-Tanning Cream-Gel.) Her days of sunbathing were over. I told her to come by and thank me again in twenty years.

To follow the guidance on self-tanning I offered to Elizabeth, please consult Chapter Ten, 'Self-Tanners', for instructions.

CLOSE-UP LOOK AT YOUR SKIN

Like Elizabeth, with DRNT skin you may experience any of the following:

- Few noticeable skin problems
- Even-toned skin
- Ease in using a wide range of skin products
- Few breakouts, if any
- Inability to tan

- High susceptibility to sunburn, especially after swimming
- Streaking with self-tanners
- Normal to dry skin in youth
- Dryness worsens for women at perimenopause and menopause
- Noticeable dryness after bathing or swimming
- Increased risk of non-melanoma skin cancers

Truthfully, I don't know how many people have this Skin Type, since DRNTs rarely consult a dermatologist unless they develop a skin disease such as psoriasis or skin cancer. Unfortunately, light-skinned DRNTs may be at a high risk of skin cancer. Since you have trouble tanning, you're more likely to abuse your skin in youth by submitting to excess sun exposure or even ultraviolet tanning beds. If you bypassed that temptation, good for you. You will likely have a lifetime of great, albeit a little dry, skin. All you have to do is moisturise, use sun protection, and enjoy your luck.

On the other hand, if gardening, tennis, fishing, golf, or other outdoor activities exposed you to frequent and unprotected sun, and you have light skin colour, make sure to go for an annual skin exam to rule out skin cancer. Your lack of pigmentation may set you up for it, the light-skinned DRNT's most significant downside. Please see Chapter Seven, 'How to Recognise a Non-Melanoma Skin Cancer', for guidelines on how to detect it so that you can also make a special trip if you develop anything that looks suspicious. Also, schedule annual checkups with your dermatologist to monitor your skin.

EFFECTIVE SELF-TANNING

As I explained to Elizabeth, DRNTs often have trouble achieving a smooth tan with a self-tanner, but I can help you get better results. All tanners, both spray and rub-on products, contain the same chemical, dihydroxyacetone, which chemically reacts with acids in the topmost level of the skin cells. The surface of dry skin consists of many dead skin cells, invisible to the naked eye (but visible under a microscope), which collect in heaps and valleys. These cells contain proteins that react to the dihydroxyacetone by turning an orange-brown colour. As a result, areas with a thicker layer of dead cells will appear darker than where cells are thinner. The self-tan will therefore look spotty.

An exfoliating scrub, used prior to self-tanner application, will remove the heaped-up skin cells, creating an even surface to permit a more consistent tan. Although this exfoliation is ideal for everyone, it's especially important for Dry Skin Types. I'll therefore be recommending self-tanners and exfoliation products in a later section of this chapter.

DRYNESS IN DARK-COLOURED SKIN

Dark-skin-toned DRNTs have the even complexion of non-pigmented skin along with the skin cancer protection of pigmented skin. But dark-toned DRNT skin does have one downside, dryness.

Tall, thin, and attractive, Gita was an elegant Indian woman who ran a public relations agency with a celebrity clientele, and she loved to show off her beautiful size 8 figure in the latest fashions. Thanks to her dark- and even-toned DRNT skin, she looked fabulous in vibrant colours, like red, turquoise and purple.

Referred by one of my celebrity clients, Gita came to me distressed by skin discolouration on her knees. 'Short skirts are in and I can't wear them,' she complained. Although her legs were shapely, her knees had dark, ashy patches, and Gita hadn't a clue what to do about them. She'd never been to a dermatologist before because she had been blessed with great skin. Since her skin was trouble free, her use of moisturiser was not that regular.

'I don't want to wear tights,' she explained, 'because it's hard to match my dark skin colour and they seem to catch and rub.' When I examined Gita's legs, I saw that she was suffering from dry skin, not a true skin disease. I reassured her that if she avoided cleansers that foam vigorously, like soaps, and moisturised frequently she would soon be proudly wearing skirts once again.

Gita followed my advice, and it worked so well for her that there was no need for a follow-up visit. But I heard from our mutual client that her skin problem had resolved and that Gita was looking great in the latest couture, and the shorter the skirts, the happier she felt.

Like Gita, with medium- to dark-toned DRNT skin you may experience any of the following:

- Even-toned facial skin
- Ease in using a wide range of skin products
- Dry, rough skin with an ashy tone
- Darkness over knees, elbows and knuckles

- Itching
- Increased dryness after bathing or swimming
- Sunscreens may appear whitish or violet on your skin

Ashiness (a greyish skin tone seen on dark skin) can be worsened by anything that dries out the skin, such as detergents, harsh hair chemicals, hotel soaps, wind or cold weather. In people with darker-toned skin, ashiness occurs because the superficial layer of the skin becomes flaky and white while the underlying dark skin peeks through. To solve this common complaint among dark-skin-toned DRNTs, moisturise. A number of fine products are marketed specifically for this condition, such as Aveeno Daily Moisturising Lotion with Natural Colloidal Oatmeal. Avoiding harsh soaps, such as hotel soaps, will help prevent this condition.

YOUR PRODUCT OPTIONS

Your skin is easy. You can use whatever you choose. Some of you prefer expensive brands because you attribute your excellent skin condition to their supposedly high-quality ingredients, while others reach for whatever's available. In many instances, the difference between the high- and low-end products is not as great as people believe, and the cheaper ones can be better for your skin. It all comes down to the right ingredients for a given type.

You have less need to seek out specialized ingredients and products (or avoid bothersome ones) than many other types. Beyond basic cleansing, your only real need is moisturising.

When it comes to shopping for products, some DRNTs will stay loyal to products they like, while others experiment with new products they find appealing due to their packaging, colour, scent or some other association. DRNTs don't need prescription products. Old-fashioned glycerin and rose water, a classic skin-hydration product, was good enough for your grandmother and can be good enough for you. Unlike sensitive types, who may react to perfumes in products, you can benefit from products with mild essential oils such as lavender, chamomile and rose.

DRNTS AND WATER

Although many health books suggest drinking water to increase skin hydration, what you drink does not impact your skin's ability to hold on to water.

Poor hydration is due to damage to the skin barrier, and drinking water makes no difference. Cells on the surface of the skin line up to form what is called the skin barrier. These cells look something like a row of bricks in a wall held together by mortar. When the mortar breaks down or weakens, the wall cannot hold, and the skin cells (acting like bricks) move and leave gaps. As a result, skin cannot hold water *in* the skin to maintain the skin's cellular integrity.

All dry types need to hydrate the skin, but this is easier for dry, resistant types, like you. Resistant skin gives you a more solid skin barrier, but you will still need to preserve and hydrate it, more than oily types. Increase the skin's ability to hold moisture with the skin care I'll recommend. The vitamin supplements recommended in 'Further Help for Dry, Resistant Skin' will also give your skin the building blocks it needs to maintain the barrier.

Interestingly, water immersion *decreases* the water content of the skin. Long baths, lap swimming or ocean sports (like snorkeling or scuba diving) that involve soaking in the water over an extended time period are harmful to your skin. First of all, research indicates that prolonged water exposure of any kind can dehydrate skin by undermining its ability to retain water. Chlorinated water, commonly found in swimming pools, is especially dehydrating. Hot water and hard water (which contains more calcium) are also rougher on the skin. For this reason, dermatologists usually suggest that dry types take a quick bath or shower (five to ten minutes) in lukewarm water. After bathing, use a soft – not rough – towel to gently pat the skin partially dry. Apply a moisturiser immediately afterwards while the skin is still damp. The oil in the moisturiser helps trap the water on the skin surface and helps the skin to absorb it.

Here's another secret: sunbathing after prolonged swimming increases your risk for harmful sunburns. Several studies have demonstrated that when exposed to either fresh or salt water, the skin's susceptibility to sunburn increases. But increased sunburn risk does not translate into increased tanning, other studies reveal. So this common practise should be avoided, especially if you're a light-skin-toned DRNT, and are more susceptible to UV ray damage due to the lack of pigment (melanin), which acts to protect skin from ultraviolet injury.

To enjoy swimming in warm weather while preventing this harmful water-sunburn synergy, after you swim, towel off, apply an ample SPF sunscreen of 30 or more, put on proper clothing, and allow your skin to dry for twenty minutes prior to sun exposure.

Many dark-skin-toned DRNTs do not use daily sunscreen because spots and wrinkles aren't a problem. However, even dark-skin-toned people can benefit from daily sunscreen application.

DRNTS AND DRYNESS

To minimise skin dryness, what you wear may be as important as the skin care products you use. Studies show that with dry skin, people are more sensitive to fabric roughness than when the skin is well hydrated. DRNTs and other dry types may feel irritated and uncomfortable wearing wool and other rough fabrics. Certain fabrics, like rough linen or polyester, may actually worsen dry skin and lead to ashiness. Wearing softer fabrics or using fabric softeners may help.

Whether it's skin care, hair care or household cleansing products, avoid anything that foams, since foaming products contain detergents. Detergents from soaps, shampoos, cleansing products and laundry detergents can increase dryness. Use non-foaming skin and hair care products. Wear gloves when washing dishes or cleaning. In laundering, use less soap and assure that it's rinsed thoroughly from clothing, bedding, towels, and other fabrics that come into contact with your skin. In addition, in certain instances, chemicals used in dry cleaning can irritate the skin. The chemicals used by ecological dry cleaners may be easier to tolerate.

YOUR SKIN TYPE'S SOLUTION

Moisturising is essential both in youth, to safeguard your skin's natural moisture, and as you age, to minimise progressive dryness. For your daily skin care, use a moisturiser for daytime and a second, richer product for nighttime.

Which products to choose? Fortunately, your resistant skin is very forgiving. Unlike Dry, Sensitive Skin Types, who must carefully avoid allergenic or inflammatory ingredients, you can use almost any product without a problem. However, to avoid hyped products of little real benefit, choose the most effective moisturisers by learning about the key ingredients you need.

There are two main categories of moisturisers: occlusives and humectants. Some ingredients belong to both categories. Occlusives 'occlude' the skin, which means they prevent water from evaporating. Plastic wrap such as cling film, which protects food by keeping it hydrated, acts in exactly the same way. Common occlusive ingredients include petrolatum (as in petroleum jelly), most types of oil (such as sesame, mineral and olive oil), propylene glycol (a popular additive in cosmetics), and dimethicone (a silicone derivative).

Humectants, such as glycerin and hyaluronic acid, act differently from occlusives. Due to their high water-absorption capabilities, humectants draw water *into* the skin. However, humectants can also act as turncoats because their water-drawing action is unidirectional. Here's how that works: although they usually draw water *from* the environment *into* the skin to hydrate it, in low-humidity conditions, that action is reversed. Instead, they may take water *from* the skin (often from the deeper epidermis and dermis) and send it out. This results in increased skin dryness. For this reason, they work better when combined with occlusives. For DRNTs, the best moisturisers contain combinations of both occlusive and humectant ingredients.

HYPOTHYROIDISM: A RISK FOR DRNTS

Dry skin may be a sign of hypothyroidism, a condition in which the body lacks sufficient thyroid hormone. Many have a thyroid deficiency without being aware of it. To rule out the possibility that your dry skin results from this condition, check out these symptoms of hypothyroidism:

- Fatigue, weakness
- Weight gain or increased difficulty losing weight
- Coarse, dry hair
- Dry, rough, pale skin
- Hair loss
- Cold intolerance (can't tolerate the cold as well as those around you)
- Muscle cramps and frequent muscle aches
- Constipation
- Depression
- Irritability
- Memory loss
- Abnormal menstrual cycles
- Decreased libido

If you suffer from two or more of these symptoms, see your regular physician for a simple blood test to check your thyroid hormone levels. If he or she diagnoses a deficiency, your levels can be treated with natural or synthetic hormone products.

Dr Baumann's Bottom Line: As a DRNT, you should avoid prolonged bathing and rough fabrics, use non-foaming, soap-free cleansers, and moisturise frequently. If you have light skin, make sure to wear sunscreen and get annual checkups to detect skin cancer.

EVERYDAY CARE FOR YOUR SKIN

The goal of your skin care routine is to address dryness and ashy skin with products that deliver occlusive and humectant moisturising ingredients. All the products I'll recommend act to do one or both of the following:

- Prevent and treat dryness
- Prevent and treat ashiness

In addition, your daily regimen will also help to address your other skin concerns by:

- Preventing skin cancer

Your skin care needs are simple: moisturise, moisturise, moisturise. With your resistant skin, you can use almost any product. However, follow my recommendations below to find the most effective moisturisers, which combine occlusives and humectants.

You don't need any prescription medications, so I've provided a one-stage nonprescription regimen for you. You are one of the few groups for whom I do not recommend a retinoid – it's too drying.

DAILY SKIN CARE

STAGE ONE: NONPRESCRIPTION REGIMEN

AM	PM
Step 1: Wash with creamy non-foaming cleanser or cleansing oil	Step 1: Wash with same cleanser as in AM
Step 2: Apply eye cream (optional)	Step 2: Spray facial water
Step 3: Apply daytime moisturiser with SPF, assuring that your combination of moisturiser, sunscreen, and foundation deliver an SPF of at least 15	Step 3: Apply eye cream (optional)
	Step 4: Apply nighttime moisturiser
Step 4: Apply a foundation with SPF (optional)	

In the morning, wash with a creamy non-foaming cleanser, or a cleansing oil. Because your skin is tight, eye cream is not a must for you, but if you wish, apply eye cream next. Then apply a daytime moisturiser that contains SPF. Finish with a foundation that also contains SPF if you wish to wear one.

In the evening, wash with the same cleanser you used in the morning. Spray facial water, then apply eye cream if you choose to. Last, apply a nighttime moisturiser.

Cleansers

Because your skin is dry, you should stay away from any soaps or cleansers that foam vigorously. Use a cream cleanser or a cold cream instead.

Did you know that using oil to cleanse the skin is quite popular in Asia? This is actually a great idea for very Dry Skin Types. Below I've listed some of my favourite cleansers, including Shu Uemura, which offers a 'collector's edition' of its Skin Purifying oils in adorable bottles.

RECOMMENDED CLEANSERS

- £ Eucerin Gentle Cleansing Milk
- £ Lutsine Gentle Cleansing Cream
- £ Neutrogena Visibly Young Facial Wipes
- £ Olay Daily Cleansng Cloths
- ££ Dr Hauschka Cleansing Cream
- ££ Estée Lauder Soft Clean Tender Creme Cleanser
- ££ Origins Pure Cream Cleanser
- ££ Prescriptives All Clean Cleanser
- ££ Topix Resurfix Ultra Gentle Cleanser
- ££ Vichy Calming Cleansing Solution
- £££ Jo Malone Avocado Cleansing Milk
- £££ Prada Purifying Milk/Face

Baumann's Choice: You can feel free to experiment!

RECOMMENDED CLEANSING OILS

£ Jojoba Cleansing Oil
££ Shu Uemura High Performance Balancing Cleansing Oil Enriched
££ SK II Facial Treatment Cleansing Oil
£££ Decléor Cleansing Oil
£££ Seikisho Cleansing Oil

Baumann's Choice: Shu Uemura High Performance Balancing Cleansing Oil Enriched. The collectable bottles are beautiful.

Facial Water

A DRNT should *never* use a toner. Toners were originally invented to help remove the residue left by soap on the skin. Non-foaming cleansers do not leave this residue, making toners unnecessary. In fact, toners strip the naturally occurring lipids that help hydrate the skin. Your aim is preserving these skin-sparing lipids, so avoid ingredients such as alcohol in your product choices.

Spraying your skin with a facial water prior to moisturising can help hydrate it. Many moisturisers contain humectants that pull water from the atmosphere. If you use a humectant in a low-humidity environment, such as in a plane, it can pull water from your skin rather than the environment. Spraying a facial water on your skin before applying a moisturiser will give the humectant water to pull *into* the skin rather than the other way around.

RECOMMENDED FACIAL WATERS

£ Evian Mineral Water Spray
££ Caudalie Grape water
££ Vichy Thermal Spa Water
££ Avène Thermal Water Spray
££ Fresh Rose Marigold Tonic Water
££ La Roche-Posay Thermal Spring Water
££ Molton Brown Skin Boost 24 Hour Moisture Mist
££ Shu Uemura Depsea Therapy
£££ Jurlique Recovery Mist MD
£££ Jurlique Rosewater Spray

Baumann's Choice: Evian is the least expensive and easiest to find. They even make a travel size great for aeroplanes.

Moisturisers

The best moisturisers contain both occlusive and humectant ingredients. You should find and regularly use two good moisturisers. The one for daytime use should contain sunscreen, while your nighttime moisturiser can be richer.

RECOMMENDED MORNING MOISTURISERS

- £ Neutrogena Visibly Young Day Cream
- £ Nivea Antiwrinkle Q10 Plus Day Cream
- ££ Elizabeth Arden Extreme Conditioning Cream SPF 15
- ££ Laura Mercier Mega Moisturiser Cream with SPF 15
- £££ Dior No-Age Age Defence Refining Crème with SPF 8
- £££ Sisley Botanical Intensive Day Cream

Baumann's Choice: Elizabeth Arden Extreme Conditioning Cream SPF 15 because it contains SPF.

RECOMMENDED EVENING MOISTURISERS

- £ Heritage Casto-Vera Cream
- £ Eucerin Lipo Balance Cream with Ceramides
- £ Nivea Soft Moisturising Cream
- ££ Atopalm MLE Cream
- ££ Avon Retroactive Repair Cream
- ££ Biotherm Aquasource Non-Stop Oligo-Thermal Cream Intense Moisturisation for Dry Skin
- ££ Elizabeth Arden Ceramide Moisture Network Night Cream
- ££ Essential Elements Shea Butter Souffle
- ££ Estée Lauder Hydra Complete Multi-Level Moisture Creme
- ££ Laura Mercier Night Nutrition Renewal Crème
- ££ Nouriva Repair Moisturising Cream
- ££ Osmotics Intensive Moisture Therapy
- £££ Dior Hydra-Move Deep Moisture Cream for Dry Skin
- £££ Lancôme Renergie Intense Lift
- £££ Natura Bisse Facial Cleansing Cream + AHA
- £££ Sisley Extra Rich for Dry Skin

Baumann's Choice: Laura Mercier Night Nutrition Renewal Crème

Eye Creams

Eye creams are not absolutely necessary, unless you have excessive dryness under your eyes. In most cases, DRNTs can use their regular daytime or nighttime moisturiser. However, many people prefer to use a separate eye cream, so I've listed some choices below.

If you suffer from puffy eyes, place wet chamomile tea bags, caffeinated tea bags, or slices of cucumber over the eyes for ten minutes. Preparation H may also reduce under-eye puffiness.

RECOMMENDED EYE CREAMS

£ Neutrogena Visibly Young Eye Cream
££ DDF Nourishing Eye Cream
££ Dr Hauschka Eye Contour Day Cream
££ Elizabeth Arden Millenium Eye Renewal Crème
££ Laura Mercier Eyedration
££ Philosophy Eye Believe
££ Relastin Eye Cream
£££ Estée Lauder Time Zone Eyes Ultra-Hydrating Complex
£££ Guerlain Issima Substantific Lip and Eye Cream
£££ La Mer Eye Balm

Baumann's Choice: I like the Neutrogena the best, and I use it on my entire face when I travel. It's not necessary to use a separate eye cream in addition to your moisturiser. I find this product especially convenient for travel because it's smaller than most day and night cream jars, which makes it easier to pack.

Exfoliation

At-home microdermabrasion creams remove the top dead skin layer that makes skin feel rough and causes it to reflect light poorly, giving you a sallow complexion. These products will help reveal a more radiant skin.

RECOMMENDED MICRODERMABRASION CREAMS

£ L'Oréal ReFinish Micro-Dermabrasion Kit
££ Clarins Gentle Exfoliating Refiner

££ Estée Lauder Idealist Micro-D Deep Thermal Refinisher
££ Laura Mercier Face Polish
£££ Dr Brandt Microdermabrasion in a Jar
£££ La Mer the Refining Facial
£££ La Prairie Cellular Microdermabrasion Cream
£££ Prada Hydrating Cream/Face

Baumann's Choice: L'Oréal ReFinish Micro-Dermabrasion Kit, but use one
of my recommended moisturisers rather then the one that comes with it.

SHOPPING FOR PRODUCTS

There are just a few specific ingredients in skin care products that you need
to avoid. But there are moisturising ingredients you should look for that will
give you the maximum benefits. Please visit me at www.DrBaumann.co.uk
to tell me your favourite products that contain the following ingredients.

RECOMMENDED SKIN CARE INGREDIENTS

Occlusive ingredients:

- Beeswax
- Dimethicone
- Grape seed oil
- Jojoba oil
- Lanolin
- Mineral oil
- Paraffin
- Petrolatum
- Propylene glycol
- Soybean oil (contains genistein)
- Squalene

Humectants:

- Alpha hydroxy acids (lactic acid, glycolic acid)
- Glycerin Sugars
- Propylene glycol
- Hyaluronic acid (HA)
- Sorbitol
- (saccharides)
- Urea

To improve the skin's barrier:

- Aloe vera
- Borage seed oil
- Canola oil
- Evening primrose oil
- Fatty acids
- Jojoba oil

- Ceramide
- Cholesterol
- Cocoa butter
- Colloidal oatmeal
- Dexpanthenol (pro-vitamin B$_5$)

- Niacinamide
- Olive oil
- Safflower oil
- Shea butter
- Stearic acid

SKIN CARE INGREDIENTS TO AVOID

Due to drying:

- Acetone
- Alcohol such as ethanol, denatured alcohol, ethyl alcohol, methanol, benzyl

alcohol, isopropyl alcohol, and SD alcohol

Sun Protection for Your Skin

You rarely have allergies to sunscreen ingredients, so you can use many of the products on the market. Cream formulations are best because they help moisturise the skin. Facial powders with sunscreen are another option if your skin is a bit more on the combination side with an O/D score above 30. However, if your skin is dry, you may not enjoy the drying feel of powder. For everyday use, SPF 15 protection is enough. However, if you expect to be out in the sun for a long period, as when playing golf or at the beach, use SPF 45 or greater. Look for a product with both UVA and UVB protection that contains Parsol (avobenzone).

RECOMMENDED SUN PROTECTION PRODUCTS

£ Cetaphil Daily Facial Moisturiser with SPF 15
£ L'Oréal Dermo-Expertise Age Perfect Anti-Sagging & Ultra Hydrating Day Cream with SPF 15
£ Nivea Sun Age Defence Moisturising Facial Sunsceen SPF 30
££ Clarins Radiance-Plus Self Tanning Cream-Gel
££ Garnier Ambre Solaire Ultra Protect Face Cream SPF 50
££ Kiehl's Face & Body Lotion SPF 40
££ Laura Mercier Mega Moisturiser cream with SPF 15
££ Origins Out Smart Daily SPF 25

£££ Erno Lazlo Hydraphel Emulsion SPF 15
£££ Lancôme Absolue Absolute Replenishing Cream SPF 15
£££ La Prairie Cellular Anti-Wrinkle Sun Cream SPF 30

Baumann's Choice: Choose any product with an SPF higher than 15 and use it every day. Your type usually prefers cream sunscreens. If you have SPF in your foundation or daily moisturiser, you can omit this step, unless you plan to have sun exposure for over one hour.

At Risk in Flight

Flying is tough on the skin and flight personnel are hit hardest. First, they're exposed to high levels of UVA through aeroplane windows. Unaware of this, they often don't apply sunscreen. Second, low humidity levels in the cabin dry skin out, making wrinkles more obvious. In the past, when smoking was allowed on the plane, the attendants were exposed to second-hand cigarette smoke as well.

For all these reasons, these jobs carry a high risk for premature skin aging. It's important to protect your skin whether you work on an airline or fly as a passenger, especially if you're a DRNT, because you have dryer skin and less skin pigmentation to protect you from sun exposure.

Here's what I recommend: always apply sunscreen prior to flying. During the flight, moisturise your skin every hour with a spritz of water, such as Evian, followed by a moisturising cream. I usually fly with no makeup on so I don't smear my makeup using this routine. Obviously, flight personnel may need to wear makeup as they are on the job, but you could choose to simplify your makeup by wearing a waterproof mascara and eyeliner, a moisturising SPF sunscreen, and a hydrating lip gloss.

Self-Tanning

Many DRNTs have trouble with self-tanners looking spotty, but using an exfoliating scrub before applying the self-tanner to remove dead skin cells will permit a more even tan.

Look for scrubs that contain alpha hydroxy acids, such as lactic acid or glycolic acid, because these help remove the dead skin cells. Read the ingredients on the label to ensure that you avoid exfoliating scrubs that contain petrolatum and mineral oil. These are occlusive moisturisers, which can keep the dihydroxyacetone from working properly. In addition, the tanners I like best contain antioxidants, which produce a more natural tan that looks less orange-yellow.

After applying your self-tanner, do not use a moisturiser for two hours, since it can interfere with the pigmentation process.

RECOMMENDED SELF-TANNERS

£ Neutrogena Build a Tan Lotion
£ Paradise Gold Sunless Streakless cream
£ Philosophy The Healthy Tan
££ Clarins Radiance-Plus Self-Tanning Cream-Gel
££ Decléor Self-Tanning Hydrating Emulsion
££ Estée Lauder Go Bronze Plus
££ Fake Bake Self-Tanning Lotion
££ Garnier Ambre Solaire Moisturising Bronzer
££ Origins Faux Glow Self-Tanner
£££ Dior Golden Self-Tanner

Baumann's Choice: All are good, but my patients rave about Decléor.

Your Makeup

Oil-free foundations are not your best bet, since your resistant, dry skin will benefit from oil rather than be harmed by breakouts. So look for cream- or oil-containing foundations.

Because your skin is dry, powders are unnecessary. Powdered blushers and eyeshadows may work, but if they feel too dry, try cream-based eye shadows and blushers. Avoid eyeshadow setting creams that contain talc, which will make the eyelid skin look drier. Remove eye makeup with mineral, almond or jojoba oil. Avoid other eye makeup removers, which may dry out your skin.

Shimmery eye shadows are often made of bismuth, mica and fish scale that can have sharp edges, which may irritate dry skin or increase a dry appearance. If you have noticed this problem, avoid these products.

RECOMMENDED FOUNDATIONS

£ CoverGirl CG Smoothers All Day Hydrating Make-Up for Normal
  to Dry Skin
£ Boots No7 Radiant Glow Foundation with SPF 15
££ Bobbi Brown Moisture Rich Foundation SPF 15
££ Chantecaille Real Skin Foundation
££ DiorSkin Liquid SPF 12
£££ Armani Luminous Silk Foundation
£££ Chanel Vitalumière Satin Smoothing Creme Makeup with SPF 15
£££ Laura Mercier Moisturising Foundation

Baumann's Choice: Boots No 7 Radiant Glow Foundation with SPF 15

RECOMMENDED BLUSHERS

£ Revlon Cream Blush
££ Bobbi Brown Cream Blush Stick
££ Fresh Blush Cream
££ MAC Cream Colour Base or Cheek Hue
££ Nars Cream Blush
£££ Clinique Touch Blush

Baumann's Choice: MAC Cream Colour Base or Cheek Hue

RECOMMENDED EYESHADOWS

£ CoverGirl Eyeslicks Gel eye colour
£ Maybelline Colour Delights Cream Shadow
£ Revlon Illuminance Creme Shadow
££ Bloom Eye Colour Cream
££ Clarins Soft Cream Eyecolour
££ Lorac Cream Eyeshadow
££ SPACENK Creamy Eyeshadow
£££ Clinique Touch Tint for Eyes

Baumann's Choice: Revlon Illuminance Creme Shadow

CONSULTING A DERMATOLOGIST

Although regular checkups to rule out skin cancer are vital for light-skinned DRNTs, there is no other reason to visit a dermatologist.

No procedures are really necessary for DRNTs. However, you might like to have a microdermabrasion procedure, instead of just using a facial scrub or at-home microdermabrasion product.

MICRODERMABRASION

In the microdermabrasion procedure, the practitioner uses a machine that sprays microcrystals to remove the upper surface layer of the skin. The procedure takes about twenty minutes and costs about £50. Many dermatologists recommend a series of these. DRNTs could have one monthly or before an important occasion to temporarily improve skin texture and increase radiance.

Though not a necessity, this is a luxury for those who can afford it. For the rest of us, facial scrubs are just fine. (I've never had microdermabrasion in my life. I don't have the time to sit there for twenty minutes when I can do the same thing myself in five minutes in the shower.)

ONGOING CARE FOR YOUR SKIN

You can't over-moisturise. Put tubes of moisturiser in your home, office, car, and carry-on bags when flying. Moisturize, moisturise, moisturise. Your skin loves moisture. Protect your skin from the sun, and decrease sun exposure. Use self-tanners if you want colour. Get annual checkups to safeguard you from skin cancer.

Further Help for Dry, Resistant Skin

In this section, you'll find follow-up information and instructions on product use and procedures for the Dry, Resistant Skin Types, as well as lifestyle recommendations, diet and supplements that can help your skin.

RETINOIDS

If retinoids are recommended in your Skin Type chapter, here's some information about how to begin using them. For more information about how retinoids work, please consult 'Using Retinoids' in 'Further Help for Oily, Resistant Skin'.

RETINOID USE

When you first start using the retinoid, apply your night cream first, then apply the retinoid. Do this every third night for two weeks. Then apply moisturiser followed by retinoid every other night.

If no redness occurs after two weeks, you can adjust your regimen and apply the retinoid after cleansing, but before your night cream. Then put on the night cream after the retinoid. Do this, using the retinoid every other day, for one week.

If you experience no redness or flaking, begin using the retinoid every night. In about twenty-four weeks you will notice smoother skin and fewer wrinkles. And beyond that, you are preventing future wrinkles.

Since retinoids speed up the rate at which skin cells divide, some flaking is normal. This flaking is not true dryness, but rather represents more dead skin cells sloughing off. You can use a facial scrub once or twice a week or before an important event to remove these flakes, allowing your skin to look radiant. Stronger products are more irritating than those with a lower percentage of retinoids, so you can switch products depending on your needs.

LIFESTYLE RECOMMENDATIONS
FOR YOUR TYPE

Your skin loves climates with high humidity and hates cold, dry and windy climates. Indoor heating and air-conditioning are drying to your skin. If you live in a dry climate, use a humidifier to add moisture to the air.

Don't be tempted by facials, because facial steaming is drying rather than hydrating. Likewise, avoid steam rooms, swimming pools, chlorinated hot tubs, and the like. Remember those old-fashioned recommendations to put your face under a towel over a pot of boiling water? Don't do it! Though I must admit that I did it myself before I knew better.

If you're a DRPW or a DRPT, avoid excessive sun, exposure to hot wax, hair removal products, hair sprays, and hair dyes that can dry your skin and provoke inflammation leading to dark spots.

Hormone replacement therapy can help to lessen skin dryness after menopause, though it will increase melasma, due to hormones stimulating pigment production. It may help prevent the wrinkles that quickly occur after menopause. Consult with your doctor to make your decision based on your family and health history.

DIET

To combat dry skin, your body needs fats to build fat-rich cells that hold on to moisture. But what fats should you eat?

Saturated, monounsaturated, and omega-3 fats are key components in the cell membranes. Vegetarians (who eat eggs and dairy products but no meat) eat about one-third less saturated fat than the average meat eater, while vegans (who eat no animal products of any kind) eat about one half as much saturated fat as the average meat-eating American. As a result, they obtain from their diet much less cholesterol than omnivores. Although cholesterol has received a bad name due to concerns about its connection with cardiovascular illness, recent studies show that it does have benefits, particularly for some postmenopausal women. It's needed for key bodily functions within the cellular membranes that impact the skin. For example, studies show that cholesterol-lowering drugs can lead to dry skin, while decreased levels of essential fatty acids have been associated with dry skin, brittle dry hair and brittle nails. If you have these symptoms and you are a vegetarian, you may want to speak to your doctor to see if you may suffer from an essential fatty acid deficiency.

The best way to assure you get a healthy diet of skin-healthy fats is by eating a wide variety of whole plant foods. You can get fats from nuts, seeds, olives and avocados. Use olive oil, replete with monounsaturated fat, for cooking and salad dressings. Coconut oil is also an excellent cooking oil, as it retains its stability at high heat. Avoid processed foods and deep-fried foods rich in trans fats and omega-6 polyunsaturated fats. These contribute to the production of free radicals, the by-products of oxidation, which is a skin aging process that antioxidant vegetables help tame. Although for many years polyunsaturated vegetable oils, like canola, corn, safflower, and soy, were recommended, canola is unstable when heated, and the process used to deodorise and stabilise it turns a certain percentage of the oil into a trans fat. Thus eating the undesirable fats found in these oils (as well as in trans fat-containing foods such as margarine, most baked goods, fried foods, processed foods, and sweets) may increase both wrinkling and the risk of developing skin and other cancers, including melanoma. Vegetarians can eat eggs and dairy to obtain saturated fats, while vegans can obtain them from coconut oil.

Fish oils are good sources of omega-3 polyunsaturated fatty acids, which can increase the lipid content of your cells. They can be obtained from fatty fish like salmon, as well as supplements like Nordic Naturals' Omega-3 Formula gelcaps, or Carlson's Arctic Cod Liver Oil capsules. In addition, Murad's Wet Suit Cell Hydrating Supplement contains ingredients that work together to help your skin retain moisture. This product includes essential fatty acids, along with phosphatidylcholine to strengthen skin cell membranes. Both these products are third-party tested to assure that they are free of environmental toxins. It's important in purchasing essential fats to ensure that you find a pure, well-tested source, as many contaminants are currently present in the environment. Omega-3s help your skin by providing healthy fats needed for cellular integrity, while they also prevent inflammation that can lead to the formation of dark spots in Pigmented Skin Types.

Antioxidants are helpful in fighting free radicals, renegade oxygen molecules that cause cellular aging and wrinkles. To find out which foods and supplements contain them, please go to the Diet and Supplement sections of 'Further Help for Oily, Resistant Skin'. Ultraceuticals Ultra Active Multi is an easy to find option with antioxidants like green tea.

Several studies have suggested that it is better to get antioxidants through natural food sources rather than supplements; however, when this is not feasible, supplements are likely to be of value.

SUPPLEMENTS

The following oral supplements can all be helpful to your skin: Murad's APS Pure Skin Clarifying Supplements with L-selenomethionine, vitamins A, C, E, B5, alpha lipoic acid, and grape seed extract; Olay's Ester-C Alpha Lipoic Collagen Support with vitamin C and alpha lipoic acid (vitamin C 500mg); Olay's Total Effects Beautiful Skin & Wellness Vitamin Pack with CoQ_{10}, lutein, vitamins C, E, and zinc. Stiefel's DermaVite Vitamin Tablets contain vitamins A, C and E, as well as zinc, selenium, copper and lycopene. Avon's VitAdvance Acne Clarifying Complex contains vitamins A, C and E, as well as zinc, selenium, and alpha lipoic acid. Take these supplements according to the manufacturer's directions. Ultraceuticals Ultra Active Age Defiance has vitamins C and E, as well as zinc, selenium and natural Fish Oil – a powerhouse combination.

Taking glucosamine supplements increases hyaluronic acid production. And don't forget vitamin C. Although it's tough to get ample quantities from supplements, every bit helps. Since this vitamin can have a slightly laxative effect, begin slowly to assure that your digestive tract can handle the dose, then increase gradually. Another option is obtaining a buffered product. Complementing your Daily Skin Care Regimen with skin supportive supplements can boost the benefits to your skin.

LOCATING RECOMMENDED PRODUCTS

To find the products recommended in your chapter, I have made it easy for you. You can log on to my website, www.DrBaumann.co.uk and enter the product that you are looking for into the search field. It will tell you how to find the product. In addition, www.Baumannstore.co.uk is a website where you can buy many of the products recommended in this book; a portion of the proceeds goes to support dermatological research. Alternatively, I suggest you go to some of my favourite websites, including www.HQhair.com, and www.skinstore.com (since they ship to the UK). All of these sites have a wide variety of products, and you can easily order from them.

Most £ products can be found at Boots and other discount pharmacies.

Most ££ products can be found at www.Baumannstore.co.uk, www. skinstore.com and in department stores such as Harrods or Selfridges. Space NK is an exciting store that sells many of the ££ and £££ choices in this book.

LOCATING SUN-PROTECTIVE CLOTHING

A good selection can be found at www.sunprecautions.com, www.coolibar. com, www.shadyladyproducts.com and www.tackletogo.com.

LOCATING A DOCTOR

I recommend using only doctors who are very experienced with botulinum toxins, fillers and peels. As a dermatologist, I feel that dermatologists have the most experience in this area. However, there are many oculoplastic surgeons, facial plastic surgeons, maxillofacial surgeons and plastic surgeons skilled at these procedures as well. Use the websites below or call these organisations to find reputable doctors in your area.

To find a board-certified dermatologist, contact:

The American Academy of Dermatology: www.aad.org. (Many European Dermatologists are also in this society.)

You can also go to www.cosmeticdoctors.co.uk and the the British Association of Dermatologists at www.bad.org.uk

The European Academy of Dermatology: is located in Belgium. Their phone number is: 32 2 650 00 90 and their website is www.eadv.org.

You may have favourite products for your skin that I have not yet discovered. To share your favourite product recommendations with me please log on to www.DrBaumann.co.uk. At this site you can also find out more information about new skin care products, sign up for updates on what is new, register for online research projects, sign up for newsletters, and share your thoughts on this book. We will have forums where you can discuss your skin concerns with others of the same skin type from around the world. Please visit me at www.DrBaumann.co.uk. I want to hear how *The Skin Type Solution* helped you!

Thanks for your participation in this exciting skin phenomenon!

Leslie Baumann, MD

NOTES

CHAPTER TWO

19. skin cracks in cold weather because the chilled lipids become stiffer: J. Leyden, A. Rawlings. *Skin Moisturization* (New York, Marcel Dekker, 2002).
20. wax esters, triglycerides and squalene: P. Clarys, A. Barel. 'Quantitative evaluation of skin surface lipids', *Clinics Dermatologic*, 1995; 13: 307–321.
20. keep moisture in the skin: D.T. Downing et al. 'Skin lipids: an update', *Journal of Investigative Dermatology*, 1987; 88: 2s.
20. non-identical twins had significantly different amounts . . . of oil production: S. Walton et al. 'Genetic control of sebum excretion and acne – a twin study', *British Journal of Dermatology*, March 1988; 118(3): 393–6.
20. sensitive skin . . . is reported by over 40% of people: E. M. Jackson. 'The science of cosmetics', *American Journal of Contact Dermatitis*, 1993; 4: 108.
21. forty to fifty million Americans are troubled with acne: G. M. White. 'Recent findings in the epidemiologic evidence, classification, and subtypes of acne vulgaris', *Journal of the American Academy of Dermatology*, 1998; 39: S34–7.
21. adult women have acne resulting from hormonal imbalance: Mitsui T. Elsevier (editor). 'Cosmetics and skin', *New Cosmetic Science*, 1993; 28.
22. bacteria that causes ulcers: C. Diaz et al. 'Rosacea: a cutaneous marker of Helicobacter pylori infection? Results of a pilot study', *Acta Dermato-Venereologica*, 2003; 83(4): 282–6.
22. treated with oral antibiotics: S. Utas et al. 'Helicobacter pylori eradication treatment reduces the severity of rosacea', *Journal of the American Academy of Dermatology*, March 1999; 40(3): 433–5.
22. facial flushing: S. B. Lonne-Rahmet et al. 'Stinging and rosacea', *Acta Dermato-Venereologica*, November 1999; 79(6): 460–1.
23. adverse reaction to a personal care product: D. I. Orton, J. D. Wilkinson. 'Cosmetic allergy: incidence, diagnosis, and management', *American Journal of Clinical Dermatology*, 2004; 5(5): 327–37.
23. allergic to at least one cosmetic ingredient: D. I. Orton, J. D. Wilkinson.

'Cosmetic allergy: incidence, diagnosis, and management', *American Journal of Clinical Dermatology*, 2004; 5(5): 327–37.

23. People with dry skin . . . will tend to have more topical skin allergies: M. N. Jovanovic et al. 'Contact allergy to Compositae plants in patients with atopic dermatitis', *Med Pregl*, May–June 2004; 57(5–6): 209–18.

23. skin barrier: for more information about sensitive skin and its causes, please see the chapters on Acne/Rosacea and Sensitive Skin in my textbook, *Cosmetic Dermatology: Principles and Practice* (New York: McGraw-Hill, 2002).

25. freckles . . . MC1R gene: M. T. Bastiaens et al. 'The melanocortin-1-receptor gene is the major freckle gene', *Human Molecular Genetics*, 2001; 10: 1701–08

25. fair skin and red hair: P. Valverde et al. 'Variants of the melanocyte-stimulating hormone receptor gene are associated with red hair and fair skin in humans', *Nature Genetics*, 1995; 11: 328–30.

25. fair-skinned redheads are at a higher risk of melanoma: R. A. Sturm. 'Skin colour and skin cancer – MC1R, the genetic link', *Melanoma Research*, October 2002; 12(5): 405–16.

29. retinoids: J. Varani et al. 'Vitamin A antagonises decreased cell growth and elevated collagen-degrading matrix metalloproteinases and stimulates collagen accumulation in naturally aged human skin', *Journal of Investigative Dermatology*, March 2000; 114(3): 480–6.

29. vitamin C: B. V. Nusgens et al. 'Topically applied vitamin C enhances the mRNA level of collagens I and III, their processing enzymes and tissue inhibitor of matrix metalloproteinase 1 in the human dermis', *Journal of Investigative Dermatology*, June 2001; 116(6): 853–9.

29. hyaluronic acid: D. Margelin et al. 'Hyaluronic acid and dermatan sulphate are selectively stimulated by retinoic acid in irradiated and nonirradiated hairless mouse skin', *Journal of Investigative Dermatology*, March 1996; 106(3): 505–9.

29. elastin: S. Tajima et al. 'Elastin expression is up-regulated by retinoic acid but not by retinol in chick embryonic skin fibroblasts', *Journal of Dermatological Science*, September 1997; 15(3)3: 166–72.

29. collagen synthesis: M. Kockaert, M. Neumann. 'Systemic and topical drugs for aging skin', *Journal of Drugs in Dermatology*, August 2003; 2(4): 435–41.

29. glucosamine: A. J. Matheson, C. M. Perry. 'Glucosamine: a review of its use in the management of osteoarthritis', *Drugs & Aging*, 2003; 20(14): 1041–60.

CHAPTER FOUR

55. sun exposure increases breakouts: H. B. Allen, P. J. LoPresti. 'Acne vulgaris aggravated by sunlight', *Cutis*, September 1980; 26(3): 254–6.

55. through intensifying oil production: T. Akitomo et al. 'Effects of UV irradiation on the sebaceous gland and sebum secretion in hamsters', *Journal of Dermatologic Science*, April 2003; 31(2): 151–9.

CHAPTER SIX

114. an *increased* number of blackheads: D. Saint-Leger et al. 'A possible role for squalene in the pathogenesis of acne. II. In vivo study of squalene oxides in skin surface and intracomedonal lipids of acne patients', *British Journal of Dermatology*, May 1986; 114 (5): 543–52.

118. making even more oily sebum: M. A. Fenske & C. W. Lober. 'Structural and functional changes of normal aging skin', *Journal of the American Academy of Dermatology*, 1986; 15: 571–85.

118. oiliness causing acne tends to decrease . . . due to menopause: P. E. Pochi et al. 'Age-related changes in sebaceous gland activity', *Journal of Investigative Dermatology*. 1979; 73: 108–11.

118. oil glands do not slow down until . . . your eighties: C. C. Zouboulis, A. Boschnakow. 'Chronological ageing and photoageing of the human sebaceous gland', *Clinical Experiments in Dermatology*, October 2001; 26(7): 600–7.

127. It helps fight bacteria: S. Nacht et al. 'Benzoyl peroxide: percutaneous penetration and metabolic disposition', *Journal of the American Academy of Dermatology*, January 1981; 4(1): 31–7.

127. moderates oiliness: J. J. Leyden, A. R. Shalita. 'Rational therapy for acne vulgaris: an update on topical treatment', *Journal of the American Academy of Dermatology*, October 1986; 15(4 Pt 2): 907–15.

CHAPTER SEVEN

145. oil production normalises at adult levels: C. C. Zouboulis. 'Acne and sebaceous gland function', *Clinical Dermatology*, September–October 2004; 22(5): 360–6.

145. sebum levels . . . fall: C. C. Zouboulis, A. Boschnakow. 'Chronological ageing and photoageing of the human sebaceous gland', *Clinical Experiments in Dermatology*, October 2001; 26(7): 600–7.

146. non-melanoma skin cancer: A. Kricker, B. K. Armstrong. 'Sun exposure and non-melanocytic skin cancer', *Cancer Causes Control*, 1994; 5: 367–392.

146. amount of wrinkling present: R. C. Brooke et al. 'Discordance between facial wrinkling and the presence of basal cell carcinoma', *Archives of Dermatology*, June 2001; 137(6): 751–4.

154. acne and folliculitis: M. Corazza et al. 'Face and body sponges: beauty aids or potential microbiological reservoir?', *European Journal of Dermatology*, November–December 2003; 13(6): 571–3.

FURTHER HELP FOR OILY, SENSITIVE SKIN

172. sunlight exposure caused a rosacea flare: James Del Rosso. 'Shining New Light on Rosacea', *Skin and Aging Supplement*, October 2003; 3–6.

172. humidity causes the skin to swell, which can lead to clogged pores and acne. J Fulton. *Acne Rx.* Published by James Fulton, Jr., 2001.

173. stress . . . can increase oil secretion: Y. Gauthier. 'Stress and skin: experimental approach', *Pathologie Biologie* (Paris), December 1996; 44(10)1: 882–7.

173. worsen acne G. G. Wolff et al. 'Stress, emotions and human sebum: their relevance to acne vulgaris', *Transactions of the Association of American Physicians,* 1951; 64: 435–44.

173. increase the production of the skin pigment melanin: K. Inoue et al. 'Stress augmented ultraviolet-irradiation-induced pigmentation', *Journal of Investigative Dermatology,* July 2003; 121(1): 165–71.

173. acne worsened during exam time: Annie Chiu et al. 'The Response of Skin Disease to Stress: Changes in the Severity of Acne Vulgaris as Affected by Examination Stress', *Archives of Dermatology,* 2003; 139: 897–900.

175. refined grain products . . . cause a rapid rise in blood glucose levels: E. Bendiner. 'Disastrous trade-off: Eskimo health for white civilization', ' *Hospital Practice,* 1974; 9: 156–189; and Diane M. Thiboutot and John S. Strauss. 'Diet and Acne Revisited', *Archives of Dermatology,* 2002; 138: 1591–1592.

175. obesity linked with acne: S. Bourne, A. Jacobs. 'Observations on acne, seborrhoea, and obesity', *British Medical Journal,* 1956; 1: 1268–1270.

175. dairy products are known to stimulate insulin production: E. M. Ostman, H. G. Liljeberg Elmstahl, I. M. Bjorck. 'Inconsistency between glycemic and insulinemic responses to regular and fermented milk products', *American Journal of Clinical Nutrition,* 2001; 74: 96–100; and Loren Cordain. 'Omega-3 Fatty Acids and Acne-Reply', *Archives of Dermatology,* 2003; 139: 942–943.

175. chocolate . . . is okay: J. E. Fulton et al. 'Effect of chocolate on acne vulgaris', *Journal of the American Medical Association,* 1969; 210: 2071–2074.

175. Vitamin A has also been shown to be associated with decreased oil secretion. Esther Boelsma et al. 'Human skin condition and its associations with nutrient concentrations in serum and diet', *American Journal of Clinical Nutrition,* February 2003; Vol. 77, No. 2: 348–355.

176. Avoiding beer . . . increased acne due to their exposure: C. Piersen. 'Phytooestrogens in Botanical Dietary Supplement: Implications for Cancer', *Integrated Cancer Therapies,* 2003; 2(2): 120–138.

176. the omega-3 fatty acids . . . may have anti-inflammatory effects: Y. I. Tomobe et al. 'Dietary docosahexaenoic acid suppresses inflammation and immunoresponses in contact hypersensitivity reaction in mice', *Lipids,* January 2000; 35(1): 61–9; and Liu Guangming et al. 'Omega 3 but not omega 6 fatty acids inhibit AP-1 activity and cell transformation in JB6 cells', *Proceedings of the National Academy of Sciences,* June 19, 2001; 98 (13): 7510–7515.

177. foods and supplements that contain antioxidants to decrease your skin cancer risk: G. Block et al. 'Fruit, vegetables, and cancer prevention: A review of the epidemiological evidence', *Nutrition and Cancer,* 1992; 18: 1–29.

177. plant phytonutrients have been shown to offer some protection against skin cancer: T. R. Hata et al. 'Non-invasive Raman spectroscopic detection of car-

otenoids in human skin', *Journal of Investigative Dermatology*, 2000; 115: 441–448.
177. spinach, kale and broccoli, contain the phytonutrient lutein: E. H. Lee et al.
'Dietary lutein reduces ultraviolet radiation-induced inflammation and immunosuppression', *Journal of Investigative Dermatology*, February 2004; 122(2): 510–7.
177. another cancer-fighting phytonutrient, lycopene: P. F. Conn et al. 'The singlet
oxygen and carotenoid interaction', *Journal of Photochemical Photobiology*, 1991;
11: 41–47.

CHAPTER TEN

237. surveyed facilities that had sunless tanning booths: J. M. Fu et al. 'Sunless
tanning', *Journal of the American Academy of Dermatology*, May 2004; 50(5)1: 706–
13.

FURTHER HELP FOR OILY, RESISTANT SKIN

276. Vitamin A has been shown to be associated with decreased oil secretion:
Esther Boelsma et al. 'Human skin condition and its associations with nutrient
concentrations in serum and diet', *American Journal of Clinical Nutrition*, February
2003; 77(2): 348–355.
277. plant phytonutrients have also been shown to offer some protection against skin
cancer: T. R. Hata et al. 'Non-invasive Raman spectroscopic detection of carotenoids
in human skin', *Journal of Investigative Dermatology*, 2000; 115: 441–448.
277. spinach, kale and broccoli, containing lutein, while tomatoes contain cancer-
fighting lycopene: E. H. Lee et al. 'Dietary lutein reduces ultraviolet radiation-
induced inflammation and immunosuppression', *Journal of Investigative Dermatology*, February 2004; 122(2): 510–7; and P. F. Conn et al. 'The singlet oxygen and
carotenoid interaction', *Journal of Photochemical Photobiology*, 1991; 11: 41–47.
277. Artichokes also have antioxidant activity, helpful in preventing wrinkles: A.
Jimenez-Escrig et al. 'In vitro antioxidant activities of edible artichoke (Cynara
scolymus L.) and effect on biomarkers of antioxidants in rats', *Journal of Agricultural and Food Chemistry*, August 2003; 51(18): 5540–5.
277. cocoa had a higher antioxidant capacity than black tea, green tea or red wine:
K. W. Lee et al. 'Cocoa has more phenolic phytochemicals and a higher antioxidant
capacity than teas and red wine', *Journal of Agricultural and Food Chemistry*,
December 2003; 3, 51(25): 7292–5.

CHAPTER TWELVE

283. treatment for their eczema would be 'the single most important improvement
to their quality of life': *ISOLATE* (International Study of Life with Atopic Eczema)
released at the European Academy of Dermatology and Venereology congress in
Florence, Italy, November 2004.

CHAPTER THIRTEEN

314. breast-fed infants have a lower incidence of atopic dermatitis: A. Schoetzau et al. 'Effect of exclusive breast-feeding and early solid food avoidance on the incidence of atopic dermatitis in high-risk infants at 1 year of age', *Pediatric Allergy Immunology*, August 2002; 13(4)1: 234–42.

314. lower incidence of eczema than breast-fed babies whose mothers were not on restricted diets: R. K. Chandra et al. 'Influence of maternal diet during lactation and use of formula feeds on development of atopic eczema in high risk infants', *British Medical Journal*, July 1989; 299(6693): 228–30.

317. Asians have a higher incidence of eczema and melasma, but a lower incidence of wrinkles and skin cancer: C. S. Lee, H. W. Lim. 'Cutaneous diseases in Asians', *Clinics Dermatologic*, October 2003; 21(4): 669–77; and A. Mar et al. 'The incidence of atopic dermatitis in the first 12 months among Chinese, Vietnamese, and Caucasian infants born in Melbourne, Australia', *Journal of the American Academy of Dermatology*, April 1999; 40(4): 597–602.

317. Japanese skin is more reactive to detergents: V. Foy et al. 'Ethnic variation in the skin irritation response', *Contact Dermatitis*, 2001; 45(6): 346–349.

324. applied to the eyelid margins, have also caused skin irritations: A. K. Bajaj et al. 'Contact depigmentation from free para-tertiary butyl phenol in Bindi adhesive', *Contact Dermatitis*, 1990; 22: 99–102.

328. problematic preservatives: E. Dastychova et al. 'Contact sensitization to pharmaceutic aids in dermatologic cosmetic and external use preparations', Ceska Slov Farm, May 2004; 53(3): 151–6.

329. Asians . . . prone to develop darkness of the skin resulting from a reaction to cosmetic products: Ronni Wolf et al. 'Cosmetics and contact dermatitis', *Dermatologic Therapy*, Vol. 14.

CHAPTER FOURTEEN

350. yucca: S. Piacente et al. 'Yucca schidigera bark: phenolic constituents and antioxidant activity', *Journal of Natural Products*, May 2004; 67(5): 882–5.

352. eye shadow(s) contain lead, cobalt, nickel, and chromium: E. Sainio et al. 'Metals and arsenic in eye shadows', *Contact Dermatitis*, January 2000; 42(1): 5–10.

352. sharp-edged particles . . . that can scratch and irritate dry, sensitive skin: Z. Draelso. *Eyelid Cosmetics in Cosmetics in Dermatology* (Churchill Livingstone, 1995, second edition; 33).

CHAPTER FIFTEEN

362. masseuses using aromatherapy oils got hand dermatitis: H. Glen et al. 'Use of Aromatherapy Products and Increased Risk of Hand Dermatitis in Massage Therapists', *Archives of Dermatology*, 2004; 140: 991–996.

362. abnormality of an enzyme that helps maintain the structure of the skin: M. Ishibashi et al. 'Abnormal expression of the novel epidermal enzyme, glucosylceramide deacylase, and the accumulation of its enzymatic reaction product, glucosylsphingosine, in the skin of patients with atopic dermatitis', *Laboratory Investigation*, March 2003; 83(3): 397–408.

363. low dietary cholesterol have been correlated to a susceptibility to dry skin: B. C. Davis et al. 'Achieving optimal essential fatty acid status in vegetarians: current knowledge and practical implications', *American Journal of Clinical Nutrition*, September 2003; 78(3 Suppl): 640S–646S.

366. immersion (over an hour) in room temperature water can disrupt the skin barrier: R. R. Warner et al. 'Water disrupts stratum corneum lipid lamellae: damage is similar to surfactants', *The Journal of Investigative Dermatology*, December 1999; 113(6): 960–6.

FURTHER HELP FOR DRY, SENSITIVE SKIN

383. hard water . . . can contribute to dryness and redness: R. Warren et al. 'The influence of hard water (calcium) and surfactants on irritant contact dermatitis', *Contact Dermatitis*, December 1996; 35(6): 337–43.

383. very high water temperatures . . . can dry the skin out and lead to redness: E. Berardesca et al. 'Effects of water temperature on surfactant-induced skin irritation', *Contact Dermatitis*, February 1995; 32(2): 8–37; and P. Clarys et al. 'Influence of temperature on irritation in the hand/forearm immersion test', *Contact Dermatitis*, May 1997; 36(5): 240–3.

383. limit immersion in the water to less than one hour so as not to impair the skin barrier: R. R. Warner et al. 'Water disrupts stratum corneum lipid lamellae: damage is similar to surfactants', *The Journal of Investigative Dermatology*, December 1999; 113(6): 960–6.

383. children with eczema who were treated with moisturisers and massaged improved: L. Schachner et al. 'Atopic dermatitis symptoms decreased in children following massage therapy', *Pediatric Dermatology*, September–October 1998; 15(5): 390–5.

383. study compared massage using essential oils versus massage without essential oils: C. Anderson et al. 'Evaluation of massage with essential oils on childhood atopic eczema', *Phytotherapy Research*, September 2000; 14(6): 452–6.

384. preservatives including formaldehyde, parabens, and others commonly used in skin, hair, and beauty products can also provoke allergic reactions: M. Gomez Vazquez et al. 'Allergic contact eczema/dermatitis from cosmetics', *Allergy*, March 2002; 57(3): 268.

385. residual detergent remaining in laundered clothing may be a prime contributor to eczema: T. Kiriyama et al. 'Residual washing detergent in cotton clothes: a factor of winter deterioration of dry skin in atopic dermatitis', *Journal of Dermatology*, October 2003; 30(10): 708–12.

386. insomnia may increase your incidence of allergic reaction: S. Sakami et al. 'Coemergence of insomnia and a shift in the Thl/Th2 balance toward Th2 dominance', *Neuroimmunomodulation*, 2002–2003; 10(6): 37–43.

387. Following a so-called Mediterranean diet . . . may help your body absorb and benefit from fat-soluble antioxidant vitamins: M. Purba et al. 'Skin wrinkling: can food make a difference?' *Journal of the American College of Nutrition*, 2001; 20: 71.

387. organic produce contains a higher level of beneficial antioxidants than conventionally raised fruits and vegetables: D. K. Asami et al. 'Comparison of the total phenolic and ascorbic acid content of freeze-dried and air-dried marionberry, strawberry, and corn grown using conventional, organic, and sustainable agricultural practises', *Journal of Agriculture and Food Chemistry*, February 2003; 51(5): 1237–41.

387. increased intake of saturated fat and monounsaturated fat in the diet has been associated with a decrease in skin hydration: Esther Boelsma et al. 'Human skin condition and its associations with nutrient concentrations in serum and diet', *American Journal of Clinical Nutrition*, February 2003; 77(2): 348–355

387. overly high ratio of omega-6 to omega-3 fats as a key contributor to cardiovascular illness: B. Henrig. *American Journal of Clinical Nutrition*, 2001.

387. increase both wrinkling and the risk of developing skin and other cancers, including melanoma: A. P. Albino et al. 'Cell cycle arrest and apoptosis of melanoma cells by docosahexaenoic acid: association with decreased pRb phosphorylation', *Cancer Research*, 1; 60(15): 4139–45.

389. Chinese herbal medicine can successfully treat eczema: M. P. Sheehan, D. J. Atheron. 'A control trial of traditional Chinese medicinal plants in widespread non-exudative atopic eczema', *British Journal of Dermatology*, 1992; 126: 179–184; and M. P. Sheehan et al. 'Efficacy of traditional Chinese herbal therapy in adult atopic dermatitis', *Lancet*, 1992; 340: 13–17.

389. herbs used in this study consisted of at least ten plant extracts: J. Koo, S. Arain. 'Traditional Chinese medicine for the treatment of dermatologic disorders', *Archives of Dermatology*, 1998; 134: 1388–1393.

CHAPTER SIXTEEN

398. MCR-1 gene is involved in red hair, freckle, and melanoma formation: M. T. Bastiaens et al. 'The melanocortin-1-receptor gene is the major freckle gene', *Human Molecular Genetics*, August 2001; 10: 1701–1708.

398. children who used sunscreen developed fewer freckles: R. P. Gallagher et al. 'Broad-spectrum sunscreen use and the development of new nevi in white children: A randomized controlled trial', *Journal of the American Medical Association*, June 2000; 283(22): 2955–60.

399. retinoids *protect* the skin from the sun by inhibiting the formation of collagenase: G. J. Fisher et al. 'Molecular mechanisms of photoaging in human

skin in vivo and prevention by all-trans retinoic acid', *Photochemical Photobiology,* 1999; 69: 154–157.

399. They also have an antioxidant effect: A. Yoshioka et al. 'Anti-oxidant effects of retinoids on inflammatory skin diseases', *Archives of Dermatological Research,* 1986; 278: 177–183.

399. retinoids do allow UVA and UVB to penetrate more deeply into the skin: D. Hecker et al. 'Interactions between tazarotene and ultraviolet light', *Journal of the American Academy of Dermatology,* 1999; 41: 927–930.

411. Rosemary: V. Calabrese et al. 'Biochemical studies of a natural antioxidant isolated from rosemary and its application in cosmetic dermatology', *International Journal of Tissue Reactions,* 2000; 22(1): 5–13.

CHAPTER SEVENTEEN

421. progestins, present in some birth control pills, can fit into receptors in hair follicles to stimulate hair growth: P. D. Darney. 'The androgenicity of progestins', *American Journal of the Medical Sciences,* January 1995; 98(1A): 104S–110S.

421. changing the birth control pill formulation can frequently resolve the problem: B. R. Carr. 'Re-evaluation of oral contraceptive classifications', *International Journal of Fertility and Women's Medicine,* 1997; Supplement 1: 133–44.

421. different people react differently to different medications: C. M. Coenen et al. 'Comparative evaluation of the androgenicity of four low-dose, fixed-combination oral contraceptives', *International Journal of Fertility and Menopausal Studies,* 1995; 40, Supplement 2: 92–7.

423. Hydroquinone . . . prolonged exposure has resulted in damage to the cornea: A. P. DeCaprio: 'The toxicology of hydroquinone – relevance to occupational and environmental exposure', *Critical Reviews in Toxicology,* 1999; 29: 283.

427. The MCR-1 gene is involved in red hair, freckle and melanoma formation: M. T. Bastiaens et al. 'The melanocortin-1-receptor gene is the major freckle gene', *Human Molecular Genetics,* August 2001; 10: 1701 1708.

CHAPTER EIGHTEEN

443. without being absorbed into the bloodstream, and causing systemic effects: L. Baumann. 'Hormones and Aging Skin' in *Cosmetic Dermatology: Principles and Practice* (New York McGraw-Hill, April 2002: 25–27).

443. use of topical creams . . . consult their physicians: Writing Group for the Women's Health Initiative Investigators. 'Risks and Benefits of Estrogen Plus Progestin in Healthy Postmenopausal Women: Principal Results From the Women's Health Initiative Randomized Controlled Trial', *Journal of the American Medical Association,* July 2002; 288: 321–333.

444. Sixty percent of non-melanoma skin cancers arise from this condition: Jeffes, 2000.

446. a sharp decline in skin thickness in women after the fifth decade of life: S. Shuster. 'The influence of age and sex on skin thickness, skin collagen and density', *British Journal of Dermatology*, 1975; 93: 639.

446. Most declines in skin collagen . . . come during the first few years after menopause: M. Brincat. 'Sex hormones and skin collagen content in postmenopausal women', *British Medical Journal*, 1983; 287: 1337.

446. Hormone replacement therapy and/or the use of topical oestrogen reverse this process: L. Baumann. 'Hormones and Aging Skin' in *Cosmetic Dermatology: Principles and Practice* (New York McGraw-Hill, April 2002: 25–27).

446. glycolic acid can increase collagen and hyaluronic acid production: E. F. Bernstein et al. 'Glycolic acid treatment increases type I collagen mRNA and hyaluronic acid content of human skin', *Dermatol Surg*, May 2001; 27(5): 429–33.

446. Vitamin C also increases collagen production: Nusgens et al. *Journal of Investigative Dermatology*, (6): 853.

446. Retinoids increase collagen production and elastin production: S. Tajima et al. 'Elastin expression is up-regulated by retinoic acid but not by retinol in chick embryonic skin fibroblasts', *Journal of Dermatological Science*, September 1997; 15(3): 166–72.

CHAPTER NINETEEN

469. prolonged water exposure of any kind can dehydrate skin: R. R. Warner et al. 'Hydration disrupts human stratum corneum ultrastructure', *The Journal of Investigative Dermatology*, February 2003; 120(2): 275–84.

469. Chlorinated water, commonly found in swimming pools, is especially dehydrating: T. Seki et al. 'Free residual chlorine in bathing water reduces the water-holding capacity of the stratum corneum in atopic skin', *Journal of Dermatological Science*, March 2003; 30(3): 196–202.

469. when exposed to either fresh or salt water, the skin's susceptibility to sunburn increases: T. Gambichler, F. Schropl. 'Changes of minimal erythema dose after water and salt water baths', *Photodermatology, Photoimmunology and Photomedicine*, June–August 1998; 14(3–4): 109–11.

469. Increased sunburn risk does not translate into increased tanning: *Journal of Photochemical Photobiology*, March 1999; 60 (3): 341–4. 'Salt water bathing prior to UVB irradiation leads to a decrease of the minimal erythema dose and an increased erythema index without affecting skin pigmentation. *Journal of Photochemical Photobiology*, March 1999; 69(3): 341–4.

469. allow your skin to dry for twenty minutes prior to sun exposure: J. Boer et al. 'Influence of water and salt solutions on UVB irradiation of normal skin and psoriasis', *Archives of Dermatological Research*, 1982; 273(3–4): 247–59.

470. Wearing softer fabrics or using fabric softeners may help: J. F. Hermanns. 'Beneficial effects of softened fabrics on atopic skin', *Dermatology*, 2001; 202(2)1: 167–70.

471. in low-humidity conditions . . . (humectant use can) result . . . in increased skin dryness: B. Idson. 'Dry skin: moisturising and emolliency', *Cosmetics Toiletries,* 1992; 107: 69.

479–80. occlusive moisturisers, which can keep the dihydroxyacetone from working properly: B. C. Nguyen, I. E. Kochevar. 'Factors influencing sunless tanning with dihydroxyacetone. *British Journal of Dermatology,* August 2003; 149(2): 332–40; and B. C. Nguyen, I. E. Kochevar. 'Influence of hydration on dihydroxyacetone-induced pigmentation of stratum corneum', *The Journal of Investigative Dermatology,* April 2003; 120(4): 655–61.

480. antioxidants, which produce a more natural tan that looks less orange-yellow: N. Muizzuddin, K. D. Marenus and D. H. Maes. 'Tonality of suntan vs. sunless tanning with dihydroxyacetone', *Skin Research and Technology,* November 2000; 6(4): 199.

FURTHER HELP FOR DRY, RESISTANT SKIN

484. (Vegetarians) obtain from their diet much less cholesterol than omnivores: B. C. Davis. 'Achieving optimal essential fatty acid status in vegetarians: current knowledge and practical implications', *American Journal of Clinical Nutrition,* September 2003; 78 (3 Supplement): 640S–646S.

484. (cholesterol has) benefits, particularly for some postmenopausal women: R. H. Knopp and B. M. Retzlaff. 'Saturated fat prevents coronary artery disease? An American paradox', *American Journal of Clinical Nutrition,* November 2004; 80(5): 1102–1103.

485. decreased levels of essential fatty acids have been associated with dry skin, brittle dry hair and brittle nails: N. N. Laha et al. 'Vegetarians dominate in dermatological disorders', *Journal of the Association of Physicians of India,* April 1992; 40(4): 285.

485. processed foods and deep-fried foods rich in trans fats and omega-6 poly-unsaturated fats . . . contribute to the production of free radicals: 'Omega 3 but not omega 6 fatty acids inhibit AP-1 activity and cell transformation in JB6 cells', Proceedings of the National Academy of Sciences of the United States, PNAS. June 19, 2001; 98(13): 7510–7515.

485. trans-fat-containing foods . . . may increase both wrinkling and the risk of developing skin and other cancers, including melanoma: A. P. Albino et al. 'Cell cycle arrest and apoptosis of melanoma cells by docosahexaenoic acid: association with decreased pRb phosphorylation', *Cancer Research,* August 2000; 60(15): 4139–45.